The Foot in Diabetes

Third Edition

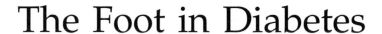

The Foot in Diabetes

Third Edition

Edited by

Andrew J. M. Boulton

Manchester Royal Infirmary, UK

Henry Connor

County Hospital, Hereford, UK

Peter R. Cavanagh

Pennsylvania State University, USA

JOHN WILEY & SONS, LTD

Chichester • New York • Weinheim • Brisbane • Singapore • Toronto

Other Wiley Editorial Offices

John Wiley & Sons, Inc., 605 Third Avenue,
New York, NY 10158-0012, USA

WILEY-VCH Verlag GmbH, Pappelallee 3,
D-69469 Weinheim, Germany

Jacaranda Wiley, Ltd., 33 Park Road, Milton,
Queensland 4064, Australia

John Wiley & Sons (Asia) Pte, Ltd., 2 Clementi Loop #02-01,
Jin Xing Distripark, Singapore 129809

John Wiley & Sons (Canada) Ltd., 22 Worcester Road,
Rexdale, Ontario M9W 1L1, Canada

British Library Cataloguing in Publication Data

A catalogue record for this book is available from the British Library

ISBN 0-471-48974-3

Typeset in 10/12pt Palatino from the authors' disks by Dobbie Typesetting Limited, Devon
Printed and bound in Great Britain by Biddles Ltd, Guildford and King's Lynn
This book is printed on acid-free paper responsibly manufactured from sustainable forestry,
in which at least two trees are planted for each one used for paper production.

Contents

Contents   vii

Contributors

Dr C. Mark Airey *Division of Public Health, Nuffield Institute for Health, 71–75 Clarendon Road, Leeds LS2 9PL, UK*

Dr David G. Armstrong *University of Texas Medical School, Health Science Center at San Antonio, 7703 Floyd Curl Drive, San Antonio, TX 78284-7776, USA*

Dr Karel Bakker *International Working Group on the Diabetic Foot, PO Box 9533, 1006 GA Amsterdam, The Netherlands*

Mr David C. Berridge *Department of Vascular and Endovascular Surgery, St James's University Hospital, Beckett Street, Leeds LS9 7TF, UK*

Professor Andrew J. M. Boulton *Department of Medicine, Manchester Royal Infirmary, Oxford Road, Manchester M13 9WL, UK*

Professor John H. Bowker *Jackson Memorial Rehabilitation Center, 1611 NW 12th Avenue, Suite 303, Miami, FL 33136, USA*

Mrs Mary Burden *Research and Development Diabetes Care, Leicester General Hospital, Gwendolen Road, Leicester LE5 4PW, UK*

Dr Gregory M. Caputo *The Center for Locomotion Studies, Pennsylvania State Diabetes Foot Clinics, Pennsylvania State University, University Park, PA 16802, USA*

Professor Peter R. Cavanagh *The Center for Locomotion Studies, Pennsylvania State Diabetes Foot Clinics, Pennsylvania State University, University Park, PA 16802, USA*

Professor Ernst Chantelau *Klinik fur Stoffwechselkrankheiten und Ernahrung, Heinrick Heine Universitat, Postfach 10 10 07, D-40001 Dusseldorf, Germany*

Mr David J. Clements   *Portsmouth Health Care NHS Trust, Kingsway House, 130 Elm Grove, Southsea, Portsmouth PO5 1LR, UK*

Dr Henry Connor   *The County Hospital, Union Walk, Hereford HR1 2ER, UK*

Dr Nicky Cullum   *Centre for Evidence-based Nursing, Department of Health Studies, University of York, York YO10 5DQ, UK*

Dr Molly Donohoe   *Department of Diabetes & Vascular Medicine, University of Exeter, Barrack Road, Exeter EX2 5DW, UK*

Dr John F. Dyet   *Hull Royal Infirmary, Anlaby Road, Hull HU3 2JZ, UK*

Dr Michael E. Edmonds   *Diabetic Department, King's College Hospital, Denmark Hill, London SE5 9RS, UK*

Dr Duncan F. Ettles   *Hull Royal Infirmary, Anlaby Road, Hull HU3 2JZ, UK*

Professor Vincent Falanga   *Department of Dermatology and Skin Surgery, Roger Williams Medical Center, Elmhurst Building, 50 Maude Street, Providence, RI 02908, USA*

Mr John Fletton   *Plymouth School of Podiatry, North Road West, Plymouth PL1 5BY, UK*

Professor Robert G. Frykberg   *3200 Grand Avenue, Des Moines, IA 50312, USA*

Dr Roger Gadsby   *Redroofs Surgery, 31 Coton Road, Nuneaton CV11 5TW, UK*

Professor Larry B. Harkless   *University of Texas Medical School, Health Science Center at San Antonio, 7703 Floyd Curl Drive, San Antonio, TX 78284-7776, USA*

Mr Patrick Laing   *Wrexham Maelor Hospital, Wrexham, Clwyd LL13 7TD, UK*

Dr Stuart Larner   *Manchester Royal Infirmary, Oxford Road, Manchester M13 9WL, UK*

Dr Mariam Majid   *NHS Centre for Reviews and Dissemination, University of York, York YO10 5DQ, UK*

Dr Kevin G. Mercer   *Yorkshire Surgical Rotation Department of Vascular and Endovascular Surgery, St James Hospital, Beckett Street, Leeds LS9 7TF, UK*

Dr Anthony A. Nicholson   *Hull Royal Infirmary, Anlaby Road, Hull HU3 2JZ, UK*

Dr Susan O'Meara   *NHS Centre for Reviews and Dissemination, University of York, York YO10 5DG, UK*

Dr Thomas P. San Giovanni   *Harvard Medical School, Boston Children's Hospital, Boston, MA, USA*

Dr Trevor Sheldon   *York Health Policy Group, Institute for Research in Social Sciences, University of York, York YO10 5DQ, UK*

Dr Maximilian Spraul   *Heinrich-Heine-Universitat Dusseldorf, Klinik fur Stoffwechsel und Ernahrung, Moorenstrasse 5, D-40225 Dusseldorf, Germany*

Dr Stephen Thomas   *Biosurgical Research Unit, Surgical Material Testing Laboratory, Princess of Wales Hospital, Bridgend, UK*

Dr Jan S. Ulbrecht   *The Center for Locomotion Studies, Pennsylvania State Diabetes Foot Clinics, Pennsylvania State University, University Park, PA 16802, USA*

Professor John E. Tooke   *Department of Diabetes & Vascular Medicine, University of Exeter, Barrack Road, Exeter EX2 5DW, UK*

Dr Ernest Van Ross   *Withington Hospital and Manchester Royal Infirmary, Oxford Road, Manchester M13 9WL, UK*

Dr Loretta Vileikyte   *Department of Medicine, M7 Records, Manchester Royal Infirmary, Oxford Road, Manchester M13 9WL, UK*

Professor John D. Ward   *68 Dore Road, Sheffield S17 3NE, UK*

Dr Grace Warren   *Westmead Hospital, Sydney, New South Wales, Australia*

Professor D. Rhys Williams   *Division of Public Health, Nuffield Institute for Health, 71–75 Clarendon Road, Leeds LS2 9PL, UK*

Dr Matthew J. Young   *Department of Diabetes, Royal Infirmary of Edinburgh, Lauriston Place, Edinburgh EH3 9YW, UK*

Preface

There can be little doubt that foot lesions and amputation represent the most important of all the long-term problems of diabetes medically, socially and economically. The risk of developing foot ulceration, which can be regarded as the end-stage complication of neuropathy and vascular disease, is much greater than that of reaching the end-stage sequelae of retinopathy and nephropathy. There have been encouraging developments in the last six years since the publication of the second edition. The International Consensus Group on the diabetic foot was founded and has already produced published guidelines on the diagnosis and management of diabetic foot problems. In 1998, the foot study group of the European Association for the Study of Diabetes was founded, and has its first main meeting prior to the Jerusalem EASD congress in 2000. In the area of treatment, we now have the first specific therapies for foot ulceration (e.g., topically applied growth factors). It is therefore clear that interest, both clinical and research, in the diabetic foot is increasing, a fact confirmed by the large number of presentations on the topic of the diabetic foot at international diabetes meetings, and also by the increasing popularity of meetings such as the Malvern Diabetic Foot Conference and the International Conference on the Diabetic Foot. However, there is always the danger of complacency, and the fact that the diabetic foot remains a major medical problem throughout the world must not be forgotten.

There are a number of new additions to this edition, including the logistics of providing a diabetic foot service, a paper on the increasingly recognized importance of psychological and behavioural issues in diabetic foot ulceration, and a chapter devoted to advances in treatment. Finally, remembering that much of what we learned about the management of the neuropathic foot originated from observations made by physicians and surgeons on the insensitive foot in leprosy, we are glad to welcome Dr Grace Warren, AM, FRCS to our team of authors. She provides a unique insight into the insensitive foot in leprosy and how this can be translated to better the future for our patients with diabetic foot problems. The question now is how these advances can be translated to routine clinical practice in every hospital and healthcare district: it is with this question that our book continues to be primarily concerned.

1

Introduction:
The Diabetic Foot—The
Good News, The Bad News

JOHN D. WARD

Royal Hallamshire Hospital, Sheffield, UK

Study of so many aspects of the diabetic foot places it as the single greatest growth area in diabetes work, both research and clinical. There have been spectacular improvements in many areas, driven by the enthusiasm and zeal of professionals, collaborating across numerous disciplines—doctors, nurses, podiatrists, orthotists, psychologists, chemists, manufacturers—the list seems endless. Success has been built on this enthusiasm and collaboration, the two essential ingredients for progress.

Understanding of the pathological processes leading to ulceration and limb disease are well documented although, sadly, the understanding of how nerves are damaged in the first place is not progressing so well and we certainly have no effective preventative treatment of nerve damage apart from effective blood glucose control. Hopefully, aggressive treatment of arterial risk factors will see that aspect of the neuro-ischaemic foot coming under control. Really positive advances have been made in the field of measurement and assessment of pressures placed on feet, both dynamic and static, with more and more sophisticated ways of assessing the foot to allow provision of suitable footwear. The ingenuity of the orthotist to study and design for the feet can only lead to admiration from those of a less practical nature. Perceptive doctors, nurses and podiatrists have for some time been aware of the devastating effects of foot problems on the lives of their patients and collaboration with psychologists is another major advance in helping patients by measuring "the effects of the disease on their daily living".

The Foot in Diabetes, 3rd edn. Edited by A. J. M. Boulton, H. Connor and P. R. Cavanagh.
© 2000 John Wiley & Sons, Ltd.

Pleasingly, much of this basic understanding of foot pathology has been translated into therapy of benefit to our patients. New dressings to assist healing abound—growth factors, colloids, fetal cells and even maggots allow professionals to be far more positive in their handling of individual patients. All this is coupled with teamwork, having raised standards year by year and continuing to do so. The diabetic foot team is now a mandatory part of every diabetic service, with attendances rising in such clinics at a pace leading one to wonder where all these patients were receiving care before. Standards must be rising as a result. Such teams now have access to a plethora of meetings, seminars, conferences, journals, books and the Internet, to keep fully up to date and up to the mark. The presence of so much information is surely a sign of a success story.

It would be unhealthy and disappointing if all this good news were not translated into prevention with a reduction in problems and amputations. Evidence is accumulating, led by such impressive studies as the North West England Diabetic Foot Study. Our masters (managers) are increasingly and rightly demanding evidence of benefits from our various strategies and we must produce such evidence at all steps in our management with particular reference to proof that preventative measures are effective. The urgency of such work lies in the answer to the question—how many diabetes centres are able to demonstrate achievement of St Vincent targets with regard to amputation? The suspicion is that not many can do this.

So with all this good news, where is the bad news? Well, in most of the world the news is bad because most of the world is poor and under-developed. This hymn of praise to diabetic foot advance is sung to the tune of the wealthy, Western and relatively affluent countries. Even in our wealthy society, deprivation is well documented as a cause of foot ulceration. A recent visit to India reinforced for me the enormous task ahead, for there, as in other third world countries, the news is not good. It is no criticism of the enthusiasm and zeal of professionals in such countries, but foot care discussion tends to centre around the site of amputation, the way of fashioning a stump and the use of skin grafting as an everyday occurrence in diabetes foot care. There are obvious reasons for this, relating to the sheer size of the problem with masses of people in deprived circumstances with relatively poor financial support for services. This is where the real challenge of the diabetic foot lies, and without vocal and positive pressure from more affluent countries through organizations such as WHO and IDF, nothing will change. Our enthusiasm and achievement must be harnessed to help those in less fortunate circumstances by persuading governments and health control agencies of the major importance and suffering relating to diabetic foot problems. Simple efforts of identification, care and education will result in massive savings for finance and patients in those countries as has occurred in the West.

2

The Size of the Problem: Epidemiological and Economic Aspects of Foot Problems in Diabetes

RHYS WILLIAMS and MARK AIREY

Nuffield Institute for Health, Leeds, UK

The impact of a particular health problem can be expressed in a number of ways, the most usual being descriptions of its prevalence and incidence. In addition, estimates can be made of the morbidity caused by the problem and, as a more general extension of this, its impact on the quality of life, not only of affected individuals but also of family members and other carers. All of these, and particularly morbidity and impact on quality of life, are important contributors to the overall economic burden of the problem. This chapter describes the impact of diabetic foot problems in terms of these five interrelated measures. They can all be substantially reduced by effective prevention, treatment and care.

Despite the difficulties of defining some of the disorders (particularly neuropathy) which lead to these problems, there are considerable published data on prevalence (the proportion of the population affected at any one time). Incidence data are harder to come by, since, in addition to defining a group and studying it once, individuals must be followed through time and re-examined to estimate the rate of occurrence of new problems. The best-worked area in terms of incidence is that of amputation—the most devastating endpoint of diabetic foot disorders—but even in this field, interpretation of the data is not without its problems, as will be explained below.

The Foot in Diabetes, 3rd edn. Edited by A. J. M. Boulton, H. Connor and P. R. Cavanagh.
© 2000 John Wiley & Sons, Ltd.

There is some information on the morbidity produced by diabetic foot problems, although this is largely confined to one particular surrogate measure of morbidity—hospital admission. In common with most chronic disorders, work on impact on quality of life is still in its infancy. In contrast, the literature contains a number of widely quoted estimates of the economic burden of diabetic foot problems—a recognition of their large contribution to the total economic burden of the disease. These estimates, however, have been almost exclusively of direct health care costs and have usually not assessed indirect costs. These are likely to be as great as, if not greater than, direct costs.

PREVALENCE

In designing studies to estimate the prevalence of diabetic foot problems there are two basic sets of questions which need to be addressed at the outset: first, how should the population be selected for study; and, second, how are these foot problems to be defined? The first of these usually involves a choice between an accessible, although possibly highly selected, population of clinic attendees and a general population sample of some kind. Both of these approaches have their merits but, if the main research question being addressed is "how frequent are these problems in people with diabetes?", then there is clearly no substitute for a general population sample. If the research questions relate more to hospital workload, associations with other metabolic characteristics or to the efficacy of clinical interventions, then a good case can be made for the study of clinic attendees.

The uncertainty surrounding these estimates is the knowledge that foot disorders are already present in some diabetic individuals at the time of diagnosis. Lehtinen et al[1] found that, although symptoms and signs of peripheral neuropathy were not common at diagnosis (in their series of 132 patients with newly diagnosed type 2 diabetes), conduction defects were present in 20 of them and not in any of their comparison subjects. Glynn et al[2] reported a series of 39 cases whose diabetes was diagnosed after they presented with foot ulceration. In a study of the incidence of amputation in Newcastle, Deerochanawong et al[3] found that seven out of 48 patients had their diabetes diagnosed during the hospital episode in which the amputation took place. Thus, prevalence estimates derived from population-based studies of individuals already diagnosed as having diabetes must be regarded as underestimates, since some of the unexamined individuals with currently undiagnosed diabetes will have detectable neurological or circulatory defects and an unknown proportion of these will have clinically detectable or symptomatic foot disorders.

Clinic-based studies of diabetic foot disorders have amply demonstrated the considerable contribution they make to the workload of the clinical team. Clinic attendees are more accessible as subjects and, in general, it is possible to carry out more comprehensive investigations in the clinic setting than in the community. This has enabled more objective criteria for the presence of foot problems to be developed and comparisons to be made between these criteria and the presence of symptoms (see e.g. Boulton et al[4]). However, to use such data to assess the burden of diabetic foot problems in epidemiological terms, the selected nature of the subjects included in these studies must be taken into account.

This selection process operates in at least two ways. First, not all patients with diabetes are clinic attendees and the probability of such attendance is likely to be biased in favour of those with complications. Although most individuals with such complications will eventually become clinic attendees, this does not always occur and may occur only when these problems are clinically quite far advanced (as reported in Glynn et al[2]). Second, such clinic series are further biased by studying consecutive attendees or random samples of patients from a number of clinics, since the presence of more advanced complications is likely to lead to more frequent attendance and, hence, to a greater probability of being sampled. This second source of bias can, to an extent, be counteracted by sampling from a complete list of current attendees (all the patients "on the books" at any one time).

The varying intensities of selection at these two levels, as well as the variable methods used for the diagnosis of disorders and the different definitions employed, probably account for much of the wide variation in prevalence estimates. In their justification for a population-based study, Franklin et al[5] mention the range of 5–60% for previous estimates of the prevalence of neuropathy derived from clinic-based studies (mainly from the USA). Nabarro[6] in the UK felt unable to give any precise estimate for the prevalence of diabetic neuropathy but suggested that up to 60% of the diabetic population might be affected, with around 20% having a clinical problem as a result.

Among the 382 insulin-treated clinic attendees studied by Boulton et al[4], 10.7% had diabetic neuropathy, as judged by the presence of symptoms and signs of peripheral nerve dysfunction. More recently, the larger, multicentre study of Young et al[7] found an overall prevalence of 28.5% for peripheral neuropathy (defined as the presence of at least moderate signs of neuropathy, with or without symptoms, or the presence of mild signs with at least moderate symptoms).

Table 2.1 summarizes six European studies of the prevalence of diabetic foot disorders which have considered samples from the general population. Where possible, the odds ratio (OR) is given as a measure of the strength of association between the presence of diabetes and each of the manifestations

Table 2.1   Results of some recent population studies of the prevalence of diabetic foot disorders

Patient group(s)	Comparison group(s)?	Selected results	Reference
Types 1 and 2 aged 20+ (n=294)	No	Amputation (3%) Foot ulceration (7%) Abnormal vibration perception (23%)	8
Types 1 and 2 aged 15–50 (n=375)	Yes (n=100)	Amputation (type 1, 1%; type 2, 0%) Foot ulceration (type 1, 3%; type 2, 0%) Hammer toes, moderate or marked (type 1, 14%; type 2, 28%); (OR[a]=2.7) Dry feet (type 1, 33%; type 2, 29%); (OR=7.4)	9
Type 2 (n=137)	Yes (n=128)	Peripheral neuropathy: abnormal temperature sensation (OR=1.7); abnormal vibration perception (OR=2.3); absent tendon reflexes (OR=6.1) Absent foot pulses (OR=4.0)	10
Types 1 and 2 (n=1077)	Yes (n=480)	Ulcers, past or present (7.4%) (OR=2.94) Amputation (1.3%) (no amputations in control group)	11
Type 2 (n=811)	No	Peripheral neuropathy: present (41.6%); symptomatic (5.3%) Peripheral vascular disease (11%) Ulcers, past or present (5.3%)	12
Type 2 (n=609)	No	Amputation (0%) Active ulcer (1.8%) Pre-ulcer (12.9%)	13

[a]OR=odds ratio (see text for explanation).

of foot disease considered. The OR is the ratio of the cross-products: (number of patients affected × number of controls unaffected)/(number of controls affected × number of patients unaffected). The null hypothesis value of the OR (i.e. when there is no association between the exposure and the manifestation) is 1.0 and those included in Table 2.1 differ significantly from this value.

Neil and colleagues[8], in their Oxford Community Diabetes Study, produced estimates of the proportions of diabetic subjects with impaired vibration perception, with existing foot ulcers and with a history of lower limb amputation. Their results suggested that 23% [95% confidence interval (CI), 18–29%] of those aged less than 75 years had impaired vibration perception (defined as a mean of three biothesiometer readings exceeding the upper 97.5% CI of the previously published age-related normal range). The proportions of their subjects who had foot ulcers or who had undergone amputations were higher than in the Swedish (Umeå) population studied by Borssen et al[9] but the subjects in the latter study were considerably younger.

Borssen et al[9], unlike the Oxford study, included a non-diabetic comparison group of 100 individuals. However, these were mainly hospital personnel and cannot, in the light of the information given, be considered as satisfactory for comparison as the groups recruited by Verhoeven et al[10] or Walters et al[11]. From the results of the Swedish study as published it is difficult to gauge the magnitude of any association between diabetes and abnormalities of vibration, spatial and pain perception. The lower frequency of foot abnormalities in subjects with type 2 diabetes compared with those with type 1 diabetes in this study was influenced by the shorter duration of diabetes in the former group (mean 4.9 vs 16.5 years).

The subjects studied by Verhoeven et al[10], although relatively few in number, can usefully be compared with a non-diabetic comparison group from the same population. Roughly one-half of both groups was aged 70 years and over and the lower extremity neurological and circulatory manifestations chosen were all significantly more common in diabetic subjects than in controls. For abnormal temperature sensation and vibration, however, this difference was confined to subjects aged less than 70 years because of the higher prevalence of these disorders in the more elderly comparison group. They found foot ulceration or a previous amputation in 5% of diabetic subjects (one assumes, although it is not stated, in none of the controls). They claim, rather mysteriously and without further explanation, that their results probably do not reflect the true prevalence of neuropathy.

The study by Walters et al[11], on the other hand, has the advantage of the inclusion of the largest number of individuals tabled here, although the comparison group was small by comparison. This may have led to an underestimate of the prevalence of foot ulceration in non-diabetic individuals (2.6%; 95% CI 1.1–3.9). The prevalence of past or present foot ulceration at 7.4% (95% CI 5.8–9.0) is in close agreement with the estimate of Neil et al[8]. Both studies included those with type 1 diabetes as well as those with type 2 diabetes.

Neither of the studies by Kumar et al[12] and de Sonneville et al[13] included comparison groups. They examined the prevalence of foot ulceration only in people with type 2 diabetes. Although both studies reported low levels of active ulceration, at 1.3% and 1.8%, respectively, the high level of peripheral neuropathy found by Kumar et al[12] (41.6%; 95% CI 38.3–44.9) and the presence of pre-ulcers (12.9%) in the Dutch study indicate the large number of type 2 patients who are risk of foot ulceration and emphasize the need for preventative measures to avoid their emergence.

The aetiology of the ulcers was described in the studies of Kumar et al[12] and Walters[11]. Of those individuals found to have ulcers, past or present, most were purely neuropathic (46% and 39%, respectively), with the majority of the remainder being of mixed aetiology (30% and 36%, respectively). These studies found 24% and 12%, respectively, to be of vascular origin without a neuropathic element. Kumar et al[12] described 12% of ulcers as not being of either neuropathic or vascular cause.

The prevalence of peripheral vascular disease (PVD) in type 2 diabetes has been described in a population-based multi-centre study in the UK[12]. The overall prevalence was 11% (95% CI 9.1–13.7) and no significant difference was found between males and females with diabetes. The relationship between smoking and PVD was confirmed, with a prevalence among smokers or ex-smokers of 15.8% vs 7.3% among non-smokers (OR=2.16). In another UK-based population study[14], comparing rates of PVD in those with diabetes and those without, odds ratios of 3.04 (95% CI 1.56–5.94) for type 1 diabetes and 2.52 (95% CI 1.76–3.61) for type 2 diabetes were reported, with prevalences of 8.7% and 23.5%, respectively. After adjusting for age there was no significant difference in prevalence between type 1 and type 2 diabetes. In this study, while both males and females with type 2 diabetes had significantly increased risk of PVD when compared to those without diabetes, for type 1 diabetes only males appeared to be at greater risk, females with type 1 seeming to retain vascular protection.

From studies such as these it is possible to make some crude estimates of the numbers of individuals with diabetes in the UK currently suffering from foot ulcers or who have already undergone an amputation as a result of their diabetes. Assuming that the number of individuals with diagnosed diabetes in the UK is around 1.5 million, that approximately 4% have already undergone an amputation and around 6% have, or have had, foot ulceration of some degree, then a predicted 60 000 people are missing a limb, part of a limb or both limbs as a result of diabetes and around 90 000 people with diabetes are likely to have, or have had, a foot ulcer problem.

There is significant ethnic variation in the prevalence of diabetic foot disease, reflecting genetic factors as well as likely differences in the availability of health services. In Japan the amputation rate is low. In a large clinic-based study[15] among 2000 patients seen in a single day throughout 35 institutions, only 0.6% had a lower extremity amputation. In another Japanese study the prevalence of gangrene and ulcers of the lower extremity was found to be 2% in outpatients and 4% among hospitalized patients[16], with the ratio of ulceration due to neuropathy being three to four times higher than ulcers due to PVD.

In contrast to these figures, data from the Indian subcontinent suggest a high prevalence of foot disease. In a study of 500 randomly selected patients with type 2 diabetes screened for neuropathy in Colombo, Sri Lanka, 4.8% (95% CI 3.0–6.8) had a history of lower extremity amputation and 30.6% (95% CI 28.0–32.0) had neuropathy[17]; 5.1 (95% CI 3.2–7) of these 500 patients had presented with neuropathic foot ulcers.

Of considerable interest is the low rate of lower extremity amputation among people with diabetes who are of South Asian origin but who are resident in the UK. In a recent study[18], incidence rates of 3.4 (95% CI 1.1–10.7) per 10 000 patient-years in people of South Asian origin compares with a rate of 14.2 (95% CI 12.6–15.9) among white Caucasians. The rate of amputation among South Asian people without diabetes is similarly low when compared to white people who do not have diabetes. This is in marked contrast to the high rates of coronary heart disease and renal disease in South Asians with diabetes.

INCIDENCE

The study of Cohen et al[19] provides information on the incidence of peripheral vascular disease in people with diabetes aged over 60. Six years after they had first been contacted in the Oxford Community Diabetes Study[8], 186 subjects were interviewed and examined again. The incidence of peripheral vascular disease in this group was calculated to be 146 per 1000 person-years (95% CI 117–174) and that of lower limb amputation to be 8 per 1000 person-years (95% CI 3–19). Six subjects were found to have foot ulcers at the time of follow-up but, as the authors point out, two examinations for a remitting and relapsing condition such as foot ulceration cannot determine its true incidence.

More recently, Currie et al[20] have studied the frequency of hospital admissions for foot ulcer in people with diabetes. Their publication is one of several highly relevant studies which have made use of complementary hospital and primary care databases in a clearly defined population in South Wales. They report a crude annual incidence of admission to hospital for the primary diagnosis of peripheral vascular disease, neuropathy, foot infection or foot ulcer in people with diabetes of 18.8 per 1000 (total) population. This compares with an overall incidence, in the general population, of between 1.9 and 2.9 per 1000. From their data it is possible to estimate the annual number of admissions for foot ulcer in people with diabetes in the UK at around 11 500[21].

A study by Boyko and colleagues[22] examined, not the incidence of foot ulceration itself but the incidence of death in people with foot ulceration. They found a relative risk of death of 2.39 (95% CI 1.13–4.58) for those with, vs those without, an ulcer at the start of the study. The average length of follow-up (of 725 people with diabetes) was just under 2 years. Over that time, the risk of death for those with an ulcer at recruitment was 12.1 per 100 person-years of follow-up compared with 5.1 in those without a foot ulcer. After adjustment for age and six other risk indicators (including cigarette smoking), a two-fold excess risk was still demonstrable. The authors do not claim to understand the mechanism for this association but it is likely that, as with retinopathy, neuropathy and nephropathy, an association exists between peripheral vascular disease and coronary artery disease. Such a clustering of complications within individuals seems to be a recurring theme in diabetes epidemiology.

Support for Boyko et al's[22] observation is given by the study of Lavery et al[23]. They identified all non-traumatic amputations in The Netherlands in 1991 and 1992. Of these (those with diabetes and those without), 9% died while they were still in hospital. The age-adjusted death rate in amputees who also had diabetes was around 30% higher than in those who did not have diabetes, although the highest death rate of all was found in patients with peripheral vascular disease and no diabetes. Within the diabetic group, the in-hospital death rate was significantly higher in those with peripheral vascular disease than in those without.

Lower limb amputation is a devastating event for individuals and their families and, as will be shown later, has important economic consequences for society. A number of estimates are available of the frequency with which these events take place. The variation in these estimates is partly explicable in terms of real differences between the morbidity experience of populations separated in time and living in different localities. Part of the variation, however, is likely to result from differences in the ways in which amputation events are recorded and differences in which rates are expressed. Given that a reduction in the incidence of amputation is one of the targets of the WHO/IDF St Vincent and other similar declarations, it is clearly important to establish the true amputation rate in people with diabetes so that progress towards this target can be measured.

Deerochanawong and colleagues[3] have, as part of the publication mentioned above, recently summarized the available studies of amputation rates and added their own information derived from a local study (Newcastle, UK). Of the European studies they summarize, that of the Danish population in 1981 and 1989[24] produced estimates of seven and 11 amputations per 100 000 (total) population per year, respectively. For Sweden (1971–1980), Lindegard and colleagues[25] published estimates of 20.5 (Gotland) and 6.5 (Umeå) (again, per 100 000 total population per year). For the population of Tayside (Scotland, UK), Waugh[26] suggested a rate of 10.1 per 1000 diabetic persons per year (which approximates to 10.1 per 100 000 total population). Deerochanawong et al's[3] own estimation of their local annual rate was 5.7 per 100 000 total population.

Since the publication of the Newcastle study a number of others have appeared, including one from the DARTS (Diabetes Audit and Research in Tayside)[27] group. Tayside and Newcastle are geographically close and, in socio-economic characteristics, not too dissimilar (at least in global terms). The DARTS study was an historical cohort study which identified, from the DARTS population-based register, a group of over 7000 people with diabetes. The age-adjusted incidence of first non-traumatic amputations in this group was 248 per 100 000 person years, compared with a similarly adjusted estimate of 20 per 100 000 person years in a non-diabetic comparison group. The incidence rate in the diabetic group was not significantly different from that in another group of patients studied in the same locality 10 years earlier, although the proportion of people with known diabetes in the locality had risen from 0.81% to 1.94% over those 10 years. Note that the "incidence density" estimates published in this DARTS study are not, in epidemiological terms, directly comparable with the "cumulative incidence" estimates given in the previous paragraph. Also, although the diabetic and non-diabetic cohorts are comparable within the DARTS study, the DARTS diabetic cohort will differ in important demographic and clinical respects from the populations studied by the researchers quoted in the previous paragraph.

The Lower Extremity Amputation Study Group[28] has suggested a standardized methodology for collection and analysis of amputation data; this would allow more valid comparisons between results from different populations. There are several important issues to be considered in the estimation and interpretation of amputation rates: (a) what constitutes an amputation—are all operations on the lower limb to be included, from the removal of individual toes to the more major below-knee and mid-thigh amputations?; (b) to what extent can routine sources of information be relied upon to identify these events accurately?; (c) should the numerator be amputation events or individuals?; (d) should the denominator be the total resident population or the number of individuals with diabetes? (if the latter, how is this number to be estimated?); and (e) when several rates are to be compared, how should these rates be standardized?

Of these issues, the most important is probably the second. The information provided by routine information systems is likely to be of variable quality and has been shown to be deficient, particularly in the recording of the presence of diabetes in surgical admissions[29]. The Newcastle[3] and Tayside[26] studies quoted above both used routine statistics, but as only one source of ascertainment, complementing this by direct access to patient records or lists of operations. The studies that investigated the accuracy of routinely collected data in diabetes hospital admissions[29] are now largely outdated. The recording system in the UK NHS has changed markedly since they were carried out, as has the context in which data are collected. (There is now much more emphasis on accuracy since the amount of money changing hands between commissioners of health care and providers of health care depends on accurate recording.) There seems to be little emphasis on the assessment of the accuracy of routine health data systems in the diabetes world in general.

MORBIDITY AND IMPACT ON QUALITY OF LIFE

The morbidity associated with diabetic foot disease places a considerable burden on both the individual and health service resources and the functional impairment due to the disease has an impact on quality of life (QoL), which may range from mild pain on walking to complete loss of mobility following amputation.

Previously, the absence of direct information on morbidity has meant that studies have used hospital admissions as a surrogate measure. For example, a recent analysis of diabetes in New Zealand by Payne et al[30], using hospital discharge data for diabetic foot disease between the years 1980 and 1993, found that the total number of discharges per 100 000 total population has increased from 13.56 in 1980 to 25.79 in 1993. The age- and sex-standardized total bed-days per 1000 total population increased from 5.02 in the earliest year to 5.85 in the most recent year of the study period.

These results contrast with those from a similarly designed study carried out on admissions in a UK region (North-western)[31], which showed that hospital admissions for diabetic peripheral vascular disease and neuropathy declined over the decade 1980/81–1990/91, the 1990/91 bed usage assigned to these two diagnostic categories being 38% lower at the end of the decade than at the beginning. For these diagnoses alone, a reduction in hospital admissions on this scale, in a region this size (4.5 million residents), had decreased hospital bed usage by around 36 000 bed-days over 10 years. Such a reduction in hospital bed usage (and, by inference, in morbidity) had previously been suggested by the advocates of specialist foot clinics[32]. One possible interpretation of the population-based data for the North-western Region is that the establishment of such clinics in several hospitals in the region over the decade had achieved a reduction in morbidity qualitatively similar to that previously demonstrated in specialist centres.

Important though it is in terms of monitoring health service activity, information on hospital activity for diabetic foot problems is probably a relatively poor surrogate for direct information on morbidity or effect on quality of life. The lack of such information must rank as the most serious deficiency in our current knowledge of the impact of these disorders. Up until several years ago there was no reliable quantitative information on the impact of foot disorders on, say, ability to work, mobility, mood, sense of well-being or any of the other recognized and measurable dimensions of quality of life (QoL)[33]. Although it is likely that concern about the immediate effects of diabetes (e.g. risk of hypoglycaemia, discomfort and inconvenience of insulin therapy, and diet) is the most important influence on the well-being of patients currently free of complications, for those who have symptomatic neuropathy or peripheral vascular disease, who have foot ulcers, or who have already undergone amputation, these must severely affect life's quality.

In this era of evidence-based medicine and limited resources, it is becoming obligatory on clinical and economic grounds to demonstrate improvements, not only in patient survival but also in the quality of patients' lives. Therefore, issues of QoL are beginning to receive greater attention in studies of treatment options for foot disease. In a recent investigation[34], the effects of infra-inguinal reconstruction for chronic critical ischaemia on QoL were examined using the Short Form 36 Health Survey Questionnaire. Chronic critical ischaemia severely impaired QoL, and reconstruction resulted in significant improvements in the domains of Physical Functioning, Pain, Vitality and Social Functioning, although not in the areas of General Health, Role Emotion or Mental Health. The study also describes some QoL improvements in those patients who had a secondary amputation following irredeemable graft occlusion, principally in the domains of Pain, Vitality and Social Functioning.

In another recent UK study by Carrington et al[35] the QoL of people with chronic foot ulceration or lower extremity amputation was compared to those with diabetes but without a history of foot ulceration, matched for age and sex. Perhaps not surprisingly, it was found that significantly poorer psychosocial adjustments to illness were present in those with ulceration or amputation than in individuals without foot problems, and that those with foot ulcers were more depressed than the diabetic controls. The study also showed that those patients with foot ulcers had a significantly more negative attitude towards their feet than either the control group or those who had undergone an amputation, suggesting that the psychological status of amputees, at least in those who had retained their mobility, was better than that of those with chronic ulcers.

The severe effect of foot ulceration on QoL has also been demonstrated by Brod[36]. This US-based study examined its impact on the lives of both patients with diabetes and lower extremity ulcers and their care givers. The patients and carers experienced a negative impact on all four domains of the QoL measure, namely social, psychological, physical and economic, and this was because of the limitations in mobility caused by the ulcer, which required the adoption of a different lifestyle. The results revealed that a reduction in social activities, increased family tensions, lost time from work and a negative impact on general health were experienced by both groups.

Advances in the area of morbidity assessment, definitions of measure and prevalence, and its ensuing QoL implications, will increase the evidence base for treatment and preventative strategies for diabetic foot disease and provide further outcome indices, other than simple functional status or mortality.

ECONOMIC IMPACT

All of the work on the economic impact of diabetic foot problems has centred on the estimation of direct health care costs—the costs of services that are involved in the identification, treatment and care of patients with these problems. In the same way that hospital admissions have served as a surrogate for morbidity, they have also served as a proxy for the estimation of health care costs. This is, to a certain extent, defensible in that the single most costly item in the treatment of people with diabetes is hospital admissions. However, focusing on admissions biases any consideration of costs towards needs that have been met, concentrates on "failures" of the system and needs some care in interpretation since, as was mentioned above, the routine information systems frequently used for this purpose underestimate the numbers of events.

Indirect costs are those of loss of life or function that result from a disease and the benefits to society which must be forgone as a result of its members ceasing to contribute their skills. For diabetes, these indirect costs are high and constitute, in studies that have estimated them, around 50% of the total costs of the disease[37]. Indirect costs have never been reliably estimated for diabetic foot problems. This is unfortunate since these costs are likely to be substantial.

A comprehensive summary of the direct costs of diabetic foot disorders in the USA has been published by Reiber[38]. She reports that the treatment of ulceration accounted (in 1986) for $150 million—1.3% of the $11.6 billion estimated direct cost for diabetes as a whole for that year—and that the average health care cost for a diabetic patient undergoing lower limb amputation (in 1985) was $24 700.

The classic Swedish study of Jönsson and Persson[39] estimated that the treatment of diabetic gangrene accounted for 25% of the institutional costs of diabetes care in the year 1977 (87.9 million out of a total of 351.6 million Swedish kronor). A more recent estimate[40], using the same methods as the original study[39], has shown, in proportional terms, very little difference in the distribution of cost between specific complications.

The work of Currie et al[20], already referred to, has provided an up-to-date estimate of hospital costs for one population in the UK. This estimate was based on 323 admissions for foot ulcer in people with diabetes which, if multiplied up on a national scale, amounts to over 24 000 admissions annually. Their cost is of the order of £1451 per case or £17 million per year nationally. This compares with an estimated cost per case of £2640 for a myocardial infarction in a person with diabetes and an annual, national cost of £64 million.

These estimates must, clearly, be accepted only with considerable caution. They rely on a number of assumptions and are based on data from one locality only. Nevertheless, in the absence of any better estimate they serve to illustrate the likely current cost of treating these disorders and to underscore the extent to which scarce resources could be reallocated if further efforts were made to prevent them.

REFERENCES

1. Lehtinen JM, Uusitupa M, Siitonen O, Pyörälä K. Prevalence of neuropathy in newly diagnosed NIDDM and nondiabetic control subjects. *Diabetes* 1989; **38**: 1307–13.
2. Glynn JR, Carr EK, Jeffcoate WJ. Foot ulcers in previously undiagnosed diabetes mellitus. *Br Med J* 1990; **300**: 1046–7.
3. Deerochanawong C, Home PD, Alberti KGMM. A survey of lower limb amputation in diabetic patients. *Diabet Med* 1992; **9**: 942–6.
4. Boulton AJM, Knight G, Drury J, Ward JD. The prevalence of symptomatic, diabetic neuropathy in an insulin-treated population. *Diabet Care* 1985; **8**: 125–8.
5. Franklin GM, Kahn LB, Baxter J, Marshall JA, Hamman RF. Sensory neuropathy in non-insulin-dependent diabetes mellitus. The San Luis Valley Diabetes Study. *Am J Epidemiol* 1990; **131**: 633–43.
6. Nabarro JDN. Diabetes in the United Kingdom: some facts and figures. *Diabet Med* 1988; **9**: 816–22.
7. Young MJ, Boulton AJM, Macleod AF, Williams DRR, Sonksen PH. A multicentre study of the prevalence of diabetic peripheral neuropathy in the United Kingdom hospital population. *Diabetologia* 1993; **36**: 150–4.
8. Neil HAW, Thompson AV, Thorogood M et al. Diabetes in the elderly: the Oxford Community Diabetes Study. *Diabet Med* 1989; **6**: 608–13.
9. Borssen B, Bergenheim T, Lithner F. The epidemiology of foot lesions in diabetic patients aged 15–50 years. *Diabet Med* 1990; **7**: 438–44.
10. Verhoeven S, van Ballegooie E, Casparie AF. Impact of late complications in type 2 diabetes in a Dutch population. *Diabet Med* 1991; **8**: 435–42.
11. Walters DP, Gatling W, Mullee MA, Hill RD. The distribution and severity of diabetic foot disease: a community study with comparison to a non-diabetic group. *Diabet Med* 1992; **9**: 354–8.
12. Kumar S, Ashe HA, Parnell LN, Fernando DJ, Tsigos C, Young RJ, Ward JD, Boulton AJ. The prevalence of foot ulceration and its correlates in type 2 diabetic patients: a population-based study. *Diabet Med* 1994; **11**: 480–4.
13. de Sonnaville JJ, Colly LP, Wijkel D, Heine RJ. The prevalence and determinants of foot ulceration in type II diabetic patients in a primary health care setting. *Diabet Res Clin Pract* 1997; **35**: 149–56.
14. Walters DP, Gatling W, Mullee MA, Hill RD. The prevalence, detection and epidemiological correlates of peripheral vascular disease; a comparison of diabetic and non-diabetic subjects in an English Community. *Diabet Med* 1992; **9**: 710–15.
15. Kuzuya T, Kanuma Y, Akazawa Y, Uehata T. Prevalence of chronic complications in Japanese diabetic patients. *Diabet Res Clin Pract* 1994; **24**(suppl): S159–64.
16. Matsuda A. Gangrene and ulcer of the lower extremities in diabetic patients. *Diabet Res Clin Pract* 1994; **24**(suppl): S209–13.
17. Fernando DJ. The prevalence of neuropathic foot ulceration in Sri Lankan diabetic patients. *Ceylon Med J* 1996; **41**: 96–8.

18. Gujral JS, McNally PG, O'Malley BP, Burden AC. Ethnic differences in the incidence of lower extremity amputation secondary to diabetes mellitus. *Diabet Med* 1993; **10**: 271–4.

19. Cohen DL, Neil HAW, Thorogood M, Mann JI. A population-based study of the incidence of complications associated with type 2 diabetes in the elderly. *Diabet Med* 1991; **8**: 928–33.

20. Currie CJ, Morgan CLl, Peters JR. The epidemiology and cost of inpatient care for peripheral vascular disease, infection, neuropathy, and ulceration in diabetes. *Diabet Care* 1998; **21**: 42–8.

21. Williams R and the International Diabetes Federation Task Force on Diabetes Health Economics. *Diabetes Health Economics: Facts, Figures and Forecasts.* Brussels: International Diabetes Federation, 1999.

22. Boyko EJ, Ahroni JH, Smith DG, Davignon D. Increased mortality associated with diabetic foot ulcer. *Diabet Med* 1996; **13**: 967–72.

23. Lavery LA, van Houtum WH, Harkless LB. In-hospital mortality and disposition of diabetic amputees in The Netherlands. *Diabet Med* 1996; **13**: 192–7.

24. Ebskov LB. Epidemiology of lower limb amputations in diabetics in Denmark. *Int Orthopaed* 1991; **15**: 285–8.

25. Lindegard P, Johnsson B, Lithner F. Amputations in diabetic patients in Gotland and Umeå counties 1971–1980. *Acta Med Scand* 1984; **687**(suppl): 89–93.

26. Waugh NR. Amputations in diabetic patients: a review of rates, relative risks and resource use. *Community Med* 1988; **10**: 279–88.

27. Morris AD, McAlpine R, Steinke D et al. Diabetes and lower-limb amputations in the community. A retrospective cohort study. DARTS/MEMO Collaboration. *Diabet Care* 1998; **21**: 738–43.

28. Unwin N and the LEA Study Group. Comparing the incidence of lower extremity amputations across the world: the Global Lower Extremity Amputation Study. *Diabet Med* 1995; **12**: 14–18.

29. Williams DRR, Fuller JH, Stevens L. Validity of routinely collected hospital admissions data on diabetes. *Diabet Med* 1989; **6**: 320–4.

30. Payne CB, Scott RS. Hospital discharges for diabetic foot disease in New Zealand: 1980–1993. *Diabet Res Clin Pract* 1998; **39**: 69–74.

31. Williams DRR, Anthony P, Young RJ, Tomlinson S. Interpreting hospital admissions data across the Körner divide: the example of diabetes in the North Western Region. *Diabet Med* 1994; **11**: 166–9.

32. Edmonds ME. Experience in a multidisciplinary diabetic foot clinic. In Connor H, Boulton AJM, Ward JD (eds), *The Foot in Diabetes,* 1st edn. Chichester: Wiley, 1987; 121–33.

33. Fitzpatrick R, Fletcher A, Jones D, Gore S, Spiegelhalter D, Cox D. Quality of life measures in health care. I: Applications and issues in assessment. *Br Med J* 1992; **305**: 1074–7.

34. Chetter IC, Spark JI, Scott DJ, Kent PJ, Berridge DC, Kester RC. Prospective analysis of quality of life in patients following infrainguinal reconstruction for chronic critical ischaemia. *Br J Surg* 1998; **85**: 951–5.

35. Carrington AL, Mawdsley SK, Morley M, Kincey J, Boulton AJ. Psychological status of diabetic people with or without lower limb disability. *Diabet Res Clin Pract* 1996; **32**: 19–25.

36. Brod M. Quality of life issues in patients with diabetes and lower extremity ulcers: patients and care givers. *Quality of Life Res* 1998; **7**: 365–72.

37. Songer TJ.   The economics of diabetes care. In Alberti KGMM, DeFronzo RA, Keen H, Zimmet P (eds), *International Textbook of Diabetes Mellitus.* Chichester: Wiley, 1992; 1643–54.
38. Reiber GE.   Diabetic foot care: financial implications and practical guidelines. *Diabet Care* 1992; **15**(suppl I): 29–31.
39. Jönsson B, Persson U.   *Diabetes. A Study in Health Economics.* Meddelande: Swedish Institute for Health Economics, 1981; 7.
40. Henriksson F, Jönsson B.   Diabetes: the cost of illness in Sweden. *J Intern Med* 1998; **244**: 461–8.

3

The Pathway to Ulceration: Aetiopathogenesis

ANDREW J. M. BOULTON

Manchester Royal Infirmary, Manchester, UK

"Coming events cast their shadows before"
Thomas Campbell

Although clearly not referring to diabetic foot problems when writing these lines, the Scottish poet's words can usefully be applied to foot ulceration in diabetes. Ulceration does not occur spontaneously, and there are many warning signs or "shadows" that may be used to predict those at risk. Joslin recognized this over 65 years ago when he stated that diabetic gangrene was not heaven-sent but was earth-born[1]. He was, of course, correct: thus, we cannot assume that a certain percentage of all diabetic patients would develop foot ulcers at some point in their life. Ulcers invariably occur as a consequence of an interaction between environmental hazards and specific pathologies in the lower limbs of patients.

The various pathologies that affect the feet and ultimately interact to increase vulnerability to ulceration will be considered in this chapter. A clear understanding of the aetiopathogenesis of ulceration is essential if we are to succeed in reducing the incidence of foot ulceration and, ultimately, amputation. The targets set in the St Vincent Declaration on Diabetes Care in Europe over 10 years ago[2]—a 50% reduction in amputations within 5 years—have not been achieved in many centres. Despite improvements in health care delivery, two reports from Germany and the UK have outlined the difficulties in achieving the St Vincent goals[3,4]. As the vast majority of amputations are preceded by foot ulcers[5], a thorough understanding of

The Foot in Diabetes, 3rd edn. Edited by A. J. M. Boulton, H. Connor and P. R. Cavanagh.
© 2000 John Wiley & Sons, Ltd.

causative pathways to ulceration is essential if we are to reduce the depressingly high incidences of ulceration and amputation. Moreover, as lower limb complications are the commonest precipitants of hospitalization of diabetic patients in most countries, there are potential economic benefits to be gained from preventative strategies, as noted in the previous chapter. Ollendorf et al[6] recently estimated the potential economic savings of a successful amputation prevention programme to be between $2 and $3 million over 3 years in a hypothetical cohort of 10 000 diabetic individuals. Finally, a successful screening programme based on early identification of those at risk should impact on the appreciable morbidity, and even mortality, of diabetic foot disease, as emphasized by Krentz et al[7].

The breakdown of the diabetic foot has traditionally been considered to result from peripheral vascular disease, peripheral neuropathy and infection. More recently, other contributory causes, such as psychosocial factors (Chapter 10) and abnormalities of pressures and loads under the foot (Chapter 4), have been implicated. The interaction between neuropathy and foot pressure abnormalities will be considered and, although covered in great detail in Chapter 16, the importance of vascular disease will be discussed briefly. There is no compelling evidence that infection is a direct cause of ulceration: it is likely that infection becomes established once the skin break occurs, so this topic will not be considered here: detailed discussion can be found in Chapter 12.

PERIPHERAL VASCULAR DISEASE

A number of large epidemiological studies have confirmed the frequency of all forms of ischaemic vascular disease[8,9]. The Framingham Study, for example, reported a 50% excess of absent foot pulses in diabetic females, with similar statistics in male patients[9]. Peripheral vascular disease (PVD) also tends to occur at a young age in diabetic patients and is more likely to involve distal vessels. Reports from the USA, UK and Finland have confirmed that PVD is a major contributory factor in the pathogenesis of foot ulceration and subsequent major amputations[10–12]. In the assessment of PVD, simple clinical assessment of the distal circulation and non-invasive tests of the circulation by a hand-held Doppler ultrasound stethoscope can be useful in the assessment of outcome[8].

In the pathogenesis of ulceration, PVD itself, in isolation, rarely causes ulceration: as will be discussed for neuropathy, it is the combination of risk factors with minor trauma that inevitably leads to ulceration (Figure 3.1). Thus, minor injury and subsequent infection increase the demand for blood supply beyond the circulatory capacity and ischaemic ulceration and risk of ulceration ensue. Early identification of those at risk and education in good foot care habits are therefore potentially protective.

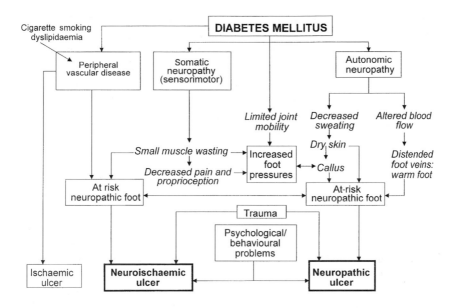

Figure 3.1 Pathways to foot ulceration in diabetic patients

Although the UKPDS suggested that tight control of blood glucose and blood pressure might influence the development of certain cardiovascular endpoints, such as stroke and sudden death, statistical evidence that these influence the progression of PVD was not forthcoming[13,14]. However, educational strategies aimed at the cessation of smoking and control of dyslipidaemia therefore remain of paramount importance. Moreover, in view of trends observed in the United Kingdom Prospective Diabetes Study (UKPDS), optimal glycaemic and blood pressure control should be aimed for.

DIABETIC NEUROPATHY

The diabetic neuropathies are a heterogenous group of conditions that may be subclassified into various polyneuropathies and mononeuropathies on clinical grounds[15]. The association between peripheral neuropathy and foot ulceration has been recognized for many years: Pryce, a surgeon working in Nottingham over 100 years ago, remarked that "it is abundantly clear to me that the actual cause of the perforating ulcer was a peripheral nerve degeneration", and "diabetes itself may play an active part in the causation of the perforating ulcers". It is the sensory and the peripheral autonomic polyneuropathies that play an important role in the pathogenesis of ulceration, and these will be discussed in some detail.

Table 3.1 Epidemiological data on diabetic peripheral sensorimotor neuropathy

Reference (Country)	Number of subjects	Type of Diabetes	Prevalence (%)	Reference
Population-based studies				
17 (UK)	811	2	41.6	17
18 (Finland)	133	2	8.3[a]	18
			41.9[b]	
Clinic-based studies				
19 (UK)	6487	1,2	28.5	19
20 (Europe)	3250	1	28.0	20
21 (Spain)	2644	1,2	22.7	21

[a]At diagnosis.
[b]After 10 years.

Sensory Neuropathy

Chronic sensorimotor neuropathy is by far the commonest of all the diabetic neuropathies, and occurs in both main types of diabetes. An internationally agreed definition is "the presence of symptoms and/or signs of peripheral nerve dysfunction in people with diabetes after exclusion of other causes"[16]. Although the quantity, and sometimes quality, of epidemiological data on the prevalence of neuropathy remains low, there have been some studies published in recent years, as summarized in Table 3.1. It can be seen however, that neuropathy is very common, and it can be safely assumed that at least half of older type 2 diabetic patients have significant sensory loss.

The onset of the chronic neuropathy is gradual and insidious and indeed, on occasions, the initial symptoms may go unnoticed by the patients. Typical symptoms include paraesthesiae, hyperaesthesiae, sharp, stabbing, shooting and burning pain, all of which are prone to nocturnal exacerbation. Whereas in some patients these uncomfortable symptoms predominate, others may never experience any symptoms. Clinical examination usually reveals a sensory deficit in a glove and stocking distribution, and signs of motor dysfunction are usually present, with small wasting and absent ankle reflexes. A particularly dangerous situation, originally described by J. D. Ward, is the "painful–painless leg" in which the patient experiences painful or paraesthetic symptoms, but on examination has severe sensory loss to pain and proprioception: such patients are at great risk of painless injury to their feet.

It must be realized that there is a spectrum of symptomatic severity in sensorimotor neuropathy: at one extreme, patients experience severe symptoms, whereas others experience occasional mild symptoms, or even none at all. Thus, whereas a history of typical symptoms is strongly suggestive of a diagnosis of neuropathy, *absence of symptoms does not exclude neuropathy and must never be equated with a lack of foot ulcer risk.* Therefore, *assessment of foot ulcer risk must always include a careful foot examination whatever the history*[16].

The ultimate diagnosis of diabetic sensorimotor neuropathy depends on the prior exclusion of other causes, such as malignancy, drugs, alcohol and many other rarer causes[15]. Optimal glycaemic control is important in the prevention and management of neuropathy[15,22] and, in addition, a number of drugs can help achieve symptomatic relief[15]. Unfortunately, none of the drugs available at the time of writing affects the natural history of this condition, which is one of gradual deterioration of nerve function. Indeed, amelioration of symptoms may indicate progression of neuropathy to the insensitive foot at risk of ulceration. Thus, again, absence of symptoms does not equate with freedom from risk of ulceration.

Autonomic Neuropathy

Sympathetic autonomic neuropathy affecting the lower limbs leads to reduced sweating and results in both dry skin that is prone to crack and fissure, and also increased blood flow (in the absence of large vessel PVD), with arteriovenous shunting leading to the warm foot. The complex interactions of sympathetic neuropathy and other contributory factors in the causation of foot ulcers is summarized in Figure 3.1.

The warm, insensitive and dry foot that results from a combination of somatic and autonomic dysfunction often provides the patient with a false sense of security, as most patients still perceive vascular disease as the main cause of ulcers (see Chapter 10). It is such patients who may present with insensitive ulceration as they have truly painless feet. Perhaps the highest-risk foot is the pulseless insensitive foot, because it indicates somatic and autonomic neuropathy together with PVD.

NEUROPATHY—THE MAJOR CONTRIBUTORY FACTOR IN ULCERATION

Cross-sectional data from established UK foot clinics in London and Manchester presented in the second edition of this volume suggested that neuropathy was present in up to 90% of foot ulcers of patients attending physician- or podiatrist-led services. Thus, most foot ulcers were considered to be of neuropathic or neuro-ischaemic aetiology. Confirmation of these facts in recent years has come from several European and North American studies.

The first single-centre study suggested that neuropathic patients had a seven-fold annual increase in the risk of ulceration in a 3 year prospective study[23]. A larger, multicentre study from Europe and North America extended these observations and reported a 7% annual risk of ulceration in neuropathic patients[24]. Other prospective trials have confirmed the pivotal role of both large fibre (e.g. proprioceptive deficit) and small fibre (e.g. loss of pain and temperature sensation) neurological deficit in the pathogenesis of ulceration[25]. Considering the above data, there can be little doubt that neuropathy causes foot ulcers with or without ischaemia, but it must be remembered that the neuropathic foot does not spontaneously ulcerate; it is the combination of neuropathy and some extrinsic factor (such as ill-fitting footwear) or intrinsic factor (such as high foot pressures; see Chapter 4) that results in ulceration. The other risk factors that are associated with ulceration will now be considered.

OTHER RISK FACTORS FOR FOOT ULCERATION

Previous Foot Ulceration

Several studies have confirmed that foot ulceration is most common in those patients with a past history of ulceration or amputation, and also in patients from a poor social background. Indeed, in many diabetic foot clinics more than 50% of patients with new foot ulcers give a past history of similar problems.

Other Long-term Complications of Diabetes

It has been recognized for many years that patients with retinopathy and/or renal impairment are at increased risk of foot ulceration. However, it is now confirmed that patients at all stages of diabetic nephropathy, even microalbuminuria, have an increased risk of neuropathic foot ulceration[26].

Race

Data from cross-sectional studies suggest that foot ulceration is commoner in Caucasian subjects when compared to groups of other racial origins, including Hispanics, Blacks and Indian-subcontinent Asians[27,28]. This may be related not only to physical factors, including limited joint mobility (LJM) and foot pressures (see below), but also to better footcare in certain religious groups, including Muslims. However, there is no suggestion that this risk is related to any geographical differences: indeed, Veves et al[29] showed no differences in risk factors for ulceration according to location at centres within Europe.

Postural Instability

Poor balance and instability are increasingly being recognized as troublesome symptoms of diabetic neuropathy, presumably secondary to a proprioceptive deficit. Studies have recently been published confirming the association between postural instability, increased body sway and foot ulceration[30,31].

Oedema

The presence of peripheral oedema impairs local blood supply and has been associated with an increased risk of ulceration[11].

Callus

The presence of plantar callus, especially in the neuropathic foot, is associated with an increased risk of ulceration: in one study, the risk was 77-fold in a cross-sectional part, whereas in the prospective follow-up, ulceration occurred only at sites of callus, representing an infinite increase in risk[32].

Deformity

Any deformity occurring in a diabetic foot, such as prominence of metatarsal heads, clawed toes, Charcot prominences or hallux valgus, increases ulcer risk.

Duration of Diabetes

Although it is well-recognized that neuropathy and vascular disease are a function of diabetes duration, a recent report highlighted the high risk of amputation (and therefore, ulceration) within the first year of diagnosis of type 2 diabetes[33]. It must be remembered that patients may present with long-term complications, and careful screening for risk of ulceration must be carried out at the time of diagnosis.

THE PATHWAY TO ULCERATION

It is the combination of two or more risk factors that ultimately results in diabetic foot ulceration. Both Pecoraro et al[10] and later Reiber et al[11] have taken the Rothman model for causation and applied this to amputation and foot ulceration in diabetes. The model is based upon the concept that a component cause (e.g. neuropathy) is not sufficient in itself to lead to ulceration, but when component causes act together, they may result in a

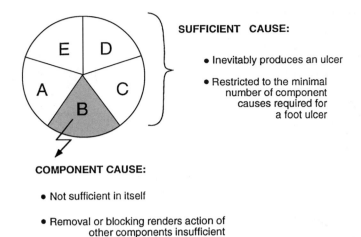

Figure 3.2 — SUFFICIENT CAUSE:
- Inevitably produces an ulcer
- Restricted to the minimal number of component causes required for a foot ulcer

COMPONENT CAUSE:
- Not sufficient in itself
- Removal or blocking renders action of other components insufficient

Figure 3.2 Diagram of sufficient and component causes of diabetic foot ulcers. A–E represent causes that are not sufficient in themselves but that are required components of a sufficient cause that will inevitably produce the effect. Reproduced by permission of the American Diabetes Association from reference 11

sufficient cause, which will inevitably result in ulceration (Figure 3.2). In their study of amputation, Pecoraro et al[10] describe five component causes that lead to amputation: neuropathy, minor trauma, ulceration, faulty healing and gangrene.

Reiber et al[11] applied the model to foot ulceration, and a number of causal pathways were identified: the commonest triad of component causes, present in 63% of incident ulcers, was neuropathy, deformity and trauma (Figure 3.3). Oedema and ischaemia were also common component causes.

Other simple examples of two-component pathways to ulceration are: neuropathy and mechanical trauma [e.g. standing on a nail (Figure 3.4); ill-fitting footwear]; neuropathy and thermal trauma; and neuropathy and chemical trauma, e.g. the inappropriate use of chemical "corn-cures".

Similarly, the Rothman model can be applied to neuro-ischaemic ulceration, where the three-component pathway comprising ischaemia, trauma and neuropathy is most often seen[10,11].

MECHANICAL FACTORS AND NEUROPATHIC FOOT ULCERATION

The insensitive neuropathic foot does not ulcerate spontaneously: traumatic or extrinsic ulcers result as a consequence of trauma to the insensitive foot, as in Figure 3.4. In contrast, intrinsic or pressure ulcers occur as a result of pressure that would not normally cause ulceration, but which, because of

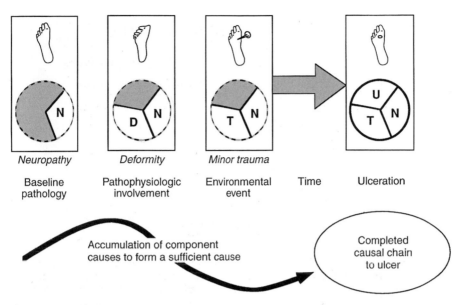

Neuropathy	Deformity	Minor trauma		
Baseline pathology	Pathophysiologic involvement	Environmental event	Time	Ulceration

Accumulation of component causes to form a sufficient cause

Completed causal chain to ulcer

Figure 3.3 The commonest causal pathway to incident diabetic foot ulcers. Reproduced by permission of the American Diabetes Association from reference 11

intrinsic abnormalities in the neuropathic foot, leads to plantar ulceration when repetitively applied. As stated in the next chapter, abnormalities of pressures and loads under the diabetic foot are very common. Both prospective[34] and cross-sectional[28,35] studies have confirmed that high plantar pressures are a major aetiological factor in neuropathic foot ulceration. Veves et al[34] observed a 28% incidence of ulceration in neuropathic feet with high plantar pressures during a 2.5 year follow-up: in contrast, no ulcers developed in patients with normal plantar pressures. These ulcers occur under high-pressure areas such as the metatarsal heads as a result of repetitive pressure application during walking. Callus tissue that forms in the dry foot (as a consequence of autonomic neuropathy) may itself further aggravate the problem. Callus tissue may cause high pressure, whereas its removal reduces pressure[36]. An example of a foot at high risk of intrinsic neuropathic ulceration, with insensitivity, prominent metatarsal heads, clawed toes and resultant high foot pressure, is provided in Figure 3.5.

The component causes for these intrinsic ulcers are greater in number than those for predominantly traumatic ulcers. Peripheral somatic and autonomic neuropathy, together with high foot pressures, are each individual component causes (Figure 3.2), as none in isolation results in ulceration.

Two additional component causes for intrinsic foot ulcers are callus and limited joint mobility (LJM). This latter abnormality, originally described in

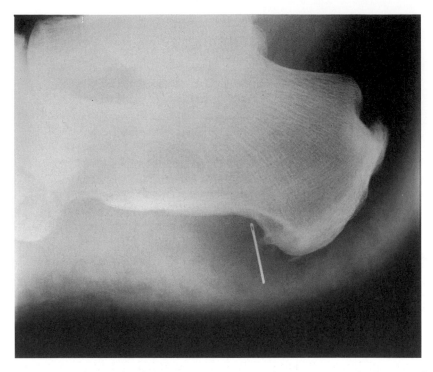

Figure 3.4 Radiograph of patient presenting with a recurrent discharging heel ulcer. On enquiry, the patient remembered some trauma to the heel but did not realize he had part of a needle in the subcutaneous tissue under the calcaneum—an example of a traumatic ulcer in the insensitive foot which could have been prevented by wearing appropriate footwear

the hand, also occurs in the foot. A strong relationship exists between LJM, insensitivity and high foot pressures[1].

The five component causes leading to intrinsic foot ulcers are, therefore: somatic peripheral neuropathy; sympathetic peripheral neuropathy; LJM; callus; and high foot pressures. There is, therefore, potential for preventing such ulcers: callus can be removed by the podiatrist; high foot pressures can be reduced by callus removal, protective insoles and hosiery; the incidence of neuropathy can be reduced by near-normoglycaemia from the time of diagnosis of diabetes. Thus, many neuropathic and neuro-ischaemic ulcers are potentially preventable.

THE PATIENT WITH SENSORY LOSS

It should now be possible to achieve a significant reduction of foot ulcers and amputations in diabetes. Guidelines now exist for the diagnosis and

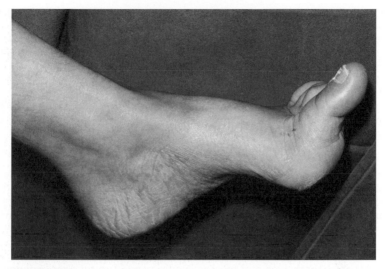

Figure 3.5 The high-risk neuropathic foot. This foot displays a marked prominence of metatarsal heads with clawing of the toes and is at high risk of pressure-induced (intrinsic) ulceration

management of neuropathy[16] and foot problems (see Chapter 21). However, much work is still required in the assessment and management of psychosocial factors (Chapter 10) and, as pointed out in an anonymous audit[4], guidelines will only be of use if properly implemented.

However, a reduction in neuropathic foot problems will only be achieved if we remember that patients with insensitive feet have lost their warning signal—pain—that ordinarily brings the patients to their doctors. It is pain that leads to many medical consultations: our training in healthcare is orientated around cause and relief of pain. Thus, the care of the patient with no pain sensation is a new challenge for which we have no training. It is difficult for us to understand, for example, that an intelligent patient would buy and wear a pair of shoes three sizes too small, and come to our clinic with an extensive shoe-induced ulcer. The explanation, however, is simple: with reduced sensation, a very tight fit stimulates the remaining pressure nerve endings and this is interpreted as a normal fit—hence the common complaint when we provide patients with custom-designed shoes is: "these are too loose". We can learn much about management from the treatment of patients with leprosy (see Chapter 22); if we are to succeed, we must realize that with loss of pain there is also diminished motivation in the healing of and the prevention of injury.

REFERENCES

1. Boulton AJM. The diabetic foot. *Med Clin N Am* 1988; **72**: 1513–31.

2. Diabetes Care and Research in Europe: the St Vincent Declaration. *Diabet Med* 1990; **7**: 360.
3. Stiegler H, Standl E, Frank S, Mender G. Failure of reducing lower extremity amputation in diabetic patients: results of two subsequent population-based surveys 1990 and 1995 in Germany. *VASA* 1998; **27**: 10–14.
4. Anon. An audit of amputations in a rural health district. *Pract Diabet Int* 1997; **14**: 175–8.
5. Larssen J. Lower extremity amputations in diabetic patients. Doctoral thesis, Lund University, 1994.
6. Ollendorf DA, Cooper T, Kotsanos JG et al. Potential economic benefits of lower extremity amputation prevention strategies in diabetes. *Diabet Care* 1998; **21**: 1240–5.
7. Krentz AJ, Acheson P, Basu A et al. Morbidity and mortality associated with diabetic foot disease: a 12-month prospective survey of hospital admissions in a single UK centre. *Foot* 1997; **7**: 144–7.
8. Young MJ, Boulton AJM. Peripheral vascular disease. In Dyck PJ, Thomas PK, Asbury AK, Winegrad AI, Porte D (Eds), *Diabetic Neuropathy*. Philadelphia: WB Saunders, 1999: 105–122.
9. Abbott RD, Brand FN, Kannel WB. Epidemiology of some peripheral arterial findings in diabetic men and women: experiences from the Framingham Study. *Am J Med* 1990; **88**: 376–81.
10. Pecoraro RE, Reiber GE, Burgess EM. Pathways to diabetic limb amputation: basis for prevention. *Diabet Care* 1990; **13**: 513–21.
11. Reiber GE, Vileikyte L, Boyko EJ et al. Causal pathways for incident lower extremity ulcers in patients with diabetes from two settings. *Diabet Care* 1999; **22**: 157–62.
12. Siitonen OI, Niskanen LK, Laakso M, Siitonen JF, Pyorala K. Lower extremity amputation in diabetic and non-diabetic patients: a population-based study in Eastern Finland. *Diabet Care* 1993; **16**: 16–20.
13. UKPDS 33. Intensive blood-glucose control with sulphonylurea or insulin compared with conventional treatment and risk of complications in patients with Type II diabetes. *Lancet* 1998; **352**: 837–53.
14. UKPDS 38. Tight blood pressure control and risk of macrovascular and microvascular complications in Type II diabetes. *Br Med J* 1998; **317**: 703–13.
15. Boulton AJM, Malik RA. Diabetic neuropathy. *Med Clin N Am* 1998; **82**: 909–29.
16. Boulton AJM, Gries FA, Jervell JA. Guidelines for the diagnosis and out-patient management of diabetic peripheral neuropathy. *Diabet Med* 1998; **15**: 508–14.
17. Kumar S, Ashe HA, Parnell L et al. The prevalence of foot ulceration and its correlates in Type II diabetes: a population-based study. *Diabet Med* 1994; **11**: 480–4.
18. Partanen J, Niskanen L, Lehtinen J et al. Natural history of peripheral neuropathy in patients with non-insulin dependent diabetes. *N Engl J Med* 1995; **333**: 89–96.
19. Young MJ, Boulton AJM, McLeod AF et al. A multicentre study of the prevalence of diabetic neuropathy in the UK hospital clinic population. *Diabetologia* 1993; **36**: 150–6.
20. Tesfaye S, Stevens L, Stephenson J et al. The prevalence of diabetic peripheral neuropathy and its relation to glycaemic control and potential risk factors: the Eurodiab IDDM Complications Study. *Diabetologia* 1996; **39**: 1377–84.

21. Cabezas-Cerrato J. The prevalence of clinical diabetic polyneuropathy in Spain: a study in primary care and hospital clinic groups. *Diabetologia* 1998; **41**: 1263–9.
22. Adler AI, Boyko EJ, Ahroni JH et al. Risk factors for diabetic peripheral sensory neuropathy. *Diabet Care* 1997; **20**: 1162–7.
23. Young MJ, Veves A, Breddy JL, Boulton AJM. The prediction of diabetic neuropathic foot ulceration using vibration perception thresholds. *Diabet Care* 1994; **17**: 557–61.
24. Abbott CA, Vileikyte L, Williamson S, Carrington AL, Boulton AJM. Multi-center study of the incidence of and predictive risk factors for diabetic neuropathic foot ulceration. *Diabet Care* 1998; **21**: 1071–4.
25. Litzelman DK, Marriott DJ, Vinicor F. Independent physiological predictors of foot lesions in patients with NIDDM. *Diabet Care* 1997; **20**: 1273–8.
26. Fernando DJS, Hutchinson A, Veves A, Gokal R, Boulton AJM. Risk factors for non-ischaemic foot ulceration in diabetic nephropathy. *Diabet Med* 1991; **8**: 223–5.
27. Toledano H, Young MJ, Veves A, Boulton AJM. Why do Asian diabetic patients have fewer foot ulcers than Caucasians. *Diabet Med* 1993; **10**(suppl 1): S39.
28. Frykberg RG, Lavery LA, Pham H, Harvey C, Harkless L, Veves A. Role of neuropathy and high foot pressures in diabetic foot ulceration. *Diabet Care* 1998; **21**: 1714–19.
29. Veves A, Uccioli L, Manes C et al. Comparison of risk factors for foot problems in diabetic patients attending teaching hospital out-patient clinics in four different European states. *Diabet Med* 1996; **11**: 709–11.
30. Uccioli L, Giacomini PG, Monticone G et al. Body sway in diabetic neuropathy. *Diabet Care* 1995; **18**: 339–44.
31. Katoulis EC, Ebdon-Parry M, Hollis S et al. Postural instability in diabetic neuropathic patients at risk of foot ulceration. *Diabet Med* 1997; **14**: 296–300.
32. Murray HJ, Young MJ, Boulton AJM. The relationship between callus formation, high pressures and neuropathy in diabetic foot ulceration. *Diabet Med* 1996; **13**: 979–82.
33. New JP, McDowell D, Burns E, Young RJ. Problem of amputation in patients with newly diagnosed diabetes. *Diabet Med* 1998; **15**: 760–4.
34. Veves A, Murray HJ, Young MJ, Boulton AJM. The risk of foot ulceration in diabetic patients with high foot pressure: a prospective study. *Diabetologia* 1992; **35**: 660–3.
35. Lavery LA, Armstrong DG, Vela SA et al. Practical criteria for screening patients at high risk for diabetic foot ulceration. *Arch Int Med* 1998; **158**: 157–62.
36. Young MJ, Cavanagh PR, Thomas G et al. The effect of callus removal on dynamic plantar foot pressures in diabetic patients. *Diabet Med* 1992; **9**: 75–7.

4

What the Practising Physician Should Know about Diabetic Foot Biomechanics

PETER R. CAVANAGH, JAN S. ULBRECHT
and GREGORY M. CAPUTO

The Center for Locomotion Studies and Pennsylvania State Diabetes Foot
Clinics, Pennsylvania State University, University Park and Hershey, PA, USA

Biomechanics is a branch of the life sciences concerned with the consequences of forces applied to living tissues. This field is clearly relevant to diabetic foot disease since the majority of foot ulcers result from mechanical stress which, because of loss of protective sensation to pain[1] is not perceived by the patient. The relevance of biomechanics to the practising physician who is treating diabetic foot problems can be stated very clearly: many of the recalcitrant diabetic foot ulcers that are seen failing to heal in a typical practice do so not because of medical issues, in which the physician is well versed (infection, impaired immunity, vascular disease, etc.), but because of simple biomechanical issues which were often not discussed during medical training. Thus, a few minutes spent becoming familiar with those biomechanical issues will pay considerable dividends in improved patient care. Biomechanical considerations are important in all three phases of care of the diabetic foot: primary prevention, healing foot ulcers, and secondary prevention (prevention of ulcer recurrence).

This chapter discusses several very practical concepts that can be applied to diabetic feet, and does not address the more quantitative areas of

The Foot in Diabetes, 3rd edn. Edited by A. J. M. Boulton, H. Connor and P. R. Cavanagh.
© 2000 John Wiley & Sons, Ltd.

biomechanics (such as tissue property characterization and modelling). It should also be pointed out that there is an entire field of foot biomechanics, which is concerned with "balancing" structural abnormalities in non-neuropathic feet. The types of interventions that are typically used by practitioners of that field (such as rigid "corrective" orthoses) are not relevant to our present discussion. Most of this chapter will concern itself with the most common diabetic foot ulcer, the neuropathic plantar ulcer. Skin breakdown due to penetrating injuries, burns, and dorsal injuries due to ill fitting footwear are all also common, but will be addressed only briefly.

STRESS AND STRESS CONCENTRATION

Because force and pressure cannot be seen without the aid of specialized instruments, it is easy to overlook the dramatic concentrations of load that can occur at bony prominences on the plantar aspect of the foot. In the single limb support phase of gait, the total force under the foot will always be approximately 110% of body weight (the extra 10% comes from the "inertial" component as the body decelerates and accelerates throughout the gait cycle). Since a typical men's size 10 foot has a total area of approximately 130 cm^2, the average pressure under the foot of a 100 kg person would be 0.77 kg/cm^2 (force/area) or, stated in the more usual units (kilopascals), approximately 75 kPa. Figure 4.1 shows an actual pressure distribution measured during barefoot walking under the foot of a patient who had a prior ulcer at a prominent metatarsal head. The actual peak pressure is almost 15 times greater than if calculated as above using the simple force/area argument. In units that might be easier to comprehend, this peak pressure under this patient's foot is approximately 160 p.s.i. (pounds per square inch) or 11.2 kg/cm^2. Pressures under the foot during running and turning while walking can be 40% greater than those encountered in walking[2].

NEUROPATHY AND HIGH PRESSURE—THE KEY COMBINATION

As discussed elsewhere in this volume (Chapter 3), peripheral neuropathy results in what has been called a "loss of protective sensation" (LOPS). The loss of sensation to touch, temperature, pain, and deep pressure can be so dense that patients, without being aware of it, can allow objects to penetrate completely through the foot from plantar surface to the dorsum, or they can burn their feet with hot water, etc.

However, most injuries or ulcers in patients with diabetes or LOPS occur at site of high plantar pressure. High pressures such as those shown in Figure 4.1 are not usually found in healthy feet and would result in extreme pain during ambulation for an individual with adequate sensation. For

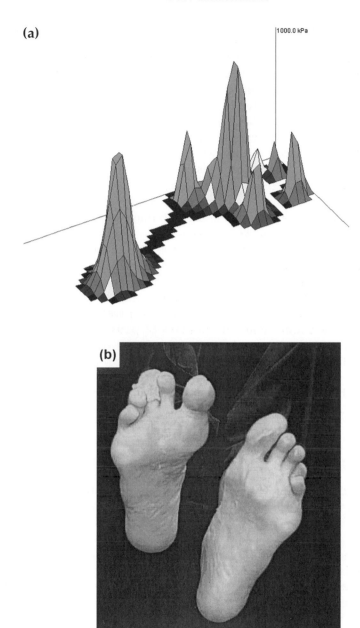

Figure 4.1 (a) Posteromedial view of a peak pressure distribution, measured during barefoot walking under the foot (b) of a patient with a prior ulcer at a prominent 2nd metatarsal head

example, patients with bony deformities from rheumatoid arthritis can experience such pressures[3] without ulceration because they adjust their gait to avoid bearing load on a prominent and painful area and/or they choose footwear that will reduce the pressure (see below).

However, the repetitive application of high pressures to the same soft tissue overlying a bony prominence in the setting of LOPS is believed to cause tissue damage which begins deep (close to the bone)[4]. Callus frequently forms at the surface, and when a patient presents with callus exhibiting a shadowy dark base to visual examination, this is usually an indication that there is a deep ulcer causing haemorrhage into callus. This "pre-ulcer" will then usually develop into an ulcer with further walking. Thus, high pressure alone is not sufficient for plantar ulceration, and neither is neuropathy—it is the combination of the two that provides the necessary and sufficient conditions for ulceration.

Since most physicians will encounter neuropathic diabetic patients who are hospitalized for non-foot-related complaints, it is important to mention here that low pressure applied for long periods of time to feet with loss of protective sensation can also cause devastating lesions. The most common manifestation is deep bilateral pressure ulcers, often penetrating to tendon and bone, on the heels of patients who have been bedridden for a period of time. A similar result can occur in just a few hours in patients who have been lying on their backs during a surgical procedure. In both situations, the ulcers are entirely iatrogenic, caused by failure of the physician to insist on load relief for neuropathic patients, and the failure of the nursing staff to either recognize, or act on the knowledge, that the patient was neuropathic.

THE MECHANISMS FOR ELEVATED PRESSURE

Over time, people with diabetes can develop abnormally high pressure under the foot during walking, and this can result from a number of intrinsic, extrinsic and behavioural factors (Table 4.1). According to Edmonds et al[5], most neuropathic ulcers occur on the toes (39%), the hallux (30%), and the metatarsal heads (24%); these areas, therefore, are of principal concern in understanding both the causes of elevated pressure and how intervention might be accomplished successfully. There is some debate about the critical magnitude of plantar pressure that is required for tissue damage. Veves et al[6] believe that a value of over 1000 kPa during barefoot walking is required while other studies report ulceration at values below 500 kPa. Armstrong et al[7] have suggested that a threshold of 700 kPa is the best compromise between sensitivity and specificity. It is, however, likely that each patient's threshold is different and that the more active a patient is, the less pressure is needed each step to cause ulceration. Also,

Table 4.1 Factors that can lead to elevated plantar pressure under the foot during walking

Intrinsic	Extrinsic	Behavioural
Foot architecture		Walking without shoes
Long second toe		
High arch		
Soft tissue alterations	Poor footwear	Poor choice of shoes
Callus	Tight or loose shoes	
Glycosylation (presumed)	Shoes with hard soles	
Migration of tissue		
Thin tissue		
Limited joint mobility	Accidents and incidents	Inadequate callus care
Foot deformity	Prior surgery	Walking patterns
Claw toes		
Hallux valgus		
Charcot fracture		

since most studies have measured barefoot pressure, the footwear chosen by an individual patient can clearly make the difference between ulceration and no ulceration.

Intrinsic Factors

Certain foot structures predispose an individual to elevated pressures. Some, like a long second metatarsal (Morton's toe) and a high arch[8,9], are not diabetes-related. Callus appears to concentrate pressure rather as if it were a foreign body under the foot. There are some indications that the properties of the plantar soft tissue may be adversely affected by glycosylation end products, although much remains to be explored in this area. Toe deformities (claw toes, hammer toes, hallux valgus) also tend to result in higher pressures[9]. Clawing of the toes appears to result in the plantar fat pads being displaced anteriorly, leaving the condyles of the metatarsal heads "exposed", and this a common finding in patients with diabetic neuropathy. Palpation of the metatarsal heads in a patient with claw toes often reveals an exquisitely thin layer of soft tissue overlying the bone, which leads directly to high pressures during walking unless counter-measures are undertaken (see below). In fact, the lack of adequate thickness of soft tissue under bony prominences has been shown to be an extremely important determinant of elevated pressure[8]. The tips of clawed toes can themselves be locations of ulcers due to concentrated pressure (Figure 4.2).

The range of motion at many joints has been shown to be decreased in patients with diabetes[10]. This is not a neuropathic complication, but probably another effect of glycosylation, whereby the collagen in joint

(a)

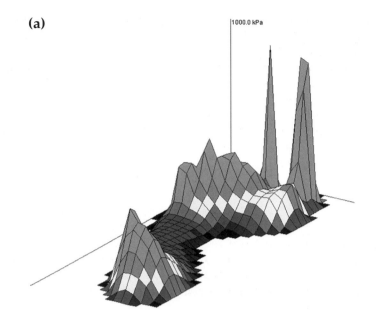

(b)

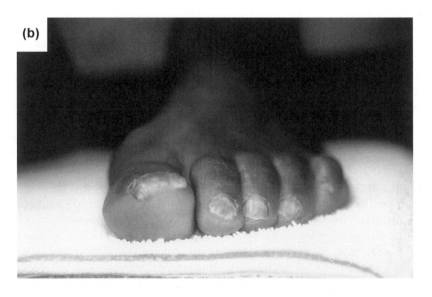

Figure 4.2 (a) Posteromedial view of a peak pressure distribution, measured during barefoot walking, showing elevated pressure at the tips of clawed second toe. Note that the pressure under toe 2 and the hallux are approximately equal. The foot is shown in (b)

capsules is stiffened by the glycosylation process. The consequence of reduced ranges of motion at the major joints of the foot and ankle, such as the first metatarsophalangeal (MTP), sub-talar and talo-crural joints, is likely to be increased plantar pressures under the forefoot[4]. The most frequently problematic joint in this regard is the first MTP[11]. Invariably, a patient with a neuropathic ulcer under the pad of the hallux will be found to have reduced capacity for dorsiflexion at this joint (Figure 4.3).

Despite the above emphasis on the forefoot, a number of conditions can cause elevated pressure in other regions of the foot. Charcot fractures of the midfoot[12,13] typically result in a "rocker bottom" foot which bears load principally on the collapsed region of the midfoot (Figure 4.4). Certain surgical procedures that are intended to reduce loads at primary areas of ulceration can have the secondary effect of increasing pressure in other areas. For example, lengthening of the Achilles tendon, which is sometimes performed following forefoot surgery, can result in what is known as a "calcaneus gait", in which elevated heel pressure occurs during much of the stance phase (Figure 4.5). Removing metatarsal heads because of ulceration in that region can lead to higher pressures under other metatarsal heads.

Extrinsic Factors

In terms of the pressures that the soft tissues are exposed to, footwear is the single most important extrinsic determinant of elevated pressure. While appropriate footwear can be of great benefit in preventing ulcers (see below), incorrect footwear can actually cause ulceration[14]. The two major deficiencies most frequently seen in shoes are incorrect sizing (too loose or too tight) and inadequate cushioning. Tight shoes can cause ulceration at a number of locations. Lesions commonly occur over dorsal deformities, such as a bunion or a dorso-lateral prominence of the fifth metatarsal head (MTH5). The tips of the interphalangeal joints on claw or hammer toes are prime at-risk sites, and ulcers in the interspace between the toes can be caused by the toes being crushed together in a shoe with incorrect contours. Loose shoes, which allow the foot to slip, can also result in ulcers.

As we shall discuss below, "cushioning" for the neuropathic foot is largely defined in static terms and can be equated with "thickness" of "soft" material under the foot. It has been shown that walking in shoes with leather soles is roughly equivalent to walking barefoot, whereas walking in simple sports shoes (trainers) can reduce pressure by up to 50% compared with barefoot walking[15]. Thus, the wrong choice or prescription of shoes can be devastating for the integrity of the diabetic foot.

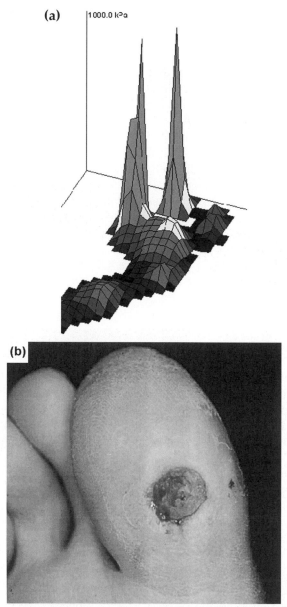

Figure 4.3 (a) Posterolateral view of peak pressure distribution, measured during barefoot walking, from a patient with a neuropathic ulcer under the pad of the hallux (b) secondary to a reduced capacity for dorsiflexion at the first MTP joint. Note that the MTH1 and hallux pressures are approximately equal, although this patient has never experienced an ulcer uner MTH2. (b) Reproduced by permission of W. B. Saunders Company from reference 30

(a)

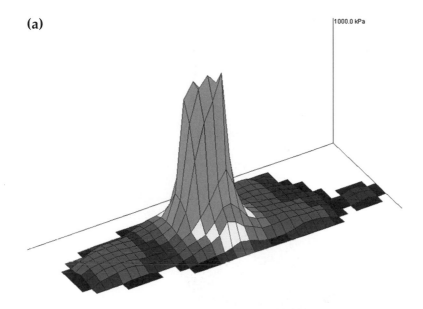

(b)

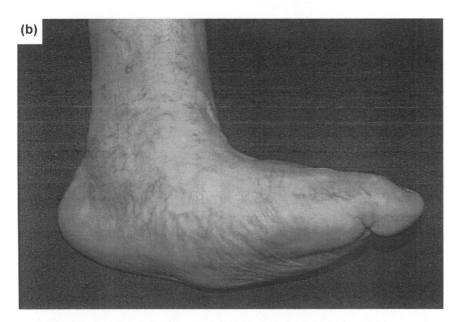

Figure 4.4 Posteromedial view of a peak pressure distribution under a "rocker-bottom" foot (b) during barefoot walking. Load is principally borne on the collapsed region of the midfoot and other regions in the rearfoot and forefoot received almost no load throughout the entire contact phase

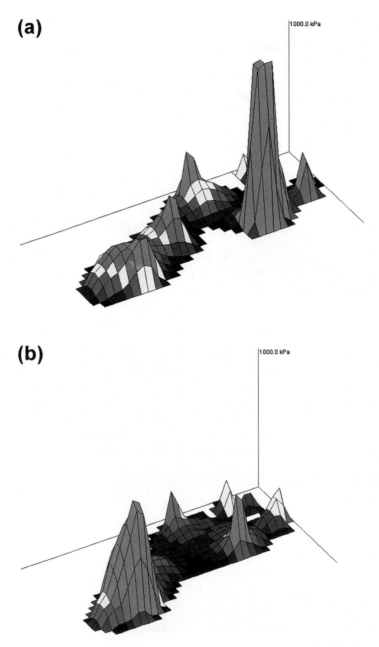

Figure 4.5 Posteromedial view of peak pressure distribution (a) before and (b) 3 months after surgery, which included an osteotomy of the first metatarsal and a lengthening of the Achilles tendon. Note the reduction in forefoot pressures and the increase in the heel peak pressures postsurgically

Behavioural Factors

It is widely believed that barefoot walking is a principal cause of plantar ulceration that is amenable to behavioural intervention. As mentioned above, we do not know the number of steps and the magnitude of pressure that will exceed an individual's threshold for ulceration. However, experience suggests that there are some patients who protect their feet adequately in footwear throughout the day, yet ulcerate because of just a few steps of barefoot walking to urinate during the night. Thus, at least for some patients, even a few steps of barefoot walking are too many. Taking showers barefoot is another dangerous behaviour. The provision of padded slippers, which can be donned easily, is a simple way to intervene in such cases.

Foot injury also occurs frequently during self-care of nails. Patients with poor eyesight should not perform self-care of nails and should be encouraged to have a family member or a chiropodist provide this care. Total neglect of nail and callus care can also be a cause of ulceration. As discussed above, callus concentrates pressure on the plantar aspect of the foot and studies have shown that the presence of callus increases the risk of ulceration by over 11 times[16]. Thus, callus should be regularly removed.

There are some indications that neuropathic patients have altered gait patterns, but it is not yet clear whether this results in elevated plantar pressure. Brand[17] hypothesized that neuropathic gait would be less variable and that this would result in continued application of stress to the same plantar location, but this has not been found to be the case[18]. Regardless, patients with LOPS will not consciously alter their gait, since they will feel no pain developing in high pressure areas from too much walking. There is also some evidence that neuropathic patients experience more falls, and injuries due to falls, than matched non-neuropathic diabetic patients[19,20]. Balance[21] and limb position sense[22] are also impaired and these two factors may lead to more frequent traumatic injuries to the feet of neuropathic patients.

PRIMARY PREVENTION: THE 30 SECOND FOOT EXAMINATION

We have established above that most foot ulcers that the practising physician will see result from mechanical insult to tissue that is deprived of normal sensation. Although we have emphasized neuropathic injury, diminished pulses identify another group of patients at risk because of ischaemia. Thus, the most important issues in prevention of foot pathology are to identify patients who have lost protective sensation and patients with significant ischaemia. Loss of protective sensation is most simply assessed with a 10 g monofilament[23] and we prefer that a forced-choice protocol be used ("Am I touching you at time A or time B?") rather than the procedure described in the International Practical Guidelines in Chapter 21. We recommend that the examination shown in Table 4.2 be performed annually. If the examination shows that the patient has protective sensation and foot pulses and, therefore, is judged not to be at risk, then 30 seconds is all the time that is needed. During this initial scan, the presence of significant deformity should also be noted, as this may affect treatment decisions even in the absence of significant neuropathy.

PRIMARY PREVENTION: THE 2 MINUTE FOOT EXAMINATION

If the initial examination determines that protective sensation has been lost, the biomechanics of the foot and shoes become critical issues in the patient's future. The examination must now be extended to look for the factors discussed above, and for other non-biomechanical factors discussed elsewhere in this volume, which could contribute to ulceration. Surprisingly, this need not be a lengthy examination—it is remarkable how much can be achieved in a short time if the clinician has a well-defined set of goals in advance of the foot examination. In approximately 2 minutes, an examination can cover all of the components shown in Table 4.3 for a patient who is at risk of foot injury.

The surface examination of the foot is fairly straightforward. The clinician must identify ulcers, callus, haemorrhage into callus, breaks or cracks in the skin, skin infection, maceration between toes, and elevated surface temperature. The latter may be an indication of infection or of an active Charcot process, as can oedema or erythema. Nail care should be assessed and the presence of ingrown or long nails, nail fungal infections, and injuries from self-care of nails should be noted. While some of these are not biomechanical issues, their importance is self-evident; most of these topics are covered elsewhere in this volume.

One does not have to be a chiropodist or a foot orthopaedic surgeon to identify the major deformities that can lead to elevated pressure. Those shown in Figure 4.6, including prominent metatarsal heads, claw or hammer toes, excessive callus, hallux valgus and prior amputation can, in combination with neuropathy, lead to ulceration (also see rocker bottom deformity in Figure 17.3). The identification of these deformities will also be important in decisions related to prescription footwear (see below).

Looking at the patient's footwear is a key component of the examination. Shoes and socks should be removed. The socks should be examined for

Table 4.2 The 30-second foot examination. On both feet, the following should be assessed:

Evaluation component	Details	Action
1. Ascertain if the patient has had any previous diabetes-related foot lesions	Ask about ulcers or blisters that were not perceived as particularly painful; ask about foot lesions that required vascular procedures to heal; look for toe or partial foot amputations	If there is a history of previous foot problems, the patient is at risk for more
2. Vascular status/pulses	Feel for: Pulse in posterior tibial artery behind medial malleolus Pulse in dorsalis pedis artery on the dorsum of the foot	If both pulses are absent in either foot, consider further evaluation, particularly if other symptoms or signs of vascular disease are present (see Chapter 16)
3. Loss of Protective Sensation: inability to feel the touch of a 10g monofilament	In a quiet room, test multiple forefoot plantar sites and in particular toes and MTHs; avoid callused areas; ask the patient to tell you every time he/she can feel the touch (do not ask for a response only when you are touching the patient); with the patient's eyes closed, bend monofilament against the skin for 1 second; repeat questionable sites; apply monofilament with random cadence; a relative can observe to reinforce abnormal findings for the patient	If the patient cannot feel the monofilament at even one site, label patient as "at risk". If you are concerned about questionable or hesitant responses, repeat the test at each clinic visit until the result is clearer, or classify the patient as "at risk"
4. Look for significant foot deformity	See the examples shown in Figure 4.6	Appropriate footwear or referral should be suggested, even in the absence of neuropathy

If the patient has no history of previous problems, can feel touch at all sites, and has *one palpable pulse in each foot*, the 30 second examination can end here. Repeat in 1 year, or sooner if findings were questionable.
If the patient has a history of previous problems, has absent pulses or cannot feel touch at even one site, then he/she is at risk for foot injury. Proceed with the additional "2 minute examination".

Table 4.3   The 2-minute foot examination. This follows on from the examination in Table 4.2 if the patient has previous foot problems, has lost protective sensation or has significant vascular disease. On both feet, the following should be examined:

Evaluation component	Details	Action
5. Examine all surfaces	Look for: Ulcer Callus Haemorrhage into callus Blister Maceration between toes Other breaks in the skin Skin infection Oedema, erythema, elevated temperature	Prescribe unweighting device to heal ulcer (see Figures 4.8 and 4.9) Remove callus (sharp debridement and/or dremmel or emery board) Treat skin infection or injury Refer if Charcot fracture suspected
6. Examine the nails	Look for: Fungal infections Ingrown toe nails Evidence of injury from self-care of nails	Consider treating fungal infections Advise against self-care of nails Suggest chiropody care
7. Identify foot deformity	Look for: Prominent metatarsal heads Claw or hammer toes Rocker bottom foot deformity Hallux valgus and bunions Prior amputation	The presence of foot deformity will dictate footwear specifications (see text and Table 4.4)
8. Examine the shoes. Have the patient put their shoes and socks on as the last component of the examination. This will show the patient's ability to examine their own feet.	Look for: Drainage into socks Worn out (flattened) insoles Shoes that are leaning badly to one side Poorly fitting shoes (too tight, too loose, too short, not enough room for the toes) Gait pattern	Prescribe appropriate footwear if necessary (see text and Table 4.4) Suggest replacement shoes if necessary
9. Establish need for education	Ask: "Why do you think I am concerned about your feet?" Do you walk without shoes at home? Who takes care of your nails?	Schedule patient for education visit with diabetes educator/ nurse if understanding is lacking or if behaviours are unacceptable

evidence of drainage from a wound, and the shoe insoles should be studied to see if they have "bottomed out" and no longer provide adequate cushioning. The size of the shoe should be compared to the size of the foot, particularly the height and curvature of the forefoot region. At the end of the examination the patient should be asked to put his/her shoes and socks on, so that the examiner can assess the patient's mobility during this process, as this will impact on the patient's ability to examine his/her own feet. At some point during the examination, the clinician should ask a few key questions, which will elicit information regarding the patient's understanding of the disease process and indicate his/her educational needs. Questions such as "Why do you think I am concerned about your feet?", "Do you walk without shoes at home?" and "Who takes care of your nails?" can be helpful in this regard. A brief observation of the patient's gait, watching for obvious abnormalities, will complete the examination. A final determination of shoe fit during weight bearing should also be performed at this time.

Action Based on the "At-risk" Examination

Appropriate actions based on the findings of the examination are listed in Table 4.2. These include referral for problems that require specialist care (e.g. symptomatic vascular impairment, suspected Charcot fracture, or periodic chiropodial care), immediate treatment for ulcers and infections (see below), the prescription of therapeutic footwear (see below) and of patient education (see Chapter 9). Callus can be trimmed by a trained health care provider in the physician's office using a number 15 scalpel and an emery board.

BIOMECHANICAL ISSUES IN TREATING A PLANTAR ULCER

One of the most often-heard complaints by specialists in diabetic foot clinics is that ulcers referred to as "non-healing" are often simply badly treated ulcers that could have been healed many months previously. This can be verified in the literature, where studies of, for example, the total contact cast (TCC, see below) show that ulcers that had existed often for more than a year were healed in approximately 6 weeks[24].

There is little doubt that the total contact cast (Figure 4.7), in combination with good wound care, is the "gold standard" for healing neuropathic ulcers[24,25]. This combination accomplishes a number of goals that are important to wound healing: reduction in oedema, load relief at the ulcer site, enforced compliance with load relief, and encouragement for the patient to keep a return appointment. However, some drawbacks of the total contact cast are that specialized staff are required to apply and remove the cast, that patients with infection should not generally be casted, and that casting can result in additional lesions, either on the other foot or on the casted foot if the cast becomes too loose.

Thus, in a typical physician practice, the TCC is not a realistic method of healing ulcers. Therefore, if referral for casting is impossible, the goals

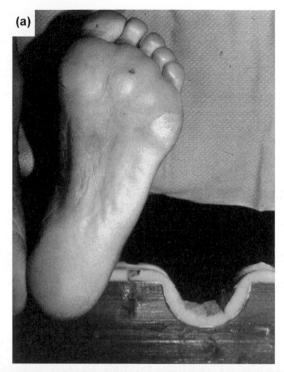

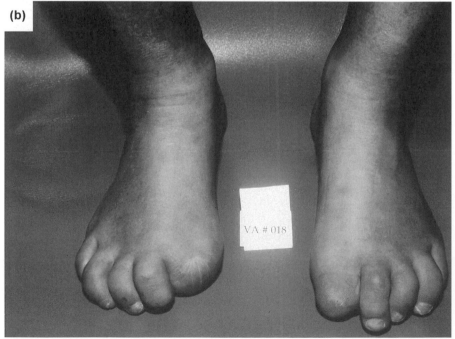

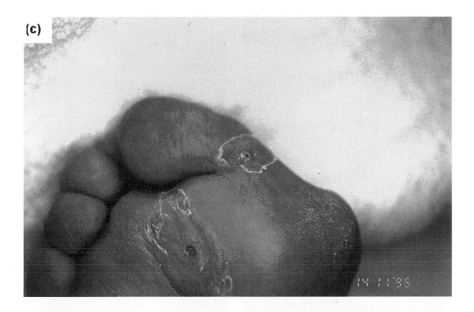

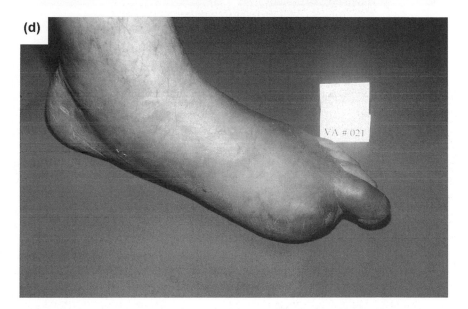

Figure 4.6 Common foot deformities that should be identified during a brief foot examination. In combination with neuropathy, these conditions can lead to ulceration. (a) Prominent metatarsal heads. (b) Clawed toes. (c) Hallux valgus and excessive plantar callus. (d) Partial amputation

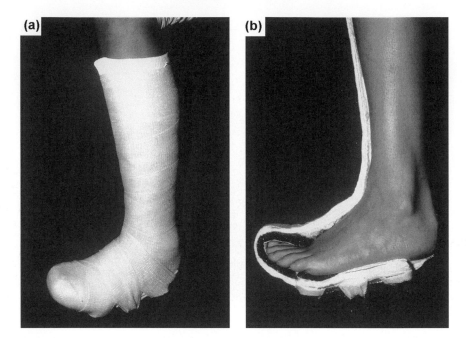

Figure 4.7   A total contact cast (a), also shown in cutaway view (b). This is the "gold standard" for wound healing. Note the soft foam wrapped around the forefoot and the way in which this mechanically isolates the forefoot from weightbearing

of wound healing in such a setting must be to provide conditions that approximate as well as possible those of the foot in a total contact cast by using some other approach. Of the various requirements discussed above for healing neuropathic ulcers, the most critical is compliance with non-weight-bearing. Bedrest would be ideal—but this is rarely realistic. The patient with an ulcer must not be allowed to walk away from an examination in the shoes that helped to cause the lesion in the first place. As obvious as this sounds, it is a rule that is frequently broken. A wound that receives continual mechanical stress will not heal, as is apparent from the duration of ulcers prior to entry in the studies mentioned above. Among the ways of achieving off-loading of forefoot ulcers are shoes that only have a rear midsole and outsole (Figure 4.8). Similar devices with heel cutouts are available for rearfoot ulcers. Braces or walkers that both take some load from the foot and transfer it to the leg, and that provide a cavity in the insole which mechanically isolates the lesion can also be useful (Figures 4.9, 17.15). All of these devices need to be used with crutches or a wheelchair if adequate unloading of the ulcer is to be achieved. Patients need to understand that they have been provided with load-relieving devices only to allow them to perform the most basic

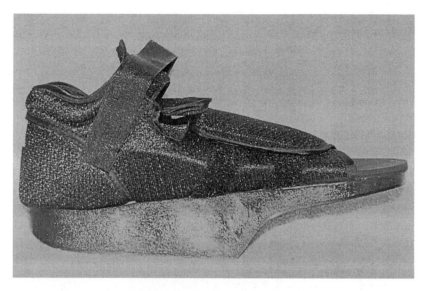

Figure 4.8 Shoe designed to provide off-loading of a forefoot plantar ulcer

activities of daily living. The foot must never touch the ground or a regular shoe until the ulcer is healed.

The way in which the footwear is used can also affect its efficacy. For example, if a patient rocks forward on the shoe shown in Figure 4.8, the forefoot can be loaded. It is likely that more off-loading is needed to heal an ulcer than is needed to prevent an ulcer. Thus, footwear in the usual sense of the word, and even "specialized" footwear, as discussed below for prevention of ulcers, is unlikely to be adequate to achieve healing.

Another key component of wound healing is debridement of the ulcer. While few studies have been performed to support this practice[26], it is widely believed that sharp debridement of an ulcer, including the removal of callus which may surround or "roof over" the ulcer, and of all devitalized tissue, is essential to healing. This process is quite distinct from surgical debridement, which often involves the removal of considerable soft tissue and possibly bone and is usually performed in the operating theatre. Sharp debridement of an ulcer can be carried out in the physician's office and a suitable wound dressing can be applied to provide a moist healing environment (see Chapter 13).

Compliance with a regimen of weight relief is likely to be the primary determinant of healing. The patient needs to understand the rationale for unloading the foot and caregivers need to be sensitized to the need to keep the foot completely clear of the ground. If a primarily neuropathic ulcer is not healing after a course of 6–8 weeks of debridement and unloading, it

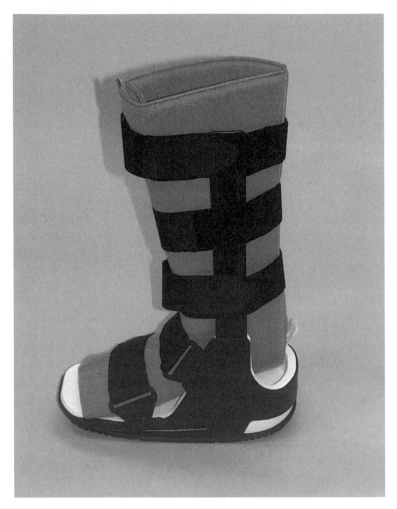

Figure 4.9   A brace designed to transfer some load to the leg and to provide space for a thick insole with mechanical relief in the ulcerated area. The outsole is of a "roller" design (see Figure 4.12)

can be assumed that the patient is not being compliant to the weight relief regimen, or that the weight relief regimen is inadequately designed. Patients in general do not believe that a few steps per day on an ulcer to get coffee or to go to the bathroom can prevent healing.

Non-plantar ulcers are easier to heal, although the principles are the same: avoidance of ongoing mechanical injury, usually from footwear or from a support surface during rest is key. Beware of the patient with a lateral malleolus or a lateral MTH5 lesion who sleeps on that side.

PRIMARY AND SECONDARY PREVENTION—THE IMPORTANCE OF FOOTWEAR

Shoes cannot heal ulcers. However, patients who have experienced a foot ulcer must pay special attention to footwear for the remainder of their lives. It is only after an ulcer has healed through one of the weight-relieving methods discussed above that definitive footwear can be provided. Specifying the details of prescription footwear is often considered to be a task that the physician delegates to others—but there are many settings in which specialized footwear assistance is not available. It is important, therefore, for the physician who is the primary provider of foot care to have a clear idea of the options available. Unfortunately, many physicians regard footwear prescription as somewhat of a mystery. This should not be the case, because more than 80% of patients can be successfully managed in either "over the counter" sports shoes (trainers) or extra-depth shoes with prescribed flat or customized insoles. Only patients with severe foot deformity or other special problems will require custom-moulded shoes (and perhaps braces), which only a specialist such as a pedorthist, orthotist or orthopaedic shoemaker can provide. This is shown schematically in the "footwear pyramid" in Figure 4.10. The approach to footwear prescription is shown in Table 4.4. Shoes are listed in order of increasing complexity and expense, and thus the clinician should aim to provide the simplest footwear solution that will keep the patient ulcer-free and active.

The clinical goals of footwear for a diabetic patient are either to prevent the development of an initial ulcer (in the case of primary prevention)[27], or

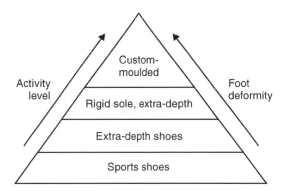

Figure 4.10 The "footwear pyramid", showing a schematic distribution of all cases of prescription footwear. Many cases can be managed in sports shoes. The next category, extra-depth shoes, can be modified to provide additional pressure relief by making the outsoles rigid and rockered. Custom-moulded shoes will need to be made by an experienced orthopaedic shoe technician, but the treating physician can provide all other categories. Reproduced by permission of W. B. Saunders Company from reference 30

Table 4.4 Footwear for the neuropathic patient (in order of complexity)

Footwear	Modification	Comment
Sports shoe (trainers)	Can replace supplied insole with flat foam insole	Make sure that there is enough dorsal room for the tops of toes
Extra-depth shoe with flat 1/4 inch insole	Often supplied with just a "spacer" insole; this should be replaced with a prescribed flat foam insole	Make sure that there is enough dorsal room for the tops of toes, particularly if thicker insole is used
Extra-depth shoe with custom insole		Insole will need to be made by a specialist technician but the mould can be made in the physician's office
Extra-depth shoe with custom insole and rigid roller or rocker outsole	Any experienced shoemaker can make the sole rigid and produce a rocker sole, as shown in Figure 4.11	Make sure that the axis of the rocker is behind the MTH of interest
Custom Footwear		This will need to be measured and made by an experienced orthopaedic shoe technician

to prevent a recurrence of ulceration at the same site or new ulceration at a different site (in secondary prevention). Footwear can also give patients the freedom to live an active life but the more active the patient is, the more "sophisticated" the footwear needs to be (see earlier discussion on the likely relationship between pressure, activity/number of steps and ulceration risk; specialized footwear can be made for golf, horse riding, etc.). The biomechanical goals are to provide load relief or "cushioning" at sites of elevated pressure and sometimes to transfer load from one site to another. These goals can often be accomplished quite simply using 1/4 inch (6.5 mm) thick flat foam insoles of various densities to accommodate to plantar deformity. Probably the most important aspect of material selection is that it should be durable and should not "bottom out" particularly. Since thick insoles require more space than is available inside a typical shoe, extra-depth shoes (Figure 4.11) are the mainstay of prescribed footwear. These shoes are built with the same shape as regular shoes, with a roomy toe box if viewed from above, but when looked at from the side, it is apparent that they have a much higher toe box, so that insoles can be worn without forcing the toes against the upper of the shoe. Thicker socks can also be accommodated in extra-depth shoes and such socks have been shown to offer additional pressure relief[28]. As discussed earlier, even the cushioning available in simple off-the-shelf sports shoes (trainers) provides significant pressure relief compared to leather-soled shoes and the use of such shoes has been shown to reduce the appearance of calluses.

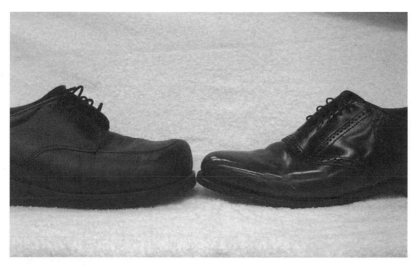

Figure 4.11   A comparison of the toe-box region of an extra-depth shoe (left) with a typical leather Oxford shoe. Note that the extra-depth shoe has sufficient space to allow a thick insole to be placed in the shoe while still leaving space to ensure that the dorsum of the toes are not pushed against the upper

Most authorities believe that moulded insoles provide a superior reduction of load compared to flat insoles. Our recent research has shown that modifications such as a build-up of the insole height behind the metatarsal heads, a high arch support, or a depression to relieve specific high pressure areas can be effective in removing load from at-risk areas and distributing it to other regions of the foot. On the other hand, simple moulding without attention to the anatomy of the particular foot may not be beneficial. While the fabrication of moulded insoles is beyond the scope of a typical office practice, several in-office methods for obtaining an impression of the shape of the foot are available (e.g. A. Alego Ltd, Sheridan House, Bridge Industrial Estate, Speke Hall Road, Liverpool L24 9HB, UK). These impressions can then be sent to an orthotic manufacturer, who will return custom moulded insoles to fit directly into extra-depth shoes.

The next level of complexity is to provide the patient with extra-depth shoes and custom insoles where the outsole of the shoe has been made rigid and contoured. This produces a "roller" or "rocker" shoe (Figure 4.12). Both these shoes allow walking without flexion of the MTP joints, thus reducing MTH plantar pressure markedly. This modification is a relatively simple one which can be performed by a local shoemaker who is given the correct instructions. The axis of the rocker shoe is generally placed approximately 2 cm behind the metatarsal head of interest. The patient

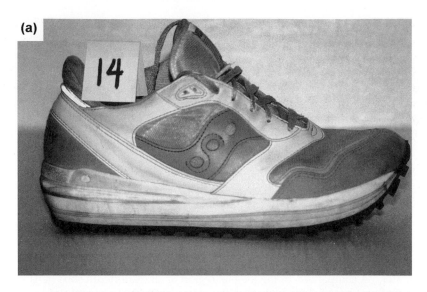

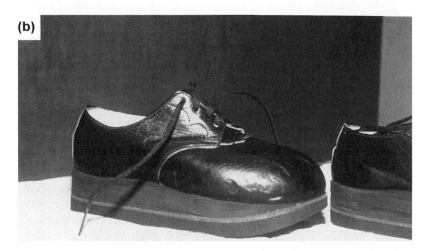

Figure 4.12 Shoes with rigid and contoured outsoles. (a) A roller shoe with a continuous curve and (b) a rocker shoe with a clear pivot point. Both these shoes allow walking without flexion of the MTP joints and this can reduce plantar pressure markedly

must be taught how to walk correctly in the shoe, allowing the shoe to rock forward during late support but not dwelling on the wedge area in the forepart. The simplest way to encourage patients to do this is to ask them to take smaller than usual strides.

Methods are available for the measurement of plantar pressure inside footwear[29], but the equipment needed is not widely available. As a result, footwear prescription is somewhat of a trial-and-error process for most physicians, who must try to discern by eye whether or not a particular shoe reduces load at a critical area. Patients with new footwear must therefore be followed very closely during the first few weeks and they should also be encouraged to increase the use of the shoes slowly and progressively during this time, starting with just one hour per day. Frequent self-examinations of the feet should also be encouraged to look for signs of tissue damage (redness, inflammation, warmth, blisters, callus, haemorrhage into callus and, in the extreme, of course, ulceration). If none of the footwear interventions described above proves satisfactory, referral of the patient to a specialized centre is warranted.

ACKNOWLEDGMENTS

The authors are grateful for the editorial assistance of Mrs Esther Y. Boone.

REFERENCES

1. Birke JA, Sims DS. Plantar sensory threshold in the ulcerative foot. *Leprosy Rev* 1986; **57**: 261–7.
2. Rozema A, Ulbrecht JS, Pammer SE, Cavanagh PR. In-shoe plantar pressures during activities of daily living: implications for therapeutic footwear design. *Foot Ankle Int* 1996; **17**: 325–59.
3. Masson EA, Hay EM, Stockley I, Betts RP, Boulton AJM. Abnormal foot pressure alone may not cause foot ulceration. *Diabet Med* 1989; **6**: 426–8.
4. Delbridge L, Ctercteko G, Fowler C, Reeve TS, LeQuesne LP. The aetiology of diabetic neuropathic ulceration of the foot. *Br J Surg* 1985; **72**: 1–6.
5. Edmonds ME, Blundell MP, Morris ME, Thomas EM, Cotton LT, Watkins PJ. Improved survival of the diabetic foot: the role of a specialised foot clinic. *Qu J Med* 1986; **60**(232): 763–71.
6. Veves A, Murray HJ, Young MJ, Boulton AJM. The risk of foot ulceration in diabetic patients with high foot pressure: a prospective study. *Diabetologia* 1992; **35**: 660–3.
7. Armstrong DG, Peters EJG, Athanasiou KA, Lavery LA. Is there a critical level of plantar foot pressure to identify patients at risk for neuropathic foot ulceration? *J Foot Ankle Surg* 1998; **37**: 303–7.
8. Morag E, Cavanagh PR. Structural and functional predictors of regional peak pressures under the foot during walking. *J Biomech* 1999; **32**(4): 359–70.
9. Ahroni JH, Boyko EJ, Forsberg RC. Clinical correlates of plantar pressure among diabetic veterans. *Diabet Care* 1999; **22**: 965–72.
10. Andersen H, Mogensen PH. Disordered mobility of large joints in association with neuropathy in patients with long-standing insulin-dependent diabetes mellitus. *Diabet Med* 1996; **14**: 221–7.

11. Birke JA, Cornwall MA, Jackson M. Relationship between hallux limitus and ulceration of the great toe. *J Orthopaed Sports Phys Ther* 1988; **10**: 172–6.

12. Myerson MS, Henderson MR, Saxby T, Short KW. Management of midfoot diabetic neuroarthropathy. *Foot Ankle Int* 1994; **15**: 233–41.

13. Pinzur MS, Sage R, Stuck R, Kaminsky S, Zmuda A. A treatment algorithm for neuropathic (Charcot) midfoot deformity. *Foot Ankle Int* 1993; **14**: 189–97.

14. Apelqvist J, Larsson J, Agardh C-D. The influence of external precipitating factors and peripheral neuropathy on the development and outcome of diabetic foot ulcers. *J Diabet Compl* 1990; **4**: 21–5.

15. Perry JE, Ulbrecht JS, Derr JA, Cavanagh PR. The use of running shoes to reduce plantar pressures in patients who have diabetes. *J Bone Joint Surg* 1995; **77**-A: 1819–28.

16. Murray HJ, Young MJ, Hollis S, Boulton AJM. The association between callus formation, high pressures and neuropathy in diabetic foot ulceration. *Diabet Med* 1996; **13**: 979–82.

17. Brand PW. The insensitive foot (including Hansen's disease). In Jahss MH (ed.), *Disorders of the Foot and Ankle and Their Surgical Management*, 2nd edn, Vol. 3. Philadelphia: WB Saunders, 1991: 2170–86.

18. Cavanagh PR, Perry JE, Ulbrecht JS, Derr JA, Pammer SE. Neuropathic diabetic patients do not have reduced variability of plantar loading during gait. *Gait Posture* 1998; **7**: 191–9.

19. Cavanagh PR, Derr JA, Ulbrecht JS, Maser RE, Orchard TJ. Problems with gait and posture in neuropathic patients with insulin-dependent diabetes mellitus. *Diabet Med* 1992; **9**: 469–74.

20. Richardson JK, Ching C, Hurvitz EA. The relationship between electromyographically documented peripheral neuropathy and falls. *J Am Geriat Soc* 1992; **40**: 1008–12.

21. Simoneau GG, Ulbrecht JS, Derr JA, Becker MB, Cavanagh PR. Postural instability in patients with diabetic sensory neuropathy. *Diabet Care* 1994; **17**: 1411–21.

22. Simoneau GG, Derr JA, Ulbrecht JS, Becker MB, Cavanagh PR. Diabetic sensory neuropathy effect on ankle joint movement perception. *Arch Phys Med Rehab* 1996; **77**: 453–60.

23. Rith-Najarian SJ, Stolusky T, Gohdes DM. Identifying diabetic patients at high risk for lower-extremity amputation in a primary health care setting: a prospective evaluation of simple screening criteria. *Diabet Care* 1992; **15**: 1386–9.

24. Mueller MJ, Diamond JE, Sinacore DR et al. Total contact casting in treatment of diabetic plantar ulcers: controlled clinical trial. *Diabet Care* 1989; **12**: 384–8.

25. Coleman WC, Brand PW, Birke JA. The total contact cast: a therapy for plantar ulceration on insensitive feet. *J Am Podiat Assoc* 1984; **74**: 548–52.

26. Steed DL, Donohoe D, Webster MW, Lindsley L. Effect of extensive debridement and treatment on the healing of diabetic foot ulcers. Diabetic Ulcer Study Group. *J Am Coll Surgeons* 1996; **183**: 61–4.

27. Chantelau E, Kushner T, Spraul M. How effective is cushioned therapeutic footwear in protecting diabetic feet? A clinical study. *Diabet Med* 1990; **7**: 355–9.

28. Veves A, Masson EA, Fernando DJS, Boulton AJM. Use of experimental padded hosiery to reduce abnormal foot pressures in diabetic neuropathy. *Diabet Care* 1989; **12**: 653–5.

29. Cavanagh PR, Ulbrecht JS. Clinical plantar pressure measurement in diabetes: rationale and methodology. *Foot* 1994; **4**: 123–35.
30. Cavanagh PR, Ulbrecht JS, Caputo GM. Biomechanics of the foot in diabetes mellitus. In Bowker JH, Pfiefer M (eds), *The Diabetic Foot*, 6th edn. Philadelphia, PA: WB Saunders, 2000.

5

Classification of Ulcers and Its Relevance to Management

MATTHEW J. YOUNG

Royal Infirmary, Edinburgh, UK

The management of diabetic foot ulceration is multidisciplinary in its most effective form, and requires communication between primary and secondary care providers. In addition, the increasing role of research-based practice, audit and clinical effectiveness in the provision of managed health care systems means that accurate and concise ulcer description and classification models are required to improve interdisciplinary collaboration and communication and to allow meaningful comparisons between and within centres[1].

The classification of an ulcer should delineate a single type of ulcer with definable characteristics which are distinct from other ulcer categories. Examples of potential classification systems are detailed below. They are often related to the risk factors which led to the ulcer and, in at least two cases, they do not use any of the descriptive characteristics of the ulcer to categorize it. As well as being a basis for clinical care, a classification should provide a guide to prognosis and should facilitate audit and research. A good example is the classification of ulcers by their suspected aetiology, such as neuropathic or neuro-ischaemic, or by their perceived severity, for example, superficial or deep. The classification of an ulcer should be applied once, based on the initial characteristics, and should not alter with the progress of therapy. A description is based upon definable characteristics but differs from a classification in that it applies to the ulcer at the exact moment it is seen. It is therefore ephemeral, changing with the progression of the ulcer. It is important to make the distinction between

The Foot in Diabetes, 3rd edn. Edited by A. J. M. Boulton, H. Connor and P. R. Cavanagh.
© 2000 John Wiley & Sons, Ltd.

classification and description of an ulcer. In the future, digital imaging and image transmission may make such systems easier, but at present descriptions are an essential part of working practice. Whilst descriptive terms such as "uninfected" or "infected" might be used to classify ulcers, most descriptive terms do not lend themselves to a classification with workable numbers of categories and are, therefore, not a basis for auditing the outcome of ulceration or for classifying an ulcer. However, descriptions are very useful in prompting adjustments to ongoing treatment as the nature of the ulcer changes. They are also essential to ensuring that health care professionals can communicate referrals and handover of care in an unambiguous way. Such referrals also need to include patient characteristics other than those of the ulcer. Where such characteristics have been shown to be important in prognosis they are also discussed below.

CATEGORIES FOR CLASSIFICATION AND DESCRIPTION OF ULCERATION

Location of the Ulcer

Ulceration of the lower limb in diabetic patients can occur at any site. However, since the aetiology and treatment of leg ulceration above the ankle is usually different from foot ulceration, this chapter will not discuss this further. It is essential to describe the site of ulceration, as this will often give clues to the cause and often the underlying aetiology for the purpose of guiding therapy. Toe ulceration is often directly shoe-induced; ulceration on the remainder of the foot is often multifactorial. Plantar ulceration is classically neuropathic; marginal ulcers are more commonly associated with ischaemia[2]. In addition, toe ulceration is significantly associated with amputation[3]. Therefore, the location of ulceration can also give a guide to prognosis, although this effect is less significant than the aetiology of the ulcer overall, or Meggitt–Wagner[4,5] grade (see below), irrespective of site[6].

Ulcers which occur in association with significant foot deformity are rarely characterized separately from other ulcers. Deformity forms the basis of a number of foot ulcer risk scoring systems, but once the ulcer has formed, deformity receives little attention as a guide to treatment or prognosis. Only Mayfield et al[7] have clearly identified deformity as an additional risk factor for amputation, but this was as part of a pre-ulceration risk stratification and not as a direct result of classifying ulcers. Despite this, ulceration and deformity continue to be reported anecdotally in many foot clinics, especially in association with neuro-arthropathy and rocker-bottom foot.

Size and Extent of Ulceration

The size of an ulcer, usually defined as either two diameters at right angles, or as surface area, is an important descriptive term. Without serial measurements of ulcer size, it is impossible to document change in any meaningful way; therefore, size measurements should be mandatory for all ulcers. However, there is less evidence that ulcer size is a guide to management or prognosis, and none of the widely applied classifications of foot ulceration uses ulcer size as a discriminator. Indeed, a recent meta-analysis of wound healing studies showed an absence of effect of ulcer size on prognosis in neuropathic ulceration.[8]

The volume of an ulcer is currently almost impossible to assess. However, ulcer depth, either measured or, more commonly, simply described, is an important factor in both descriptive and classification systems. Exposure of bone and tendon is a feature of all classifications derived from the Meggitt–Wagner classification.[4,5] The use of sterile blunt probes to fully explore the extent of an ulcer is a useful tool to identify bone and deep tissue involvement in ulcers that do not appear to be extensive upon initial inspection. Probing to bone was shown to identify osteomyelitis with a positive predictive value of 89% in one series[9]. The identification of deep tissue involvement, and in particular deep infection or osteomyelitis, is strongly associated with an increased risk of major amputation[10]; therefore, probing should be performed in all but the most obviously superficial ulcers.

Aetiology

In many classification systems the categorization of foot ulceration is based logically upon the aetiological factors. The management of ulceration has common features, namely pressure relief, debridement and infection control, although these vary depending on the nature of the ulcer. Patients with neuropathy who develop foot ulcers have a significantly better prognosis than patients with vascular insufficiency. The simple absence of pulses doubles amputation risk[11]; ankle pressure indices are lower in patients who have had or will have amputations[12]; transcutaneous oxygen tensions are associated with delayed healing and amputation if less than 30 mmHg[13]; and the number of lesions detected on peripheral arteriograms is directly proportional to amputation risk[14]. Therefore, it is clearly important to identify vascular insufficiency, so that revascularization can be attempted where appropriate. Even in the absence of these criteria, an ulcer which is not healing despite optimal care should be investigated for vascular insufficiency.

The coexistence of neuropathy in patients with peripheral vascular disease[15] has led to the use of the term "neuro-ischaemic foot" and at least one classification is based on this distinction[2]. Some patients with peripheral vascular disease do have intact peripheral sensation, which is manifest as rest pain or as pain during ulcer debridement or in the presence of infection. Pain is, itself, an independently poor prognostic indicator in patients with diabetic foot ulceration[11]. However, given the relative paucity of purely ischaemic lesions in diabetic patients and the frequency of coexisting sensory or motor neuropathy, the term "neuro-ischaemic" is probably a good one for these patients and will be referred to again later in this chapter.

The presence of gangrene is the significant turning point in the Meggitt–Wagner classification system[4,5], separating the primarily neuropathic from the primarily ischaemic foot. However, the realization that localized gangrene in the toes can occur as a result of infective vasculitis in a foot with normal peripheral pulses highlights the fact that this may be an unduly simplistic approach. The presence of tissue necrosis and gangrene in infected feet should not be taken to imply failure of peripheral circulation without other supporting evidence. Resection of infected tissue necrosis or toe auto-amputation may allow a foot to heal without surgical amputation in an otherwise well-perfused limb. Extensive gangrene, from either peripheral arterial occlusion or infection, is usually a precursor to major amputation, regardless of aetiology. However, it is not clear how much gangrene must be present for it to be defined as extensive. Whilst it might appear clinically obvious when a foot needs amputating, the wide disparity in amputation rates between centres suggests that a stricter definition might be required.

Infection

As has been implied above, infection has a significant adverse effect on the diabetic foot with ulceration. Unfortunately, in many cases it is very difficult to detect infection in diabetic foot ulcers and to gauge its extent and severity. Few of the descriptive or classification systems that include infection as a parameter give any definition as to what constitutes infection. Bacterial colonization of diabetic foot ulcers is the norm in bacteriological surveys and yet it is generally accepted that the classical signs of inflammation that typify infective processes elsewhere are significantly reduced in the diabetic foot. For this reason, whilst some regard the presence of bacteria as insignificant in the absence of signs of infection, many advocate treating all ulcers as if potentially superficially infected and use systemic antibiotics in most, if not all patients[16]. However, when osteomyelitis is present, most clinicians, especially surgeons, will advocate surgery[17], although two recent papers have reported good outcomes with conservative management[18,19] and this approach should be probably used more frequently.

Even extensive infection may be difficult to detect. The presence of swelling, heat and pain could indicate a neuro-arthropathic foot (although it is more common to make the converse error). Even if infection is present, there may be little or no supporting systemic features, such as fever or raised white cell count[17,20]. Even the erythrocyte sedimentation rate can be normal. Features such as lymphangitis, frank pus and foul drainage suggest that a foot is severely infected.

Osteomyelitis is also difficult to detect in the diabetic foot. The typical systemic features of infection may be absent, and radiological and other imaging techniques may be inconclusive or misleading (see Chapters 15 and 17). Therefore, it is important to have a high index of suspicion, to use the probe-to-bone test, and to examine serial radiographs of deep ulcers, which take a long time to heal. If osteomyelitis develops then it is a significant risk factor for amputation, regardless of vascular status[10].

Other factors

A number of patient characteristics can be identified from epidemiological surveys as having a significant effect on the outcome of treatment of diabetic foot ulceration. Very few of these are actually independent predictors of amputation but most form part of a multivariate regression. A history of previous foot ulceration, and in particular of previous amputation, is one such independent indicator that there is a high risk of amputation during a subsequent event. In addition there is a need for further evaluation of post-ulcer care if the foot heals[21]. One of the reasons for this is the strong association between patient non-compliance with therapy and amputation in a number of studies. Inability to comply with off-loading strategies and antibiotic therapy, and failure to attend the clinic, may all compromise the foot. In addition, late presentation to clinic with an ulcer carries a high risk of subsequent amputation, although this may be as much due to primary care delays as patient delays[22].

Irrespective of these factors it is more common for men to have foot ulcers and to have amputations compared to women. The elderly, especially if they live in institutionalized care or have a low walking tolerance, and patients with longer duration of diabetes, are at greater risk of major amputation[23]. Although one study did not identify end-stage renal disease as a factor that influenced healing[24], in most studies, amputation risk is generally higher in patients with other major diabetes complications, particularly renal impairment and visual impairment[7,12,20,21,23,24].

Type 2 patients on insulin, higher glycated haemoglobin, and random glucose levels are also associated with a greater risk of amputation or re-ulceration in some studies, and may again reflect a lower degree of patient compliance with therapy[21].

THE MYTH OF THE NON-HEALING ULCER?

Many reports have tried to categorize ulcers as "healing" and "non-healing". It is important to be able to identify those patients in whom treatment is failing and for whom a new approach should be used. This is particularly true with the advent of very expensive advanced wound-healing technologies, such as growth factors or skin replacements, which are targeted at the chronic non-healing primarily neuropathic foot ulcer. If no objective measure of ulcer healing is used, there is no possibility that such patients will be detected and, once again, the need for measurement and standardized descriptions of ulcers cannot be stressed too highly. Based on a review of all of the studies included in the discussion above, it is clear that the primary reasons for failure of the diabetic foot ulcer to heal are inadequate or inappropriate pressure relief, inadequate debridement and infection control, failure to recognize or treat vascular insufficiency and patient non-compliance. An ulcer can truly be described as non-healing only when all of these factors have been addressed, including angiography and reconstruction where necessary, or by the implementation of non-weightbearing regions, using inpatient bed-rest or a non-removable cast. Such ulcers will be rare. This is discussed further in a review by Cavanagh et al[25].

CURRENT CLASSIFICATION SYSTEMS

The most widely used and validated foot ulcer classification system is the Meggitt–Wagner classification[4,5], which divides foot ulcers into five categories. Grade 1 ulcers are superficial ulcers limited to the dermis. Grade 2 ulcers are transdermal with exposed tendon or bone, and without osteomyelitis or abscess. Grade 3 ulcers are deep ulcers with osteomyelitis or abscess formation. Grade 4 is assigned to feet with localized gangrene confined to the toes or forefoot. Grade 5 applies to feet with extensive gangrene. A significant problem with the Meggitt–Wagner classification is that it does not differentiate between those Grade 1–3 ulcers which are associated with arterial insufficiency and might be expected to heal less well, or those Grade 1 and 4 ulcers which are significantly infected and which might also be expected to have a poorer prognosis. Despite this, the Meggitt–Wagner classification has been shown to give an accurate guide to risk of amputation in a number of studies and remains the standard by which other classifications have to be judged[6,26].

In an effort to improve upon the Meggitt–Wagner classification, Harkless et al[27] proposed an expansion of the grading system to allow for ischaemia in the early grades[27]. Each of the original Meggitt–Wagner Grades 1–3 are subdivided into A (without ischaemia) or B (with significant ischaemia).

Although the prognosis of the various foot lesions is postulated, there does not appear to be any validation of this system or the newer Texas system[28] which has superseded it.

CLASSIFICATIONS BASED ON FOOT ULCER DESCRIPTION CATEGORIES

The limitations of the Meggitt–Wagner classification were demonstrated by Reiber et al[29], who tried to classify their patients retrospectively using a number of different systems and found that between one-fifth and a half of their patients could not be categorized satisfactorily. To accommodate this, a number of descriptive systems have been devised, most notably from the Nottingham group[30,31]. However, as they state in their most recent version[31], these are descriptions rather than classifications. Their proposed system has three main categories—the person, the foot, and the lesion—together with 14 variables. To classify an ulcer on such a basis would lead to at least 2×10^{14} categories, even if they were only dichotomous variables, and indeed, many are multifactorial. Therefore, most systems based on descriptions concentrate on the ulcer and aetiological factors alone. The Gibbons classification includes ulcer depth and infection but ignores aetiology and, in particular, vascular impairment[32]. The most validated of this type of system is the classification proposed by Lavery et al[28]. This classification excludes factors other than those influencing the wound, since the authors felt such parameters were difficult to measure or categorize, despite the fact that some of those factors are known to influence outcome at least as much as the parameters they chose to include[33]. Indeed, the authors have addressed the outcome problem elsewhere[34]. The three main categories are related to the relative depth of the ulcer. Grade 1 is a superficial ulcer not involving capsule or bone. Grade 2 is an ulcer which extends to tendon or joint capsule. Grade 3 is a lesion which extends into joint or bone. Each of these grades is then subdivided into one of four stages: (a) uninfected and not ischaemic; (b) infected but not ischaemic; (c) ischaemic but not infected; (d) ischaemic and infected. Thus, an ulcer could be placed into one of 12 categories. Two years later the same group reviewed their classification in practice and demonstrated that amputation risk was clearly and independently linked to both increasing depth and grade of ulcer. No uninfected and non-ischaemic patients had an amputation in the follow-up period, whereas patients with both infection and ischaemia were 90 times more likely to have a midfoot or higher amputation than patients with lower-graded lesions, despite following clearly defined treatment protocols which are described in this paper[33].

CLASSIFICATIONS BASED ON FOOT ULCER RISK CATEGORIES

The third main type of foot ulcer classification system relies on the underlying foot ulcer risk categories of peripheral neuropathy, peripheral vascular disease and deformity. These have been used in various combinations in a number of classifications which are further reviewed by Harkless et al[27]. Ultimately these are screening tools for education and pre-ulcer intervention. Patients with ulcers are grouped together in the final category as the highest risk of amputation in population surveys, but this method of classifying foot lesions gives little information as to how to approach an individual ulcer or about the variable prognoses between ulcers.

A minimalist approach to foot ulcer classification was proposed by Edmonds and Foster[2] in the previous edition of this book. Foot ulcers were divided into neuropathic and neuro-ischaemic on the basis of clinical tests, monofilaments and Doppler ultrasound, understanding the limitations of this test in the diabetic foot[35]. This has the advantage of simplicity and also identifies patients with vasculopathy, which is the principal adverse prognostic indicator for amputation of the diabetic foot and which may require revascularization. This classification approach provides a very simple means for rapid comparison of outcomes across clinics, but it may be limited if used for more detailed prognostication and treatment planning.

CAN THE CURRENT CLASSIFICATION SYSTEMS BE IMPROVED?

With such a variety of classification systems available, it is clear that no one system offers an ideal compromise between comprehensive applicability and simplicity. The reviewers of classification systems usually want each system to include their own particular facet. For example, the Texas system was reviewed by Levin[36], who noted that site of ulceration was missing, despite the fact that this has been shown to be an uncertain predictor of outcome[36]. A good classification system would seem to require some allowance for patient factors and inclusion of a deformity index, particularly in relation to ulceration in association with Charcot feet. At present, most of the current classifications force the user to become totally foot-centred at the expense of the patient as a whole. Whilst this is not likely to create problems in multidisciplinary practice, it is a possible cause of fragmented care when the foot clinic is separate from diabetology and other support. Addressing the social as well as the diabetes related issues of patients is likely to improve foot ulcer outcomes[29].

At present, the definitions of neuropathy, ischaemia, infection, deep ulceration, etc. are still open to interpretation. Clear and explicit standards for these parameters in the context of foot ulceration would aid the evolution of classifications and improve their prognostic reliability. Such a classification might then form the basis of an integrated care pathway for foot ulceration for each patient.

THE VALUE OF CLASSIFICATION SYSTEMS IN CLINICAL PRACTICE

At the beginning of this chapter, a distinction was made between descriptions and classifications of ulcers. At times the boundaries are blurred, but descriptions in general are more detailed and apply to individuals, while classifications are pigeonholes which facilitate research and audit in groups of patients. Individuals within the same classification grade will have other characteristics, principally the presence or absence of other diabetes complications, diabetic control, social factors and treatment compliance levels, which may influence their treatment and outcome. In general, however, increasing severity of ulceration has been clearly shown in most systems to influence prognosis and amputation rate. It is a major step from that premise to a decision to amputate on the basis of a poor classification grading. Despite various multi- and univariate analyses of potential risk factors, no classification yet devised can aid such decision making and all decisions have to be made on an individual basis[23].

Treatment regimens are in many ways the same for all ulcers and should not normally be influenced by classification grade alone. Some principles of management—for example, pressure relief (including pressure from shoes) and debridement—apply to all ulcers. The value of scoring and grading systems in planning treatment is that they prompt the clinician to search for the depth of the ulcer, to consider whether infection is present, and to seek evidence of vascular insufficiency. Thus, the care of the patient is improved simply because all the major relevant factors in the healing of the ulcer are considered during classification[1]. For this reason alone it should be the standard practice for all clinicians treating diabetic foot ulcers to adopt a classification system, either their own or one chosen from those outlined above.

Unfortunately, none of the present foot ulcer classifications discussed above has been validated prospectively outside of their originating centre. A multicentre prospective study of diabetic foot ulceration, using one or more classifications or examining a number of potential candidate criteria for inclusion in a final classification, would be of immense help in answering the question of whether or not the classification of diabetic foot ulceration could bring about the improvements in foot ulcer care that we all seek.

Ultimately, the use of one classification system would allow audits to be corrected for case mix and would allow the process and outcome to be examined purely on the basis of treatment. In the first instance, and within one system of health care, or in smaller clinics with relatively few ulcer patients, a simple approach such as the Edmonds and Foster neuropathic vs neuro-ischaemic classification may usually suffice[2]. This would also be easy to apply to retrospective audits of care. Overall, the case mix of ulcer depth and infection between centres and within the categories should be relatively even and the numbers of amputations in purely neuropathic patients could be compared. In addition, the effects of vasculopathy could be separated out and the effects of vascular interventions could be assessed. There are few universally comparable data for these outcomes over the past decade, but applying this system would be a major step forward and could quickly allow comparison with historical studies, using Meggitt–Wagner grades[4,5]. This would also provide the answers to the question posed by the St Vincent target on whether amputation rates for diabetic gangrene are falling.

In international comparisons, in which referral patterns vary widely, such as between the UK and the USA, a more detailed classification would be required. However, as the classification increases in complexity the number of patients required to validate it increases exponentially. Therefore, a system like the Texas classification is really applicable only to large clinics, which are likely to have sufficient numbers in each category, so that one or two amputations or non-compliant patients will not skew the results. Even with the 360 patients used by Armstrong et al in the validation study, there were a number of categories with less than five patients[33]. Irrespective of reservations about the absence of patient-related factors, the refinements of the Texas system over the Meggitt–Wagner classification offer a significant improvement and represent the best system that has been devised to date. In the absence of a prospective multicentre study, the Texas system could be adopted more widely and used in future prospective data collections for the purposes of audit and clinical research into foot ulcer outcomes and treatment[33].

CONCLUSIONS

The use of classifications ensures a systematic approach to the evaluation of patients with foot ulceration. This in turn should lead to improved treatment on the basis of a full and thorough assessment. If the classification system that is adopted does not take into account patient factors such as co-morbidities, social factors and levels of treatment compliance, some local arrangements should be made to ensure that these are not overlooked. Following a care plan based upon the patient's classification should not preclude regular reassessment, particularly if the ulcer is not healing as expected. The truly non-healing neuropathic ulcer probably does not exist, but failures in care still do.

REFERENCES

1. American Diabetes Association. Consensus development conference on diabetic foot wound care. *Diabet Care* 1999; **22**: 1354–60.
2. Edmonds ME, Foster AVM. Classification and management of neuropathic and neuroischaemic ulcers. In Boulton AJM, Connor H, Cavanagh PR (eds), *The Foot in Diabetes*, 2nd edn. Chichester: Wiley, 1994; 109–20.
3. Isakov E, Budoragin N, Shenhav S, Mendelevich I, Korzets A, Susak Z. Anatomic sites of foot lesions resulting in amputation among diabetics and non-diabetics. *Am J Phys Med Rehab* 1995; **74**: 130–33.
4. Meggitt B. Surgical management of the diabetic foot. *Br J Hosp Med* 1976: **16**; 227–32.
5. Wagner FW. The dysvascular foot: a system for diagnosis and treatment. *Foot Ankle* 1981; **2**: 64.
6. Apelqvist J, Castenfors J, Larsson J, Stenstrom A, Agardh C-D. Wound classification is more important than site of ulceration in the outcome of diabetic foot ulcers. *Diabet Med* 1989; **6**: 526–30.
7. Mayfield JA, Reiber GE, Nelson RG, Greene T. A foot risk classification system to predict diabetic amputation in Pima Indians. *Diabet Care* 1996; **19**: 704–9.
8. Margolis DJ, Kantor J, Berlin JA. Healing of diabetic neuropathic foot ulcers recieving standard treatment: a meta-analysis. *Diabet Care* 1999: **22**; 692–5
9. Grayson ML, Gibbons GW, Balogh K, Levin E, Karchmer AW. Probing to bone in infected pedal ulcers. A clinical sign of underlying osteomyelitis in diabetic patients. *J Am Med Assoc* 1995; **273**: 721–3.
10. Balsells M, Viade J, Millan M, Garcia JR, Garcia-Pascual L, del Pozo C, Anglada J. Prevalence of osteomyelitis in non-healing diabetic foot ulcers: usefulness of radiologic and scintigraphic findings. *Diabet Res Clin Pract* 1997; **38**: 123–7.
11. Apelqvist J, Larsson J, Agardh C-D. The importance of peripheral pulses, peripheral oedema and local pain for the outcome of diabetic foot ulcers. *Diabet Med* 1990; **7**: 590–4.
12. Hamalainen H, Ronnemaa T, Halonen JP, Toikka T. Factors predicting lower extremity amputations in patients with type 1 or type 2 diabetes mellitus: a population-based 7-year follow-up study. *J Intern Med* 1999; **246**: 97–103.
13. Adler AI, Boyko EJ, Ahroni JH, Smith DG. Lower-extremity amputation in diabetes. The independent effects of peripheral vascular disease, sensory neuropathy, and foot ulcers. *Diabet Care* 1999; **22**: 1029–35.
14. Faglia E, Favales F, Quarantiello A, Calia P, Clelia P, Brambilla G, Rampoldi A, Morabito A. Angiographic evaluation of peripheral arterial occlusive disease and its role as a prognostic determinant for major amputation in diabetic subjects with foot ulcers. *Diabet Care* 1998: **21**; 625–30.
15. Hoeldtke RD, Davis KM, Hshieh PB, Gaspar SR, Dworkin GE. Are there two types of diabetic foot ulcers? *J Diabet Comp* 1994; **8**: 117–25.
16. Foster A, McColgan M, Edmonds M. Should oral antibiotics be given to 'clean' foot ulcers with no cellulitis? *Diabet Med* 1998; **15**(suppl 2): A27.

17. Armstrong DG, Lavery LA, Sariaya M, Ashry H. Leukocytosis is a poor indicator of acute osteomyelitis of the foot in diabetes mellitus. *J Foot Ankle Surg* 1996; **35**: 280–3.

18. Venkatesan P, Lawn S, Macfarlane RM, Fletcher EM, Finch RG, Jeffcoate WJ. Conservative management of osteomyelitis in the feet of diabetic patients. *Diabet Med* 1997; **14**: 487–90.

19. Pittet D, Wyssa B, Herter-Clavel C, Kursteiner K, Vaucher J, Lew PD. Outcome of diabetic foot infections treated conservatively: a retrospective cohort study with long-term follow-up. *Arch Int Med* 1999; **159**: 851–6.

20. Eneroth M, Apelqvist J, Stenstrom A. Clinical characteristics and outcome in 223 diabetic patients with deep foot infections. *Foot Ankle Int* 1997; **18**: 716–22.

21. Mantey I, Foster AV, Spencer S, Edmonds ME. Why do foot ulcers recur in diabetic patients? *Diabet Med* 1999; **16**: 245–9.

22. Fletcher EM, Jeffcoate WJ. Foot care education and the diabetes specialist nurse. In Boulton AJM, Connor H, Cavanagh PR (eds), *The Foot in Diabetes*, 2nd edn. Chichester: Wiley, 1994; 69–75.

23. Larsson J, Agardh CD, Apelqvist J, Stenstrom A. Clinical characteristics in relation to final amputation level in diabetic patients with foot ulcers: a prospective study of healing below or above the ankle in 187 patients. *Foot Ankle Int* 1995; **16**: 69–74.

24. Griffiths GD, Wieman TJ. The influence of renal function on diabetic foot ulceration. *Arch Surg* 1990: **125**; 1567–9.

25. Cavanagh PR, Ulbrecht JS, Caputo GM. The non-healing diabetic foot wound: fact or fiction? *Ostomy Wound Manage* 1998; **44**(suppl 3A): 6-12S.

26. Calhoun JH, Cantrell J, Cobos J, Lacy J, Valdez RR, Hokanson J, Mader JT. Treatment of diabetic foot infections: Wagner classification, therapy, and outcome. *Foot Ankle* 1988; **9**: 101–6.

27. Harkless LB, Lavery LA, Felder-Johnson K. Diabetic ulceration: classification and management. In Bakker K, Nieuwenhuijken-Kruseman AC (eds), *The Diabetic Foot. Proceedings of the 1st International Symposium on the Diabetic Foot, May 1991*, Amsterdam: Excerpta Medica, 1991; 78–82.

28. Lavery LA, Armstrong DG, Harkless LB. Classification of diabetic foot wounds. *J Foot Ankle Surg* 1996; **35**: 528–31.

29. Reiber GE, Pecoraro RE, Koepsell TD. Risk factors for amputation in patients with diabetes mellitus. *Ann Intern Med* 1992: **117**; 97–105.

30. Jeffcoate WJ, Macfarlane RM. The description and classification of diabetic foot lesions. *Diabet Med* 1993; **10**: 676–9.

31. Macfarlane R, Jeffcoate WJ. How to describe a foot lesion with clarity and precision. *Diabetic Foot* 1998; **1**: 135–44.

32. Gibbon GE, Ellopoulous GM. Infection of the diabetic foot. In Kozak GP, Hoar CS Jr, Rowbotham JL, Wheelock FC Jr, Gibbons GW, Campbell D (eds), *Management of Diabetic Foot Problems*. Philadelphia, PA: WB Saunders, 1984; 97–102.

33. Armstrong DG, Lavery LA, Harkless LB. Validation of a diabetic wound classification system. The contribution of depth, infection, and ischemia to risk of amputation. *Diabet Care* 1998; **21**: 855–9.

34. Armstrong DG, Harkless LB. Outcomes of preventative care in a diabetic foot specialty clinic. *J Foot Ankle Surg* 1998; **37**: 460–66.

35. Kalani M, Brismar K, Fagrell B, Ostergren J, Jorneskog G. Transcutaneous oxygen tension and toe blood pressure as predictors for outcome of diabetic foot ulcers. *Diabet Care* 1999; **22**: 147–51.

36. Levin ME. Classification of diabetic foot wounds. *Diabet Care* 1998; **21**: 681.

6

Providing a Diabetes Foot Care Service
(a) Barriers to Implementation

MARY BURDEN

Leicester General Hospital, Leicester, UK

An ideal diabetic foot care service has informed people to know when and how to access appropriate care. This implies a structure of trained health care professionals in the right place at the right time, ready to administer the appropriate care. Implementation of an effective foot care service, then, relies on the integration of the various professionals concerned. The aim of this chapter is to explore some of the barriers to implementing such a foot care service and to encourage readers to identify barriers in their own areas and seek to overcome them. The barriers discussed in this chapter include failure to diagnose diabetes before foot problems arise, lack of recognition that foot care is important, funding and managerial barriers, lack of integration of services, failure to implement agreed care, and deficiencies in the measurement of outcomes. Although the discussion is based on experience in a health district in the UK, many of the problems are equally applicable to health services in other countries.

WHAT IS NEEDED FOR AN IDEAL SERVICE?

An underlying philosophy to which everyone can subscribe is an important initial step. If everyone is working towards different goals, then it should not be a surprise that little is achieved. One philosophy could be "prevention of loss of limb, or, when this is inappropriate, achievement

The Foot in Diabetes, 3rd edn. Edited by A. J. M. Boulton, H. Connor and P. R. Cavanagh.
© 2000 John Wiley & Sons, Ltd.

Table 6a.1 Suggested stepped care for the diabetic foot: a similar method adopted
in primary care has reduced amputation rates in an observational study[4]

Risk group	Identification	Action
Low-risk foot	Normal examination findings	Advise annual medical review General preventative measures
At-risk foot	Presence of one or more risk factors	Patient or carer to inspect daily Health Care Worker to inspect at each visit Referred to chiropodist for continuing care Prescribed footwear if needed Opportunistic surveillance by health care professionals
High-risk	Previous ulceration, amputation in other leg; no peripheral pulses	As before, but with planned multi-disciplinary assessment and surveillance. Emergency contact numbers and self-referral to specialist care
Active ulceration	Visible loss of epithelium of the foot	Urgent referral to specialized care (telephone call, seen within 48 hours), or hospital admission

of optimum mobility". This accords with the St Vincent Declaration target
of reducing by one-half the rate of limb amputations for diabetic gangrene[1],
but says nothing about how this can be achieved.

A further requirement is to identify those who are at risk. This does not
only involve those people with diagnosed diabetes, because many are
undiagnosed and some of these are only diagnosed when they present with
foot complications[2,3].

Having diagnosed diabetes, identification of the "at risk foot" and staged
education about footcare[4] (see Table 6a.1) then come into play. The at-risk
foot patient includes those with peripheral vascular disease, neuropathy,
foot deformities and visual and social problems. The population at risk are
mainly elderly[5] and treatment must be accessible to this group. Movement
between the "identification and education" and the "provision of
treatment" aspects of care are often problematic and are the areas where
patients fall through the net, either failing to receive appropriate referral or
being lost to follow-up.

So, what are some of the barriers to implementing the ideal
service?

BARRIERS TO IMPLEMENTING THE IDEAL SERVICE

Cultural Barriers

Traditionally, preventative care has a low priority in health care, but individuals may also put a low priority on footwear and are often embarrassed about their feet. Some cultures are explicit about this; for example, in India cobblers are rated lowly within society because they deal with feet[6], but in other cultures this is not as open.

Foot care appears to have a low priority among the complication of diabetes, despite the cost of providing care for those suffering foot ulcers. Government and charities have encouraged mobile retinal screening programmes[7], yet there are no initiatives for foot examination vans! People with diabetes themselves sometimes seem to accept that foot problems are inevitable. Health professionals compound this if they detect sensory neuropathy and can explain why it happened, yet do nothing to put preventative care in place. These cultural barriers need to be acknowledged before they can be addressed.

Funding Barriers

Some Health Authorities in the UK have no clearly defined diabetes budget, let alone a diabetic foot care budget. Diabetes is included under such budget headings as "medicine", "obstetrics", "renal", "chiropody" and "district nursing". In effect this means that "diabetes" is often tagged onto the end of budget priorities. Despite the recognition that diabetes and its complications are a large part of the total NHS budget[8], the funding to structure and organize services is not available. Funding and planning responsibility for provision of care is fragmented and can be an easy target for the manager who is required to reduce expenditure.

Managerial Barriers

Management of the diabetic foot is complex, both clinically and organizationally. It involves many different types of health care professionals working in different settings under different management systems. The foot care team is usually defined as "the multi-disciplinary specialist team" and includes individuals from different disciplines who regularly meet to plan and provide a service. The team is often dominated by hospital-based specialists, and it is easy to forget the many others who are involved in diabetic foot care outside the hospital and who must also be considered as part of the team. If, as Knight has pointed out[9], the inter-relationships between members of a hospital team are often complex, the

Table 6a.2　The foot care team: who manages or employs them

Team member	Usual agency
The person with diabetes	
Medical:	
Diabetologist	Directorate of medicine in hospital trust
General practitioner	District health authority
Surgeons (vascular and orthopaedic)	Directorate of surgery in hospital trust
Nursing:	
Plaster nurse	Outpatient directorate in hospital trust
Diabetes specialist nurse	Directorate of medicine/community trust
Practice nurse	General practitioner
District nurse	Community trust
Ward staff	Various
Nursing/residential home staff	Various
Podiatrists	Community trust
Orthotists	Private contractor/health trust

organizational requirements for success on a district-wide scale are even more complicated.

Some diabetic services date back to the 1950s[10]. These have often developed without the benefit of formal planning, whereas newer services may have the organizational machinery to ensure integration of the different elements. However, in the ever-changing National Health Service it is easy to overlook important sections: vigilance and team communication are needed to prevent this. Recent examples in the UK include the threat to orthotic services in different parts of the country.

In the UK the various agencies involved in the provision of diabetic foot care services (Table 6a.2) used to work together in a spirit of cooperation and harmony, but much of this has been lost since the introduction of the purchaser–provider split and of competition between provider health service trusts. It is, as yet, too soon to evaluate what effect the introduction of primary care groups and trusts in 1999 will have upon foot care services. As suggested by Donohoe and colleagues elsewhere in this chapter, it might represent a golden opportunity to provide an integrated seamless service, but there is also the potential for some components of the service to be curtailed or even lost altogether.

To integrate services, it is important to find out how the various elements work and how they inter-relate. Who manages whom? Where does the funding come from? Is there central planning or does everybody do their own thing? The podiatrists may be employed and managed by a community trust, yet work in the hospital; if so, they may have little influence over what happens within the hospital, which provides them with facilities. Similarly, a hospital-based foot clinic may find it impossible to arrange additional podiatry time if funding for podiatry is controlled by a community-based manager who may have other priorities, because his budget also has to provide for services which are unrelated to diabetes.

Other parts of the service (e.g. the orthotist and the provision of orthotic footwear) may be managed through external contracting processes and this can make them vulnerable, without the impact being fully appreciated until it is too late. Even the hospital members of the team are managed by different directorates: e.g. out-patients, medicine, surgery. The orthopaedic and vascular surgeons play an important part in foot care but their involvement is not always structured or built into their work patterns.

These managerial barriers make it difficult to move forward towards an integrated service.

Incompatible Frameworks of Care and Working Practices

Although many districts have developed the major components of a diabetic foot care service, few have yet managed to unify these components into a comprehensive district service, such as the one in Exeter which is described later in this chapter.

Using Leicestershire (UK) as an example, with its population of nearly a million, the elements of prevention, treatment and follow-up fall within the remit of different disciplines and it is difficult to get the "diabetic foot" recognized as a speciality in its own right. There are several different frameworks for delivery of care in Leicestershire. For example, the podiatrists are divided into three divisions, each with a manager. These divisions, however, do not correspond to the framework for district nurses, who work in clusters around a health centre. This makes it difficult for podiatrists and district nurses to work together, especially in identifying who does what and when. There is little communication and liaison between the different professional disciplines in the community (nursing, podiatry and tissue viability), each developing their own working methods. The community disciplines do not involve the hospital foot care team in the planning and delivery of diabetic foot care and the hospital does not involve the community. Working practices do not necessarily complement each other.

Good communication is essential, as the decision making of each individual health professional may be crucial in deciding outcome in the diabetic foot. The problem is compounded by the large numbers of health professionals involved. In Leicestershire there are over 400 general practitioners, four diabetologists, 10 diabetes specialist nurses, 48 podiatrists and 10 chiropody assistants, three orthotists, 377 whole-time equivalent (WTE) district nurses, 173 WTE practice nurses and the many nurses and care assistants who care for people in residential and nursing homes.

Barriers to Integration of Services

Integration of services has been recognized as important in the delivery of diabetic services[11]. This is usually thought of as integration between primary and secondary care, to allow movement "seamlessly" between these two aspects of care, as need dictates. However, the situation in relation to the diabetic foot is particularly complex because of the many different types of health professionals, working in many different settings under different management systems.

In the *Shorter Oxford English Dictionary*[12] integration can mean "to combine elements into a whole", "to render entire or complete" or "to complete (what is imperfect) by the addition of the necessary parts". Depending on the circumstances in which health professionals find themselves working, one or two, or indeed all three, of these activities are required. To understand the barriers to integration of services, it is necessary to have information about the size of the population for which the service is provided, where the hospitals, clinics and service providers are located and how they are organized, and it is also important to have data on health care outcomes. It is essential to understand the existing service from the perspective of each of the many different disciplines involved in providing the service.

THE PERCEPTION OF SERVICE PROVIDERS

A local study was undertaken in Leicestershire to identify perceived gaps in the service and problems in developing an integrated service[13]. Fifteen service providers were interviewed and all disciplines were represented. The majority (73%) considered that the existing service was not adequately integrated; 53% considered that the delivery of care was not equitable; and the same number thought that insufficient priority was given to prevention. Commonly identified issues included poor communication, lack of joint planning initiatives, and a lack of agreed policies and guidelines. Provision of care was often inappropriate, with some low-risk patients receiving frequent chiropody but some higher-risk individuals getting none at all.

Suggested potential solutions included a joint planning mechanism, uniform policies, guidelines and documentation, structured training that acknowledged the fast turnover rate in a large health care team, and the need to publicize how the service was provided.

There was concern that if a more structured framework was used the service would lose its flexibility, which all agreed was its strength. This flexibility included the ability to contact any member of the specialist hospital team (not just the doctor) and arrange for a patient to be seen urgently. The mechanisms for self-referral were also perceived as important. The participants felt that the priority was to introduce common documentation and communication.

Local studies such as this are essential to identify deficiencies in the service and to inform the planning process.

MEASURING THE QUALITY OF CARE

Audit of the process and outcome of care are essential components of the service. Without such information we have no objective measurement of the quality of care and of improvement or deterioration in that quality. The importance of collecting and analysing data (whether on amputations, as for the St Vincent Declaration target monitoring, or other information, such as quality of life measures) using a standardized methodology to allow comparison with other districts has been emphasized in Chapter 2. Even if this is done, it is not always easy to relate outcomes to particular components of the service, and it is essential to audit, and to keep re-auditing, the process of care in different parts of the service against agreed guidelines. In Leicestershire, research- or consensus-based guidelines have been agreed over a period of time, and yet these are often ignored or challenged by those who are unaware of, or who have misunderstood, the evidence. For example, long-term antibiotic therapy for osteitis may be stopped prematurely by general practitioners who are unaware of the importance of a prolonged course or who are concerned that it will lead to antibiotic resistance, and some nurses may use inappropriate dressings because they have been taught, in another context, that "moist" dressings are better than "dry" in all circumstances.

CONCLUSION

Potential barriers to implementation of an integrated foot care service include issues relating to culture and tradition, funding, managerial and organizational structure and established working practices. Each of these must be identified and addressed. Barriers can only be identified if representatives of all disciplines involved in service provision are asked about their perceptions of the service and, as discussed in the next section, the issues are only likely to be successfully addressed if there is a team leader who has overall responsibility for planning and coordination. Monitoring the quality of the process and outcome of care is an essential component of the service.

REFERENCES

1. Department of Health/British Diabetic Association. *St Vincent Joint Task Force for Diabetes: the Report*. London: British Diabetic Association, 1995.

2. Glynn JR, Carr EK, Jeffcoate WJ. Foot ulcers in previously undiagnosed diabetes mellitus. *Br Med J* 1990; **300**: 1046–7.
3. New JP, McDowell D, Burns E, Young RJ. Problem of amputations with newly diagnosed diabetes mellitus. *Diabet Med* 1998; **15**: 760–4.
4. Rith-Najarian S, Branchaud C, Beaulieu O, Gohdes D, Simonson G, Mazze R. Reducing lower extremity amputations due to diabetes. Application of the staged diabetes management approach in a primary care setting. *J Family Pract* 1998; **47**: 127–32.
5. Kald A, Carlsson R, Nilsson E. Major amputation in a defined population: incidence, mortality and results of treatment. *Br J Surg* 1989; **76**: 308–10.
6. Seth V. *A Suitable Boy*. London: Orion Books, 1993.
7. Taylor R, Broadbent DM, Greenwood R, Hepburn D, Owens DR, Simpson H. Mobile retinal screening in Britain. *Diabet Med* 1998; **15**: 344–7.
8. British Diabetic Association/King's Fund. *Counting the Cost: the Real Impact of Non-insulin Dependent Diabetes*. London: British Diabetic Association, 1996.
9. Knight AH. The organization of diabetes care in the hospital. In Pickup J, Williams G (eds), *Textbook of Diabetes*, 2nd edn, vol 2. Oxford: Blackwell Science, 1997; 2–3.
10. Walker J. *Chronicle of a Diabetic Service*. London: British Diabetic Association, 1989.
11. British Diabetic Association. *Recommendations for the Management of Diabetes in Primary Care*, 2nd edn. London: British Diabetic Association, 1997.
12. *Shorter Oxford English Dictionary*, 3rd edn. Oxford: Oxford University Press, 1973.
13. Burden ML. Barriers to integration of foot care services. *Diabet Foot* 1999; **2**: 27–32.

6

Providing a Diabetes Foot Care Service
(b) Establishing a Podiatry Service

DAVID J. CLEMENTS

Portsmouth HealthCare NHS Trust, Portsmouth, UK

The podiatrist has a major role in the specialist multi-professional diabetic foot care team[1,2] and it is imperative that the whole podiatry service is structured to support this input. It is essential that the service is adequately funded with support from local purchasers and commissioners of services. In the UK this involves lobbying directors of public health and chairmen of primary care groups and enlisting the support of the local diabetes services advisory group[3]. Useful evidence to support the case for adequate podiatry services is available from various sources in the UK[4,5,6], USA[7,8] and internationally[9]. It is essential that podiatry services, which are commonly under-resourced, should be urgently upgraded if they are to cope with the rapidly increasing prevalence of diabetes and its complications, which is affecting all continents and most countries[10].

Podiatry departments have traditionally been based in the community, with relatively little contact with district general hospitals. However, the current trend, clearly supported by the literature[11,12], is for podiatrists to contribute to highly skilled multiprofessional hospital-based teams, while still providing a more general service in the community. Because podiatry is a community-based specialty but with increasing representation in hospital-based specialist foot care teams, the podiatry department is particularly well placed to provide a good quality service that spans the gaps between community, primary and secondary care for those patients presenting with diabetic foot problems.

The Foot in Diabetes, 3rd edn. Edited by A. J. M. Boulton, H. Connor and P. R. Cavanagh.
© 2000 John Wiley & Sons, Ltd.

STRUCTURE—GENERAL PRINCIPLES

It would be wrong to suggest there is any one perfect way to structure local podiatry services. Differences in service provision, size of podiatry teams, levels of funding and size of local population will vary greatly. That being said, I do believe that the following principles should be borne in mind when developing a podiatry service for people with diabetes.

People with diabetes access podiatry services with a variety of different needs and problems ranging from initial advice at diagnosis through basic foot care and minor foot problems to severe ulceration and gangrene. The structure of the service has to reflect these differing needs and provide the appropriate level of expert care for each patient. To this end, all podiatrists working for the local podiatry department should be clear about their role within the team and identified as specialist, advanced or general practitioners in diabetes, as described below, and trained accordingly. The structure should also ensure that the department is not reliant upon any one individual—however talented—to carry out all the specialist diabetes work. Organizational learning and training, rather than individual learning, is key to the long-term success of the service.

The service should have a clearly identified lead clinician who has experience of working closely with the hospital-based diabetes care team and an ability to communicate well with other health professionals. The lead clinician should have a high level of clinical skill which is respected by other members of the team. The role should also include elements of research, audit and training in addition to a willingness to be innovative. Ideally, the specialist clinician will also work in community clinics to ensure good liaison with the community-based podiatry staff. Communication is an essential role, informing members of the primary care team of developments and ensuring integration of services.

Training

The quality of training of podiatrists varies greatly from one country to another. For example, in Germany there is no requirement for a structured education (see Chapter 9), whereas in the UK all state registered podiatrists receive basic training in the care of the diabetic foot as part of their professional training; however, the level and quality of this is varied and limited. As there is no mandatory requirement for continuing professional development (CPD), relatively few podiatrists will have updated their knowledge and skills. Unfortunately, some believe themselves capable of providing a higher level of care than their training allows, and they often work in isolation with little reference to other professional carers. The proper management of diabetes requires a multidisciplinary approach, and all staff must understand that no aspect of diabetes should be considered in isolation. The requirement to train podiatrists who wish to practise at specialist or advanced practitioner level is clear, but it is imperative that all podiatrists should be trained in the assessment of diabetic foot problems and should know when to refer to a practitioner with more advanced training and expertise. Where possible, training should be multi-professional rather than uniprofessional to emphasize the multi-disciplinary nature of clinical practice, and courses should be provided locally to improve interaction and networking between professionals. Funding from local education consortia is sometimes available for multiprofessional courses and specialist conferences, and is worth pursuing. All staff should be supported in writing for publication and actively encouraged to attend relevant conferences. The service should ensure that all relevant and current periodicals are available to staff.

ASSESSMENT

One of the prime criteria of success is that patients get to the right part of the service at the right time. To ensure that this happens, the use of an assessment tool or form is very helpful[13]. If possible, the assessment tool should have a scoring system to allow year-on-year comparisons and to facilitate audit. It should be widely accepted and uniformly used in community, primary and secondary care. It should provide clear triggers for referral. There are a large number of assessment tools available and many departments have produced their own. It is important that these are developed multidisciplinarily and are based firmly on current research evidence wherever possible. In Portsmouth, a Baseline Diabetic Podiatric Assessment form, which allocates scores for known risk factors for diabetic foot problems, is used by the podiatry service, diabetes centre, general practitioners and practice nurses at annual diabetic review and prompts referral of those with high scores for an in-depth "at-risk" assessment by more highly trained staff.

ACCESS

Most people with diabetes do not need specialist attention to their feet and can safely be left to access routine community podiatry services near their own homes[4]. In most areas of the UK people with diabetes are still able to self-refer for treatment or advice, and they should generally be seen for initial assessment with a higher priority than other patients. When known to be suffering from some form of foot complication or to be "at risk", patients should be referred to an appropriately experienced podiatrist. Patients who are at risk of developing complications should be placed on an "at-risk" register[2] and regularly advised about direct access to the specialist team.

SPECIALIST TEAM

The specialist team is made up of podiatrists who have wide experience of working with diabetic foot complications. Its members should have regular update sessions on all aspects of diabetes, and are identified as part of the multiprofessional diabetic foot care team where they share in the treatment of severe diabetic foot complications. This role includes the use of more specialist treatment modalities and wound care regimens at the diabetes centre. Members of the team work primarily in the community, where they review non-healing ulcers and look after patients designated as at "high risk". Additionally, a significant presence in the secondary care sector is essential, with adequate flexibility to respond to urgent need. They also act as a resource for other staff and professional groups, providing advice and training. The current recommendation for staffing levels is two whole-time-equivalent specialist podiatists for every 250 000 of population served[2].

ADVANCED PRACTICE TEAM

This team is made up of staff who have a special interest in diabetes and have undergone further training, but who have limited experience of working with severe diabetic foot complications. The members of this team work in the community alongside, and in close liaison with, the primary health care team[14], carrying out risk assessments, participating in the care of healing ulcers and looking after patients designated as "medium-risk". Advanced practitioners should attend some joint specialist clinic sessions to gain experience of the diabetic foot care team approach and the care of more severe problems.

GENERAL PODIATRY TEAM

All general podiatrists see people with diabetes and routinely carry out baseline diabetic assessments and look after "low-risk" patients. They need to be aware of the indications for early referral to advanced or specialist practitioners should the need arise.

GUIDELINES

It is essential to agree on unambiguous protocols for assessment and referral, and on guidelines for interventions, treatment, wound care and prevention strategies. Although these relate to the foot and are often seen (by podiatrists) as the podiatrist's prerogative, it is important for the patient that all health professionals agree to these guidelines and work to the same agenda. The multiprofessional specialist diabetic foot care team will have particular responsibility for some of these issues; for example, referrals to vascular surgeons, the use of biomechanical investigations, arterial imaging techniques and referral for specialist footwear. Other guidelines, such as antibiotic and wound care regimens, must be agreed more widely with general practitioners and community and practice nurses. Where applicable, involvement in the production of locally written integrated care pathways[15], for example an amputation pathway, is essential to ensure that referral triggers and systems are included and that standards of care are specified.

CONCLUSIONS

A high-quality and adequately funded podiatry service is an essential component of proper diabetic foot care management. General podiatry services should be readily accessible to patients in local communities, with specialist care provided as part of a multidisciplinary specialist foot care team, which will usually be hospital-based. There must be a lead clinician who has overall responsibility for service provision. All podiatrists must be adequately trained for their particular roles, and must be clear about their roles within the team structure. A system of continuing professional development is essential and training, like clinical practise, should be multiprofessional. Good communication is essential. There should be uniform assessment documentation, which should contain clear prompts for more specialist assessment. Guidelines for all aspects of the service should be agreed and these should form the basis for regular auditing of the service.

REFERENCES

1. Rännemaa T, Hämäläinen H, Toikka T, Liukkonen I.   Evaluation of the impact of podiatrist care in the primary prevention of foot problems in diabetic subjects. *Diabet Care* 1997; **20**: 1833–7.
2. British Diabetic Assocation.   *Recommendations for the Structure of Specialist Diabetes Care Service*. London: British Diabetic Association, 1999; 6, 8, 11.
3. British Diabetic Association.   *Guidance on Local Diabetes Services Advisory Groups*. London: British Diabetic Association, 1997.
4. Edmonds M, Boulton A, Buckenham T et al.   Report of the UK St. Vincent Diabetic Foot and Amputation Group. *Diabet Med* 1996; **13**(suppl 4): S27–42.
5. Clinical Standards Advisory Group.   *Standards of Clinical Care for People with Diabetes: Report of a CSAG Committee and the Government Response*. London: HMSO, 1994; 1–40.

6. NHS Executive Health Service Guidelines. *Key Features of a Good Diabetes Service* (HSG[97]45), 1997.
7. American Diabetes Association. Position statement. Preventative foot care in people with diabetes. *Diabet Care* 1998; **21**: 2178–9.
8. Mayfield JA, Reiber GE, Sanders LJ et al. Preventative foot care in people with diabetes (American Diabetes Association Technical Review). *Diabet Care* 1998; **21**: 2161–77.
9. International Working Group on the Diabetic Foot. International Consensus on the Diabetic Foot and Practical Guidelines, 1999. PO Box 9533, 1006 GA Amsterdam, The Netherlands.
10. Amos AF, McCarty DJ, Zimmet P. The rising global burden of diabetes and its complications: estimates and projections to the year 2010. *Diabet Med* 1997; **14**(suppl 5): S25–34.
11. Frykberg RG. The team approach in diabetes foot management. *Adv. Wound Care*, 1998; **11**: 71–7.
12. Sibbald RG, Knowles A, Tyrrell W. Special foot clinics for patients with diabetes. *J Wound Care* 1996; **5**: 238–43.
13. Plummer ES, Albert SG. Foot care assessment in patients with diabetes: a screening algorithm for patient education and referral. *Diabet Educ* 1995; **21**: 47–51.
14. Gadsby R, McInnes A. The "at risk" foot: the role of the primary care team in achieving St. Vincent targets for amputation. *Diabet Med* 1998; **15**(suppl 3): S61–4.
15. Currie L, Harvey G. Care pathways development and implementation. *Nursing Standard* 1998; **12**(30): 35–8.

6

Providing a Diabetes Foot Care Service
(c) The Exeter Integrated Diabetic Foot Project

MOLLY DONOHOE, JOHN FLETTON* and JOHN E. TOOKE

Royal Devon and Exeter Hospital, Exeter and *Plymouth School of Podiatry, Plymouth, UK

A number of local and general issues relating to diabetes foot care in the Exeter District stimulated us to introduce an integrated diabetic foot care programme. As the approach we were proposing required considerable organizational change as well as resources, it was elected to introduce a programme as a pragmatic randomized controlled trial of a model of integrated foot care for people with diabetes, a project that became known as the Exeter Integrated Diabetic Foot Project. Amongst the factors leading to this work were the realization of the enormous economic impact on finite resources of the chronic complications of diabetes[1]. In addition the changes set out in the UK National Health Service (NHS) White Paper[2], which aimed at replacing the internal market in health care delivery with a partnership-based, performance-driven concept of patient-focused inte-grated care, provided the framework for the sort of initiative we anticipated. Thirdly, the St Vincent Declaration[3] commits us to reduce amputation in people with diabetes which, from our previous survey, appeared to be relatively high in the Exeter District. Investigation of the cause of the relatively high amputation rate led us to believe that an apparent misappropriation of chiropody/podiatry provision in diabetes foot care may have been partly responsible, resulting in the fact that a

The Foot in Diabetes, 3rd edn. Edited by A. J. M. Boulton, H. Connor and P. R. Cavanagh.
© 2000 John Wiley & Sons, Ltd.

significant proportion of patients with high-risk feet were not receiving podiatric care, whilst a high proportion of low-risk patients were[4].

Although there is good evidence from studies conducted in secondary care settings[5,6,7] that improvements in outcome can be achieved for the diabetic foot, there is little evidence for the effectiveness of community-based initiatives. Furthermore, there is a relative lack of controlled studies evaluating integrated care, which has been promoted as a means of delivering health needs at both individual and population level for a number of conditions, including diabetes[8,9].

The clinical management of 75% of people with diabetes in the Exeter district takes place in the community, emphasizing the need for a primary care-based study. Previous research has demonstrated that the prevalence of neuropathic ulceration can be reduced by accurate and timely identification of high-risk factors, in combination with appropriate strategies for patient education and the provision of effective podiatry services[5,6,7]. However, the relevant evidence stems largely from dedicated, hospital-based "centres of excellence". A local study amongst a group of podiatrists showed that understanding of high-risk status was incomplete in a number of respondents[10]. This was not entirely surprising, as continuing professional education, particularly relating to diabetic foot complications, was singularly lacking. In addition, the study indicated poorly developed relationships between the participating podiatrists and their colleagues in primary and secondary care, particularly with respect to referral processes.

Against this background, it was hypothesized that the implementation of a fully integrated model of foot care, which included the provision of an educational programme relating to foot complications in diabetes, for all members of the primary health care team, would improve patients' and health professionals' knowledge of, and attitude towards, the management of the diabetic foot, appropriation of clinical resources and, ultimately, health costs and outcomes.

THE STUDY

An intervention period of 6 months was considered an appropriate compromise in balancing the requirement for sufficient time to achieve measurable outcomes with the need to restrict potential cross-contamination of control group practices. Furthermore, previous work has shown that knowledge and attitude change can be achieved in a relatively short interval of time[11].

Ten general practices, in different localities of a Devon health district, were invited to participate in the project. They were matched on a number of important general variables, which included the number of practice partners, patient list size, geographic location and distance from a district general hospital. A number of variables specific to diabetes were also taken into account, for example, the maintenance of a practice register, the existence of a structured approach to patient care, and the presence of a defined relationship with a chiropodist/podiatrist. Each of the paired practices was randomly allocated either to receive the integrated model of care, or to continue with its existing diabetes foot care protocol. In addition, control practices received an alternative educational intervention on a diabetes complication unrelated to the foot.

Clearly, the most compelling outcome measure for a study of this type would have been the demonstration of a reduction in amputation rates. It was recognized at the outset, however, that such evidence was unlikely to be forthcoming in a time-scale of only 6 months.

It was therefore necessary to identify appropriate alternative outcome measures[12]. Recognizing the key role played by a well-informed and cooperative patient in the management of foot disease in diabetes[13], primary end-points were defined as an increase in patients' knowledge about, and attitude towards, their foot care. Aware of the importance of a co-ordinated team-centred approach to prevention and management of foot complications[14], secondary end-points focused on an increase in the knowledge of primary health care professionals, together with the effect of the model on the appropriateness of patient referrals to both the specialist diabetes foot clinic and the community podiatry service.

Questionnaires were used to evaluate the impact of the model of care on patients' knowledge and attitudes, and similarly knowledge about diabetic foot complications amongst the health professionals. These questionnaires, based on previously validated models[15], were modified to incorporate contemporary information concerning various aspects of foot care in diabetes. These were piloted locally to ensure acceptable levels of validity and reliability. Questionnaires were then administered, immediately prior to the intervention, to 1939 patients and 150 health professionals in the 10 matched practices.

THE INTEGRATED DIABETIC FOOT CARE MODEL

The integrated model of care that was evaluated is an organizational framework focusing on the primary care-based annual review (Figure 6c.1). It includes educational initiatives, aimed at clarifying management of the diabetic foot, criteria for referral and health professional responsibilities. At the start of the 6 month study period, general practitioners, practice and district nurses, together with podiatrists, employed in the subserving community NHS clinics of intervention practices, were invited to attend an initial practice visit by members of the specialist diabetic foot care team. At

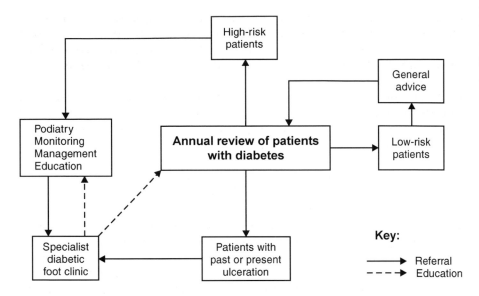

Figure 6c.1   Integrated model of foot-care in diabetes

this visit, the model of care was discussed and guidelines given regarding referral to the specialist diabetic foot clinic (Table 6c.1) and community chiropody/podiatry services. The roles and responsibilities of patients were emphasized and patient information leaflets circulated. Education was given regarding identification of the high-risk foot in diabetes and each practice was supplied with a Semmes–Weinstein monofilament, known to be an objective and reliable method of establishing the presence of sensory neuropathy in a community context[16].

A single member of the diabetic foot care team made three visits to the intervention practices over the ensuing 6 months to visit practice nurses, district nurses and at least one representative of the district nursing team. All general practitioners were contacted by telephone and sent a

Table 6c.1   Criteria for referral to a specialist diabetic foot clinic

- Ulcer with spreading infection/cellulitis, gangrene or digital necrosis—urgent same-day referral
- Ulcer defined as any full-thickness penetration of the dermis on the plantar surface of the foot, not responding after 1 week of treatment
- Suspected Charcot's arthropathy
- Patients with high-risk feet wearing inappropriate footwear—referral for footwear provision, pressure-relieving insoles or specialist footwear advice, as appropriate
- Patients with a past history of diabetic foot ulceration, to ensure optimal risk factor management

written summary of the initiatives discussed at the initial practice visit. The five general practices in the control group continued with their existing foot care arrangements and also received an initial visit at which an unrelated educational component dealing with diabetic nephropathy was presented.

At the end of the 6 month intervention period, the knowledge and attitude questionnaires were re-administered to the respective patient and health professional groups. Paired questionnaire response rates were over 65% in both patient groups, and 80% in both health professional groups.

THE IMPACT OF THE MODEL OF CARE

What impact did the integrated model of care have in terms of changing knowledge levels and attitudes amongst the intervention patient groups? It was not surprising to find no difference between the groups in patients' knowledge scores at the baseline assessment. It was unexpected, however, to discover that knowledge scores were significantly higher in both patient groups on completion of the study, with no significant difference between them. One possible explanation for this apparent phenomenon is the presence of a Hawthorne effect[17] whereby the very activity of conducting a study or survey may raise awareness and interest, and emphasizes the importance for controlled study design if valid conclusions are to be drawn in health services research of this type.

Patients' attitudes towards foot care in diabetes is arguably a more important factor in determining their subsequent health-related behaviour than the precise level of knowledge held about potential complications. Prior to the intervention, there was no difference in attitude scores between the patients in either group. On completion of the study, however, there was a significantly greater mean change in attitude amongst those patients in the intervention group. In addition, intervention patients were significantly more likely to have had their feet examined, to have received foot-care education and to have found that education useful.

There was no difference between the groups in the knowledge scores of the health professionals at the pre-intervention assessment, and at completion scores improved only in the intervention group. Even though preliminary data leading to the study suggested that community podiatrists' knowledge was suboptimal, it was higher than the other professional groups involved at the outset of the study and predictably, therefore, exhibited the smallest increase at follow-up.

What were the implications of the model of care for the appropriateness of patient referrals? With respect to the specialist diabetic foot clinic, a significant increase was found in the number of appropriate referrals made from the intervention practices, but not from the control practices.

In contrast there was, however, no observable difference between intervention and control groups in the appropriateness of patient referrals to community podiatry clinics at the end of the study. This latter finding may have been a consequence of the relatively short study time scale, combined with a waiting period for community podiatry services.

CONCLUSIONS

In summary, the community-based Exeter Integrated Diabetic Foot Care Project demonstrated that patients' knowledge of and attitudes towards their foot care, and the knowledge and behaviour of health professionals, can be measurably enhanced, relatively inexpensively, in a fairly short period of time. These findings have positive implications for improved patient outcomes and efficient utilization of resources. In light of the proposals contained in the recent NHS White Paper[2], particularly regarding the formation of primary care groups, the concept of an integrated approach to patient care in the community is fundamental.

What changes are imminent as a direct result of the study? These are currently confined to a local level. Three new posts are being created, enabling key podiatry staff to coordinate both the implementation of the integrated care model, and the education of community podiatrists in the three localities of the health district. It is envisaged that the appointees will liaise closely with the specialist diabetic foot care team to discuss patient management issues, plan and implement regular educational initiatives and provide a structured forum for communication between the community podiatrists, who often work in relative isolation, and their colleagues in the primary care team. The principal aim is to optimize the local contribution that podiatry can make in the management of foot complications in diabetes but, in addition, it has the potential to enhance job satisfaction within that professional group. Furthermore, rational utilization of existing podiatry services will be facilitated by the abolition of patients' self-referral. By so doing, it is envisaged that those patients at greatest risk of foot complications, and therefore those most likely to benefit from podiatry care, actually do receive that care in a consistent way, as and when they need it. Having introduced the integrated care model to all practices in the Exeter Health Care District, we plan to assess prospectively the impact on amputation and foot ulceration.

REFERENCES

1. Williams DRR. The size of the problem: epidemiological and economic aspects of foot problems in diabetes. In Boulton AJM, Connor H, Cavanagh P. (eds), *The Foot in Diabetes* 2nd edn. Chichester: Wiley, 1994; 15–24.

2. Department of Health. *The New NHS, Modern, Dependable*. London: HMSO, 1997.
3. Krans HMJ, Porta M, Keen H, Johansen S (eds), *Diabetes Care and Research in Europe: the St Vincent Declaration Action Programme*. Copenhagen: World Health Organization, 1995.
4. Fletton JA, Perkins J, Jaap AJ, Brash PD, Tooke JE. Is community chiropodial/podiatric care appropriately targeted at the "at-risk" diabetic foot? *Foot* 1995; **5**: 176–9.
5. Bild DE, Selby JV, Sinnock P, Browner WS, Braveman P, Showstack JA. Lower extremity amputation in people with diabetes: epidemiology and prevention. *Diabet Care* 1989; **12**: 24–31.
6. Edmonds ME, Blundell MP, Morris ME, Thomas EM, Cotton LT, Watkins PJ. The diabetic foot: impact of a foot clinic. *QJ Med* 1986; **232**: 761–3.
7. Thomson FJ, Veves A, Ashe H, Knowles EA, Gem J, Walker MG et al. A team approach to diabetic foot care—the Manchester experience. *Foot* 1991; **2**: 75–82.
8. Carruthers I. Personalized care for people with diabetes—a Health Commission Perspective. *Pract Diabet Int* 1995; **12**: 250.
9. Churchman-Liffe BL. Integrating the health care system: lessons across international borders. *Frontiers of Health Service Management* 1994; **11**: 3–48.
10. Fletton JA, Robinson IM, Tooke JE. Community chiropodial/podiatric care and the "at risk" diabetic foot: a case for professional updating? *J Brit Pod Med* 1996; **51**: 4.
11. Sykes J. The Education of Diabetic Patients by Practice Nurses. MSc Thesis, University of Exeter, 1993.
12. Reiber GE, Pecoraro RE, Koepsell TD. Risk factors for amputations in patients with diabetes mellitus. *Ann Int Med* 1992; 97–102.
13. McInnes AD. The role of the chiropodist. In *The Foot in Diabetes*, Boulton AJM, Connor H, Cavanagh P (eds), 2nd edn. Chichester: Wiley, 1994; 77–91.
14. Connor H. Prevention of diabetic foot problems: identification and the team approach. In Boulton AJM, Connor H, Cavanagh P (eds), *The Foot in Diabetes* 2nd edn. Chichester: Wiley, 1994; 55–67.
15. Meadows KA, Fromson B, Gillespie C, Brewer A, Carter C, Lockington T, Clark G, Wise PH. Development, validation and application of computer-linked knowledge questionnaires in diabetes education. *Diabet Med* 1988; **5**: 61–7.
16. Klenerman L, McCabe C, Cogley D, Crerand S, Laing P, White M. Screening for patients at risk of diabetic foot ulceration in a general diabetic outpatient clinic. *Diabetic Med* 1996; **13**: 561–3.
17. Roethlisberger FJ, Dickson WJ. *Management and the Worker*. Cambridge, MA: Harvard University Press, 1939.

7

The Diabetic Foot in Primary Care: a UK Perspective

ROGER GADSBY

Warwick University, Warwick, UK

GENERAL PRACTITIONER INVOLVEMENT IN DIABETES CARE

Traditionally, many people with diabetes in the UK had their care supervised by hospital doctors, but there was no organized system of care for those who did not attend hospital clinics. In the 1970s a few systems of "shared care" between hospital clinics and general practitioners were developed, and by the 1980s a number of general practitioners with a particular interest in, and enthusiasm for, diabetes care began to develop diabetes mini-clinics in their practices. Published evidence suggests that these mini-clinics can provide a standard of care equivalent to that achieved in hospital practice[1]. In 1990 a new contract for the provision of care in general practice introduced incentive payments for the provision of "chronic disease management programmes", and within a few years more than 90% of general practitioners were claiming these for diabetic care programmes.

It is interesting to note that in the USA in recent years there have been changes in the organization of health care with the development of "managed care". In this system the provider faces increased accountability in the nature and frequency of interactions with patients who have chronic diseases such as diabetes. The requirements for foot care are that a documented foot examination (including an assessment of deformity, sensation and vascular status) be recorded each year. In the near future this is expected to become more specific, requiring assessment of the presence or absence of protective sensation, foot pulses and training in self-care of

The Foot in Diabetes, 3rd edn. Edited by A. J. M. Boulton, H. Connor and P. R. Cavanagh.
© 2000 John Wiley & Sons, Ltd.

the foot[2]. It is to be hoped that recently introduced changes in the organization of primary care in the UK will also produce more specific requirements.

ST VINCENT DECLARATION TARGET
FOR REDUCING AMPUTATION

The St Vincent Declaration target for diabetes foot care is to reduce the number of amputations from diabetic gangrene by 50% in 5 years[3]. In the UK a joint task force with representation from the British Diabetic Association (BDA) and the Department of Health was established to develop strategies to achieve this target. The report of the Diabetic Foot and Amputation subgroup of the Task Force[4] offers several strategies to achieve this 50% reduction in amputations in the UK. These include:

1. Screening for the "at-risk foot" in primary care.
2. Special review and extra education for those at risk.
3. Prompt referral to a multidisciplinary diabetes foot care team should ulceration or infection occur.

RECOGNITION OF THE "AT-RISK" FOOT
IN PRIMARY CARE

The detection of risk factors for ulceration and amputation requires regular visual inspection of the feet, assessment of foot sensation, and palpation of foot pulses by a trained health care professional, and this must be done as part of the individual diabetic patient's annual review. The examination can be performed by any suitably trained member of the primary health care team; in some practices it may be carried out by the general practitioner, in others by a practice nurse, podiatrist or foot care nurse.

The important parts of the examination are: a *history* of previous ulceration or amputation; *inspection* of the feet for deformity and callus; *examination* of the feet for ischaemia and loss of sensation; and checking that the shoes fit and are in good condition.

Previous Ulceration or Amputation

A history of previous ulceration puts the foot at risk. Following amputation, the remaining limb is particularly at risk; this may be due to increased plantar pressure loading and the fact that most pathophysiological processes are bilateral[5].

Foot Inspection to Detect Deformity and Callus

The deformities of claw and hammer toes, prominent metatarsal heads, Charcot arthropathy, overriding toes, hallux valgus and hallux rigidus may all contribute to a high-risk foot. The motor component of peripheral neuropathy gives rise to small muscle wasting, resulting in imbalance of flexor and extensor muscles which can cause deformity[6]. Hard skin in the form of callus may arise at points of abnormally high repetitive pressure in the foot, and is a powerful predictor of ulceration[7].

Detection of Ischaemia

The posterior tibial and dorsalis pedis pulses should be palpated. Absence of these pulses indicates ischaemia and puts the foot in the "at-risk" category[4]. The advanced ischaemic foot characteristically feels cold and may be pale or cyanosed. Further assessment of the degree of ischaemia may need to be carried out by the district foot care team, as described in Chapter 16.

Detection of Neuropathy

The role of impaired vibratory perception in the pathogenesis of foot ulceration has been well documented[8]. Objective measurement of this sensory parameter with a biothesiometer has been used to identify those at risk of developing ulceration[9]. However, this instrument is not widely available in general practice, since it can weigh 2.5 kg, requires a power source and may cost £400. The assessment of vibration sensation using a tuning fork is very unreliable, and so other instruments have been assessed for their usefulness in detecting neuropathy. These include the tactile circumferential discriminator[10], the graduated tuning fork[11] and thermal discrimination devices [12]. These have not been prospectively evaluated, and have not become widely used in general practice.

Identification of neuropathy based on insensitivity to a 10 gm (5.07) nylon monofilament is convenient and appears to be cost-effective[13]. This device was developed for use in screening for insensitivity due to peripheral neuropathy in leprosy. Procedures for the use of the monofilament are described in Chapters 4 and 21. If the pressure cannot be detected by the patient, then protective pain sensation is lost[14]. Testing with the 5.07 monofilament has been shown to have excellent inter- and intra-observer reproducibility and good specificity for the detection of peripheral neuropathy[15]. In a recent study in an outpatient clinic, which examined the reproducibility of screening using a monofilament, biothesiometer and palpation of pedal pulses, only the monofilament gave adequately reproducible results (over 85%) for measurements repeated after 2 weeks[16].

The ability to identify feet at risk of ulceration has been demonstrated prospectively in two studies using the biothesiometer[9,17] and in one study using the monofilament[18]. In this latter study, conducted in primary care in the USA, 358 people with diabetes were screened and then monitored over 32 months. Risk was graded using three parameters: sensitivity to the 5.07 monofilament; presence or absence of foot deformity; and history of previous ulceration or amputation. Insensitivity to the monofilament was associated with a 10-fold increased risk of ulceration and a 17-fold increased risk of amputation, but no data was given for the sensitivity, specificity or predictive value of the test. Risk stratification was improved by inclusion of the other parameters. The importance of a past history of ulceration or amputation was emphasized by the finding of a 78-fold increased risk of further ulceration. Forty-eight per cent of patients with a past history of ulceration or amputation retained sensation to the monofilament, which indicates that use of the monofilament alone does not have good predictive value, probably because, as Warren points out in Chapter 22, protective pain sensation may be lost while sensation to touch and pressure are still preserved.

Other Factors Associated with Increased Risk of Foot Disorders

These include poor glycaemic control, long duration of diabetes, poor vision, social deprivation, social isolation, smoking and being resident in a care home[19]. The general practitioner should be aware of these factors in the patient's history and be alert to the risk of ulceration.

Numbers at Risk

Information on the prevalence and incidence of amputation, ulceration and neuropathy is given in Chapter 2. However, the numbers of patients at risk of developing ulcers or requiring amputations are much greater than those who actually suffer these complications. In the North West of England Diabetes Foot Care Study, of 9710 adults with diabetes, only 33% had no risk factors in their history or examination and 55% had two or more factors putting them at high risk[20]. In this study 1.7% had ulcers present and 1.3% had had amputations. In my own practice, using the four parameters of previous history of ulceration, foot deformity, absent foot pulses and insensitivity to the monofilament, we have found that 30% (75 of 252 screened) are at risk (unpublished results). Those with no risk factors for their feet receive basic foot education and are re-screened yearly as part of their annual diabetes review. Those with "at-risk" feet receive more detailed foot education and 3 monthly review.

SCREENING AND INTERVENTION IN PATIENTS WITH "AT-RISK" FEET

McCabe and colleagues have described a strategy for screening and intervention which they tested in a trial of 2001 patients attending a hospital clinic[21]. Patients were randomized to a control group (*n*=1000), who continued to receive standard care in the routine diabetic clinic, and an index group (*n*=1001). The index group were screened for risk factors and the 13% who were judged to be at high risk (defined as foot deformities, a history of foot ulceration, or an ankle:brachial index of $\leqslant 0.75$) were offered open access to a weekly foot protection clinic which provided foot care (chiropody and hygiene maintenance), support hosiery, protective shoes and additional education. Those patients in the index group who were not defined as at high risk continued to receive standard care in the routine clinic. At 2 year follow-up there was a significant reduction in major amputations in the index group compared with the control group ($p < 0.01$). There were fewer minor amputations and new ulcers in the index group, but the differences were not statistically significant, possibly because any patients who developed new ulcers during the study were automatically transferred to the foot protection clinic. The foot protection clinic was cost-effective in terms of major amputations prevented (cost of clinic, £100 372; savings from avoiding 11 major amputations at £12 000 each, £132 000). Cost-effectiveness might have been improved if it had been possible to improve compliance with attendance at the foot protection clinic, and with the use of chiropody services and of protective footwear in the high-risk group.

EDUCATION OF STAFF IN PRIMARY CARE

Few primary care clinicians will have had much teaching on the current management of diabetic foot problems. Some may still believe, as was often taught in former years, that there was little that could be done to prevent what was regarded as an inevitable progression from neuropathy to ulceration and from ulceration to amputation. They may be unaware that preventative foot care and footwear can reduce the risk of a first ulcer, and the suggestion that radical debridement of dead tissue from around a neuropathic foot ulcer to leave a freshly bleeding surface (of healthy tissue!) could be of benefit may be anathema to some of those in primary care. Such thinking could mean that the value of, and need for, early referral might not be appreciated.

All primary care staff involved in diabetes care must be given up-to-date information about foot care management. Practice nurses are especially important, as they have a central role in diabetes foot education and screening in many general practices. The arrangements for providing the education and training will vary from one country to another, and even within countries depending on local circumstances. In parts of Germany, reimbursement for diabetic care by family physicians and their staff is dependent on attendance at an approved, structured educational programme (Chapter 9). As suggested by Clements (Chapter 6b), there is much to be said for education being provided on a multiprofessional basis to emphasize the importance of multidisciplinary clinical management in diabetes care and to promote team working. At least some of the training should be provided at a local level, so that staff are familiar with local guidelines for management and referral. However, it is not always practicable to provide all training locally, and in some countries there are now a number of assessed and accredited courses in primary diabetes care. In the UK these include the Certificate in Primary Diabetes Care (CIPDC), which is a 6 month distance learning course with 5 university-taught days at Warwick University.

Nationally, the BDA has recently formed a primary care section— Primary Care Diabetes (UK)—which has organized foot care workshops. These have proved to be very popular, although it can be argued that those who attend are the enthusiastic minority. Making appropriate education available to the majority of primary care physicians may best be accomplished at a local level, and in the UK this can be provided through interactive lectures and workshops organized by tutors in general practice.

Experiential learning by staff in the primary care diabetic clinic through the attendance and advice of a district diabetes facilitator, a post with a number of different functions and one which is recommended by the BDA[22], is another helpful method of education.

REFERRAL TO SPECIALIST CARE

To Whom to Refer

The Diabetic Foot and Amputation Group of the St Vincent Task Force in the UK has recommended that a diabetes foot care team, comprising a named podiatrist, diabetologist and nurse, with assistance from an orthotist and surgeon, be set up in each district general hospital[4]. The report outlines their roles and responsibilities and summarizes these by saying that the team will be treating ulceration and sepsis in the neuropathic and neuro-ischaemic foot using techniques which include debridement, special dressings, plaster casting and the provision of insoles and orthotic shoes. This team would be the first point of referral for the general practitioner when someone with diabetes presents in primary care with ulceration, infection or symptomatic ischaemia; hence, their contact details should be published and known to those working in primary care. However, many local hospitals do not yet have such a team, and the general practitioner may then be uncertain as to whom the patient should be referred. In these circumstances the patient may be sent to the hospital casualty department or emergency room, or admitted under the care of whichever surgeon or physician happens to be on call for emergencies on that particular day. The outcome of non-specialist care may be less than satisfactory and even if no structured multi-disciplinary foot care team exists, there should be local guidelines, with contact names and telephone numbers, to ensure that the patient can be referred to an appropriate specialist.

When to Refer

Those patients who are detected at routine screening as being at significant risk of foot problems should be referred, according to advice given in national or local guidelines, to the specialist foot care team before complications occur.

When ulceration does present to the general practitioner, there may be a temptation to refer to the practice nurse for a dressing, with a prescription for an antibiotic if infection is suspected. The practice nurse will then arrange to see the patient every few days to change the dressings. Such a "wait and see" policy may go on for several weeks before referral is contemplated, and may prove disastrous. In a study of 669 ulcers presenting to a specialist multidisciplinary foot clinic[23], the median time between ulcer onset and first professional review was 4 days (range 0–247), and the median time from first professional review and first referral to the specialist clinic was 15 days (range 0–608). Only 30% of patients were referred to the specialist team within 1 week of onset, 48% within 4 weeks and 78% within 6 weeks. It was considered that the condition of 25 ulcers may have deteriorated as a result of delayed referral from primary care to the specialist clinic. This study shows that there is still much to be done to teach patients with diabetes to check their feet for ulcers every day, and to educate the primary care team about the need for rapid referral to the specialist team.

Recent international guidelines on the management of diabetic neuropathy advise that patients presenting with ulceration, blistering, bleeding into callus, cellulitis or acute ischaemia should be referred immediately, usually on the day of presentation unless this is impossible for any reason[24].

PATIENT EDUCATION MATERIALS

It is very helpful to give people with diabetes a written leaflet about foot care to reinforce the verbal teaching that has been given. It also enables them to have something to refer to at home to remind them of the key educational messages that were shared.

There are many foot care advice leaflets available from national diabetes associations and from the pharmaceutical industry. It is important to read them thoroughly before giving them to patients, to ensure that they give appropriate and relevant information which does not conflict with any verbal advice. It is useful to have a simple leaflet for those at low risk and a more detailed one for those at higher risk who need to take more precautions; the European Association for the Study of Diabetes has produced one leaflet giving general instruction and a separate one for the at-risk foot[25]. It is best to use leaflets from one source, as a review of eight examples suggested that five contained contentious and sometimes contradictory statements[26].

GUIDELINES FOR DIABETES FOOT CARE

It is good practice to ensure that all aspects of management conform with currently accepted guidelines. Wherever possible these should be evidence-based, although gaps in the evidence inevitably mean that some are derived from expert consensus. Care must be taken if the expert opinion contains only token representation from those working in primary care, as there might then be a risk that actions which would be appropriate in secondary care are inappropriately recommended for primary care. Some guidelines, especially those on referral practices, may need adaptation to suit local circumstance. Existing guidelines include those based on the International Consensus on the Diabetic Foot (Chapter 21), and in some countries guidelines are available from national diabetes associations and clinical audit groups.

REFERENCES

1. Greenhalgh P. *Shared Care for Diabetes—a Systematic Review*. Royal College of General Practitioners Occasional Paper 67. London: Royal College of General Practitioners, October 1994.
2. Cavanagh P. Care of the diabetic foot: an American perspective. *Diabet Foot* 1998; **1**: 124–6.
3. World Health Organization (Europe) and International Diabetes Federation (Europe). Diabetes care and research in Europe: the St Vincent Declaration. *Diabet Med* 1990; **7**: 360–70.
4. Report of the Diabetic Foot and Amputation Group. *Diabet Med* 1995; **13**: (Suppl 4) S27–43.
5. Veves A, Van Ross E, Boulton AJM. Foot pressure measurements in diabetic and non-diabetic amputees. *Diabet Care* 1992; **15**: 905–7.
6. Cavanagh PR, Ulbrecht JS. Biomechanical aspects of foot problems in diabetes. In Boulton AJM, Connor H, Cavanagh PR (eds), *The Foot in Diabetes*, 2nd edn. Chichester: Wiley, 1994; 25–36.
7. Murray HJ, Young MJ, Hollis S, Boulton AJM. The association between callus formation, high pressure and neuropathy in diabetes foot ulceration. *Diabet Med* 1996; **13**: 979–82.

8. Boulton AJM, Kubrusly DB, Bowker JH et al. Impaired vibratory perception and diabetic foot ulceration. *Diabet Med* 1986; **3**: 335–7.
9. Young MJ, Breddy JL, Veves A, Boulton AJM. The prediction of diabetic neuropathic foot ulceration using vibration perception thresholds. *Diabet Care* 1994; **17**: 557–60.
10. Vileikyte L, Hutchings G, Hollis S, Boulton AJM. The Tactile Circumferential Discriminator: a new, simple screening device to identify diabetic patients at risk of foot ulceration. *Diabet Care* 1997; **20**: 623–6.
11. Thivolet C, El Farkh J, Petiot A, Simonet C, Tourniare J. Measuring vibration sensations with a graduated tuning fork: simple and reliable means to detect diabetic patients at risk of neuropathic foot ulceration. *Diabet Care* 1990; **13**: 1077–80.
12. Liniger C, Albeanu A, Assal J-P. Measuring diabetic neuropathy: "low tech" vs "high tech". *Diabet Care* 1990; **13**: 180.
13. Gadsby R, McInnes A. The at-risk foot: the role of the primary care team in achieving St Vincent targets for reducing amputation. *Diabet Med* 1998; **15**: Supplement S61–4.
14. Young M, Matthews C. Neuropathy screening: can we achieve our ideals? *Diabet Foot* 1998; **1**: 22–5.
15. Valk G, de Sonnaville J, Van Houtum W et al. The assessment of diabetic polyneuropathy in daily clinical practice. *Muscle Nerve* 1997; **20**: 116–118.
16. Klenerman L, McCabe C, Cogley D et al. Screening for patients at risk of diabetic foot ulceration in a general diabetic outpatient clinic. *Diabet Med* 1996; **13**: 561–3.
17. Abbott CA, Vileikyte L, Williamson S, Carrington AL, Boulton AJ. Multicentre study of the incidence of and predictive risk factors for diabetic foot ulceration. *Diabet Care* 1998; **21**: 1071–5.
18. Rith-Najarian SJ, Stolusky T, Gohdes DM. Identifying diabetic patients at high risk for lower extremity amputation in a primary health care setting. A prospective evaluation of simple screening criteria. *Diabet Care* 1992; **15**: 1386–9.
19. Royal College of General Practitioners. *Clinical Guidelines for Type 2 Diabetes. The Prevention and Treatment of Foot Ulcers.* London: Royal College of General Practitioners, January 2000. www.rcgp.org.uk
20. Carrington AL, Abbott CA, Kulkarni J et al. Prevalence and prevention of diabetic foot ulceration and amputation in North West England. *Diabetes* 1996; **43**: 52.
21. McCabe CJ, Stevenson RC, Dolan AM. Evaluation of a diabetic foot screening and protection programme. *Diabet Med* 1998; **15**: 80–4.
22. British Diabetic Association. *Recommendations for the Structure of Specialist Diabetes Services.* London: British Diabetic Association, 1999.
23. Macfarlane RM, Jeffcoate WJ. Factors contributing to the presence of diabetic foot ulcers. *Diabet Med* 1997; **14**: 867–70.
24. Boulton AJ, Gries FA, Jervell JA. Guidelines for the diagnosis and outpatient management of diabetic peripheral neuropathy. *Diabet Med* 1998; **15**: 508–14.
25. EASD Leaflets. *Prevention of Foot Lesions and Loss of Pain Sensation.* In St Vincent Declaration Newsletter. Copenhagen: WHO (Europe), Summer 1995.
26. Connor H. Footcare advice: what do we tell our patients and what should we tell them? *Pract Diabet Int* 1997; **14**: 75–7.

8

Podiatry and the Diabetic Foot: An American Perspective

LARRY B. HARKLESS and DAVID G. ARMSTRONG

University of Texas Medical School, San Antonio, TX, USA

Podiatry as practised in the USA is different from the practice of chiropody in the UK, although some British chiropodists are now also trained as podiatrists[1]. While chiropodists provide basic care, podiatrists provide complete foot care. The scope of podiatric practice, as defined by the American Podiatric Medical Association, includes the diagnosis and treatment of the human foot and ankle and their governing and related structures, including the local manifestations of systemic conditions by any system or means. The scope of podiatry practice includes all aspects of diabetic foot pathology. American podiatrists practise comprehensive foot care, concentrating not only on surgical treatment, but also on conservative palliative care. They debride ulcers, incise and drain abscesses and perform ablative procedures where needed. Podiatrists treat neuropathic arthropathy from early immobilization through to surgical reconstruction. They can prescribe medication for symptomatic neuropathy or amelioration of ischaemic disease[2].

To provide this level of care, podiatry training in the USA usually includes an undergraduate Bachelor's degree followed by a 4-year doctorate programme in podiatry and, for 99% of students in the 1999 graduating class, subsequent residency training. Residences vary in duration from 1 to 3 years, with those receiving shorter training typically concentrating on non-surgical therapy. Beyond this residency training,

The Foot in Diabetes, 3rd edn. Edited by A. J. M. Boulton, H. Connor and P. R. Cavanagh.
© 2000 John Wiley & Sons, Ltd.

several centres have added additional diabetic foot study in the form of fellowship programmes. These include the Beth Israel Deaconess/Joslin Clinics at Harvard Medical School and the University of Texas Health Science Center at San Antonio, and typically offer a fourth year of postdoctoral training.

In the USA, podiatrists are considered primary foot care providers, receiving patients directly or by referral from other specialists. Commonly, the podiatrist will be the first practitioner to recognize the pedal signs and symptoms of diabetes mellitus in the undiagnosed patient and be in a position to make timely referrals to the diabetologist or vascular surgeon. In the ideal practice scenario, the podiatrist is a central member of a team which includes the diabetologist, vascular surgeon, orthopaedic surgeon, infectious disease specialist, specialist in physical medicine and rehabilitation, pedorthist/orthotist, social worker, and nurse educator. When presented with a patient having a severe diabetes-related foot infection, podiatrists commonly admit or co-admit the patient with the diabetologist.

While vascular and general medical follow-up for the high-risk patient is scheduled about once every 4 months, podiatrists will see these high-risk patients more frequently, usually about every 2 months. This level of contact allows timely updating of shoe wear and inlays, and identification of evolving risk areas. On the surface, the podiatry provider in the USA seems well positioned to deliver high-level front-line diabetes-related foot care. However, podiatry is not completely accepted as the primary foot care source in all parts of the USA, but rather in pockets, usually near academic centres. In addition, while podiatrists have a higher level of training than the chiropodists of the UK, training in the USA is not thoroughly consistent. This is particularly evident when comparing the type, quality and duration of post-graduate training. In August of 1998, the American Podiatric Medical Association (APMA) House of Delegates accepted the recommendations of the Educational Enhancement Project (EEP) committee, which was mandated to address the issues of uniformity and quality. One of the central themes of this project was further integration of pre- and postgraduate podiatric medical education into allopathic teaching institutions. Specific recommendations from the EEP include absolute standardization of core curricula at each podiatric medical college. Additionally, EEP sets clear expectations for podiatric medical residents to function on many of their clinical rotations at the level of their allopathic or osteopathic counterparts.

In the fee-for-service and managed care systems coexistent the USA, there is occasionally a greater incentive for given practitioners of any specialty to treat the patient rather than to make a referral to the most qualified practitioner, who in some instances would be the podiatrist. It is not uncommon for podiatrists to see a patient late in the process, after other treatments have failed. Too frequently this example may involve a patient with neuropathic ulceration and secondary abscess formation, which might have been resolved promptly with early debridement and local wound care, but which was protracted by treatment attempts using antibiotic therapy alone. Edelson and co-workers[3] evaluated 255 subjects admitted with a diabetic foot infection to a university teaching hospital without a dedicated diabetic foot referral pathway, such as a multidisciplinary team approach to care. In that study, patients' wounds were evaluated with minimal competency less than 14% of the time, regardless of the specialty of the admitting physician. This phenomenon appears to be true in the outpatient setting as well, where diabetic patients presenting for primary care have their feet evaluated between 10% and 19% of the time[4]. It has been our experience that a multidisciplinary system emphasizing consistent, treatment-based wound[5] and risk[6,7] classification and open communication between specialties yields the most consistent short- and long-term results.

In an effort to alleviate some of the aforementioned problems surrounding both fee-for-service and managed care models (even when resource availability is limited), some centres have adopted successful disease management designs intended to provide care in a holistic manner to persons with diabetes[8–11]. Peters and Davidson[8] reported a significant improvement in overall glucose control among patients followed in a comprehensive diabetes care service, compared with those followed in a standard health maintenance organization model. More specifically, we have noted that patients followed in a diabetic foot care centre which is part of a comprehensive disease management programme may also see their risk of foot disease mitigated[12]. In this 3 year longitudinal study of 341 persons, enrolled into a programme which stratified patients' follow-up appointment, education, shoe gear, and other resources based on risk, those at highest risk for ulceration were over 54 times less likely to re-ulcerate and 20 times less likely to receive an amputation if they were compliant with the care instituted in this model.

Although the highest prevalence of diabetes (and its commensurate complications) is in minority populations (African–American, Mexican–American, Native American, etc.), these groups are the least likely to have health care access or adequate resources to care for their maladies[13–17]. Unfortunately, it is the exception rather than the rule to find a podiatry service in the teaching hospitals that serve indigent minority populations.

In the USA, the provision of routine professional foot care and specialist shoewear are limited to those who can afford them or else are restricted by the bureaucratic process with respect to the care of indigent persons. A minority of providers know the necessary paper pathways or devote the time and effort required by the system. It is our contention that the cost of proper footwear would be paid for many times over by reduction in the frequency of lower extremity amputations[12,18–20]. Over the past decade, a shoewear demonstration project passed by the US Congress has allowed reimbursement for therapeutic shoes and appliances to those patients eligible for federally funded health insurance (Medicare).

Podiatry plays an important role in diabetes-related foot care. The involvement of podiatry care into the mainstream of diabetes management has been a component of the reduced incidence of lower extremity ulcerations and subsequent amputations[20–23]. As a profession, there remains a strong need to integrate more completely with the mainstream medical delivery system, to participate in basic research, and to ensure a consistent supply of highly trained providers, competent in the management of diabetes-related foot pathology.

REFERENCES

1. Berry BL, Black JA. What is chiropody/podiatry? *Foot* 1992; **2**: 59–60.
2. Harkless LB, Dennis KJ. The role of the podiatrist. In Levin ME, O'Neal LW, (eds), *The Diabetic Foot*, 4th edn. St. Louis, MI: CV Mosby, 1988; 249–72.
3. Edelson GW, Armstrong DG, Lavery LA, Caicco G. The acutely infected diabetic foot is not adequately evaluated in an inpatient setting. *Arch Intern Med* 1996; **156**: 2373–8.
4. Wylie-Rosett J, Walker EA, Shamoon H, Engel S, Basch C, Zybert P. Assessment of documented foot examinations for patients with diabetes in inner-city primary care clinics. *Arch Family Med* 1995; **4**: 46–50.
5. Armstrong DG, Lavery LA, Harkless LB. Validation of a diabetic wound classification system. The contribution of depth, infection, and ischemia to risk of amputation. *Diabet Care* 1998; **21**: 855–9.
6. Rith-Najarian SJ, Stolusky T, Gohdes DM. Identifying diabetic patients at high risk for lower-extremity amputation in a primary health care setting: a prospective evaluation of simple screening criteria. *Diabet Care* 1992; **15**: 1386–9.
7. Armstrong DG, Lavery LA. Diabetic foot ulcers: prevention, diagnosis and classification. *Am Family Physician* 1998; **57**: 1325–32.
8. Peters AL, Davidson MB. Application of a diabetes managed care program. The feasibility of using nurses and a computer system to provide effective care. *Diabet Care* 1998; **21**: 1037–43.
9. McDonald RC. Diabetes and the promise of managed care. *Diabet Care* 1998; **21**(suppl 3): C25-8.
10. Rubin RJ, Dietrich KA, Hawk AD. Clinical and economic impact of implementing a comprehensive diabetes management program in managed care. *J Clin Endocrinol Metabol* 1998; **83**: 2635–42.
11. Chicoye L, Roethel CR, Hatch MH, Wesolowski W. Diabetes care management: a managed care approach. *Ukr Biokhim Zh* 1998; **97**: 32–4.
12. Armstrong DG, Harkless LB. Outcomes of preventative care in a diabetic foot specialty clinic. *J Foot Ankle Surg* 1998; **37**: 460–6.
13. Pugh JA, Tuley MR, Basu S. Survival among Mexican–Americans, non-Hispanic whites, and African–Americans with end-stage renal disease: the emergence of a minority pattern of increased incidence and prolonged survival. *Am J Kidney Dis* 1994; **23**: 803–7.

14. Lavery LA, van Houtum WH, Armstrong DG, Harkless LB, Ashry HR, Walker SC. Mortality following lower extremity amputation in minorities with diabetes mellitus. *Diabet Res Clin Pract* 1997; **37**: 41–7.

15. Lavery LA, Ashry HR, Basu S. Variation in the incidence and proportion of diabetes-related amputations in minorities. *Diabet Care* 1996; **19**: 48–52.

16. Fishman BM, Bobo L, Kosub K, Womeodu J. Cultural issues in serving minority populations: emphasis on Mexican–Americans and African--Americans. *Am J Med Sci* 1993; **306**: 160–6.

17. Nelson RG, Gohdes DM, Everhart JE, Hartner JA, Zwemer FL, Pettitt DJ, Knowler WC. Lower extremity amputations in NIDDM: 12 year follow-up study in Pima Indians. *Diabet Care* 1988; **11**: 8–16.

18. Davidson JK, Alogna M, Goldsmith M, Borden J. Assessment of program effectiveness at Grady Memorial Hospital, Atlanta, GA. In Steiner G, Lawrence PA, *Educating Diabetic Patients*. New York: Springer Verlag 1981; 329–48.

19. Edmonds ME, Blundell MP, Morris ME, Thomas EM, Cotton LT, Watkins PJ. Improved survival of the diabetic foot: the role of a specialized foot clinic. *Qu J Med* 1986; **60**: 763–71.

20. Litzelman DK, Marriott DJ, Vinicor F. The role of footwear in the prevention of foot lesions in patients with NIDDM. *Diabet Care* 1997; **20**: 156–62.

21. Crane M, Werber B. Critical pathway approach to diabetic pedal infections in a multidisciplinary setting. *J Foot Ankle Surg* 1999; **38**: 30–3.

22. Hamalainen H, Ronnemaa T, Toikka T, Liukkonen I. Long-term effects of one year of intensified podiatric activities on foot-care knowledge and self-care habits in patients with diabetes. *Diabet Educ* 1998; **24**: 734–40.

23. Ronnemaa T, Hamalainen H, Toikka T, Liukkonen I. Evaluation of the impact of podiatrist care in the primary prevention of foot problems in diabetic subjects. *Diabet Care* 1997; **20**: 1833–7.

9

Education—Can It Prevent Diabetic Foot Ulcers and Amputations?

MAXIMILIAN SPRAUL

Heinrich Heine Universität, Düsseldorf, Germany

A number of studies have shown that the prevalence of diabetic foot ulcers and amputations can be reduced by the introduction of multidisciplinary specialized foot clinics and services[1–5]. Patient education featured strongly in these programmes, but always as part of multifaceted interventions, and it is not therefore possible to determine to what extent education contributed to their success. There have been few studies which have attempted to examine the importance of education *per se*, and little is known about which components of an educational programme are important for success. Moreover, although the prevention of diabetic foot ulcer and amputations requires input from many different health care professionals working in different areas of the health care system, the education of these professionals has received little attention.

STUDIES OF EDUCATIONAL PROGRAMMES FOR PATIENTS

Despite the established role of foot care education for patients with diabetes, the existing data provide conflicting results.

In a prospective randomized study, Malone et al[6] have shown that the incidence of foot ulcers and amputations can be considerably reduced using a simple 1-hour educational programme. Patients who did not receive the

The Foot in Diabetes, 3rd edn. Edited by A. J. M. Boulton, H. Connor and P. R. Cavanagh.
© 2000 John Wiley & Sons, Ltd.

education had rates of ulceration and amputation that were three times higher than in the educated group, even though the median follow-up was longer in the group who received education (12 months vs 8 months). All patients had an active foot lesion or had had an amputation prior to enrolment in the study. The educational intervention consisted of the provision of a simple set of patient instructions for diabetic foot care and a review of slides depicting infected diabetic feet and amputated limbs. Such fear-inducing techniques may be effective in patients with active lesions, but whether it is appropriate to a wider diabetic population is debatable (see Chapter 10). Moreover, this report lacks important information such as the ages and sex distribution of the patients in the two groups.

Litzelman et al[7] demonstrated a reduction in lower extremity clinical abnormalities, and improvement in patients' foot care knowledge and performance of appropriate foot care, using a 12 month intervention programme that targeted both patients and health care providers. The patients entered into a mutually agreed behavioural contract for foot care and this was reinforced by telephone and postcard reminders. Healthcare providers were given written guidelines and algorithms on foot-related risk factors for amputation. In addition, the folders for patients in the intervention group had special identifiers, which prompted providers to examine patients' feet and to reinforce education. This intervention caused a change in the behaviour of providers, who were more likely to examine the feet of patients in the intervention group in contacts during normal office hours (68% vs 28%) and to refer them for chiropody (11% vs 5%).

Barth et al[8] compared a conventional (1 hour) educational session with an intensive (9 hours spaced over four weekly sessions) programme which used cognitive motivational techniques and in which three of the sessions were conducted by a podiatrist and one by a psychologist. The intensive group showed significantly greater improvements in knowledge, compliance with recommended foot care practice, and compliance with advice to consult a podiatrist. At the first follow-up visit, after 1 month, patients in the intensive group were significantly less likely to have foot problems requiring treatment than those in the conventional group, but this difference was not apparent at the 3 month and 6 month visits.

Bloomgarden et al[9] found no beneficial effect on foot lesions in a group who had received a single foot care session compared with a group who did not receive the intervention. However, the session was based only on the use of films and card games to provide the knowledge, and patients were not actively involved in the motivational process, neither were they trained in the necessary practical skills of foot care.

Pieber et al[10] evaluated the efficacy of a treatment and teaching programme for patients with type 2 diabetes in general practice. Patients in the intervention group showed improved knowledge of appropriate foot care and evidence of better foot care (e.g. less callus formation and better nail care), but the evaluation period was too short to determine whether these improvements resulted in any change in diabetic foot problems.

There are many reasons why most of these studies may have failed to show significant benefits. An effective educational programme must be properly structured, as will be discussed later in this chapter, and must also address the barriers that inhibit patients from implementing their knowledge, a topic which is discussed in Chapter 10. However, even if patients have appropriate knowledge and the motivation to apply that knowledge, benefits may not occur unless their health providers also take appropriate actions.

THE EDUCATION OF HEALTH CARE PROVIDERS AND CARERS

Litzelman et al[7] reported that, without specific prompting, only 28% of health providers regularly examined the feet of their diabetic patients. In a study by our own group of the evaluation of a structured education programme for elderly insulin-treated patients[11] we found that regular foot inspection by family physicians was carried out in less than 25% of patients. Moreover, none of the patients in this study who came to amputation had been referred to a specialist diabetic foot clinic before the amputation was performed. In a study which attempted to define the precipitating factor leading to foot ulceration, Fletcher et al[12] found that 12% were attributable to lack of care by patients, but professional mismanagement was judged to have caused or contributed to the ulceration in 21%. They concluded that the thrust of current educational efforts should be reassessed, with greater attention being given to the education of health care providers.

Primary Care Physicians

The majority of type 2 diabetic patients, especially if elderly, are treated exclusively by family physicians. Education must target these doctors and their practice personnel. We have developed a structured patient education programme for type 2 diabetes enabling the office personnel of general practitioners to perform patient education[13]. This programme has already reached more than 150 000 patients all over Germany. A concurrent aim was to educate general practitioners and their personnel about the care of their diabetic patients. More than 14 000 general practitioners and their office personnel had to participate in a special course, since only participation entitled them to reimbursement. In addition, for family doctors in private practice with a special interest in the diabetic foot, seminars have been set up where the doctors and their personnel are taught in detail about screening, prevention and treatment of the diabetic foot.

In a model project, an annual check for diabetic complications, focusing on a detailed examination of patients' feet, was created to improve the detection of diabetic complications in primary health care[14]. Complete documentation is the prerequisite for remuneration of the physicians. This has led to a nearly complete check of the feet of the diabetic patients, but has also provided important data which will permit the provision of shared-care programmes (e.g. referral for specialized foot care for high-risk patients).

Surgeons

Many surgeons, at least in Germany, are unaware of the principles of adequate surgical treatment of infected diabetic feet. The huge benefit of conservative treatment, especially for the infected neuropathic foot, is not generally known in the surgical disciplines. Moreover, the provision of adequate preventative measures after an amputation, to prevent the recurrence of lesions in these high-risk patients, is not generally acknowledged. In our experience, the introduction of a weekly ward round of the internists together with the surgeon, the vascular surgeon and the team of the diabetic foot clinic is instrumental in improving the knowledge and cooperation of the different medical professions.

For the improvement of the surgical treatment of the diabetic foot, we have recently started a project to document prospectively all amputations in North Rhine (9.7 million inhabitants). The 192 surgical departments in this region are asked to complete a standardized questionnaire for each amputation, giving detailed information about diabetes, pre-operative diagnosis and treatment, etc. This project has already provided essential information about the reality of amputations in North Rhine and will enable the participating surgeons to perform quality control[15]. We hope that completion of these questionnaires will also help to remind surgeons of the importance of appropriate management.

Chiropody

The quality of the training of chiropodists differs in European countries. For example, in the UK and The Netherlands a high-quality education is mandatory for chiropodists, whereas in Germany chiropody is the only paramedical profession without any structured mandatory education. Moreover, the reimbursement for chiropody for diabetic patients was discontinued 5 years ago, so there is little incentive for chiropodists to undertake any specialist education.

Health Carers

Many patients are unable to perform adequate foot care because of poor vision, limited mobility or cognitive problems. Crausaz et al[16] reported that 71% of the patients in a high-risk foot clinic had poor vision. Thomson and Masson[17] studied the ability of elderly patients to identify foot lesions and to perform routine foot care. Despite good vision in 75% of their elderly subjects, 39% of the patients were unable to reach their toes and only 16% could identify plantar lesions. The authors conclude that many elderly diabetic patients may be better served by regular provision of foot care rather than by intensive education. In another study[18], 39% of foot lesions were first noted by health care professionals, and a further 5% by a relative or friend. It is therefore important that relatives, friends and staff in nursing and residential homes are taught the principles of diabetic foot care in such cases.

THE CONSTRUCTION OF AN EDUCATIONAL PROGRAMME

Education cannot improve outcomes if there are barriers to behavioural change. Psychological barriers are discussed in Chapter 10 and structural barriers, such as a lack of easy access to chiropody services, must be removed. Educational programmes which are based solely on issues which are perceived as important by health care providers are unlikely to succeed. Programmes must address the beliefs and priorities of people with diabetes, and they must include strategies to facilitate behavioural change. If an educational programme is to be successful it must incorporate certain principles.

The Curriculum

There must be a written, structured curriculum comprising concrete learning objectives, teaching methods and a description of the necessary educational material[19]. An example of a structured curriculum is given in Table 9.1.

The Programme

This must be as short as is practicable, precise, relevant and understandable, especially with elderly patients. It must encompass all those generic learning objectives that are relevant to all patients, and must also include modules tailored to the needs of individual patients; for example, patients at high risk of diabetic foot problems need more detailed information about specific risks. An overview of the whole programme

Table 9.1 Example of a structured curriculum

Learning objectives: patients should:	Foot Care/motivation		Material/ media
Be motivated for adequate foot care	*Ask*	What—from your point of view— are the benefits of adequate foot care?	Flip-chart, pens
	Summarize Complete	Answers on the flip-chart • Lower risk of foot lesions and ulceration • Well-groomed feet • Feel that you can control your diabetes and not vice versa • You feel safe and protected (self-confidence) • Better relationship with health care provider	
Reflect on barriers to foot care	*Ask*	What—from your point of view— are the barriers to or potential disadvantages of adequate foot care?	Flip-chart, pens
	Summarize Complete	Answers on the flip-chart • Need to spend more time on diabetes care • Greater expenses for footwear, podiatrist, etc • Restrictions (e.g. walking barefoot, etc)	
Reflect on how the barriers can be overcome	*Ask*	How can we deal with these barriers?	Flip-chart, pens
	Summarize	Answers on the flip-chart	
Perform a cost–benefit analysis	*Request*	Please weigh the benefits of adequate foot care against the potential barriers Do you think the benefits outweigh the barriers?	
Form an intention		Do you want to optimize your foot care?	
Reflect on how negative outcome expectancies can develop	*Explain*	Patients sometimes think that even if they don't follow the recommended foot care, they will not develop foot complications. It may be that those patients have frequently walked barefoot on the beach, used heating pads, etc but have never encountered foot problems	
Reflect on their own point of view	*Ask*	What do you think about this perception? Do you have similar ideas?	
Understand why it is worth acting preventatively	*Emphasize*	It is like crossing a street with a red traffic light. It may turn out well for you several times but there is no guarantee that it will turn out well in future. So why leave it to fate?	

should be given to patients at the start. The most important aspects, for example, danger signs which require prompt action by the patient, should be summarized and repeated. Education, like other elements of diabetic care, is a team effort and all members of the team must agree to abide by the content and methodology of the programme, because inconsistent or contradictory messages are counter-productive.

The Educational Process

This must follow the psychological principles of adult learning. It must be an active process with opportunities for participation by the patient. It is helpful if patients are asked:

- To reflect on the pros and cons of their own vulnerability to both minor and severe foot problems.
- How they care for their feet at present, before explaining how it should be done.
- What they think about the information they are given.
- What they would have to do differently in future to implement the recommended standards of foot care.
- Whether they consider it feasible to incorporate such changes into their daily lifestyle.
- Whether they perceive any barriers to carrying out the recommendations and, if so, what additional support might help them to achieve adequate foot care.
- What they consider to be their responsibilities and what they view as the responsibilities of the health care team.
- Whether they have had previous ulcers and, if they have, why those ulcers occurred and how any preventable factors might be avoided in the future (it is often helpful if the teaching sessions include patients who have had an ulcer and who have experienced the benefits of subsequent preventative foot care).

The more that patients have to work with the information provided during the programme, the more likely it is that information will result in behavioural change. In this respect, group education has advantages over individual teaching because the interaction between patients supports the learning process[20,21]. Patients pass through different stages of motivation and every educational programme should use specific strategies to help patients pass through these stages. Barriers to motivation and behavioural change must be addressed, because the perception of risk of ulceration or amputation will not in itself result in behavioural change unless patients believe themselves able to carry out the recommended practice.

Educational Aids

Retention of spoken information can be enhanced by visual aids (pictures, posters, flip-charts, overhead transparencies and videos) because coding of information employs both verbal and visual systems. The benefit of visual media can depend on patients' attitudes to a particular medium; for example, those accustomed to viewing videos as a form of entertainment may not adapt to use it as a medium for serious learning. Books or leaflets may be useful as an *aide-mémoire* after participation in a teaching programme, but, used alone, are less likely to influence behaviour because of the lack of active participation.

Practical Skills

These should be taught in practical training sessions in the same way as techniques for the injection of insulin or home glucose monitoring are taught.

CONCLUSIONS

If educational programmes are to result in improved health outcomes, the programmes must:

- Be properly structured with written curricula and defined learning objectives.
- Take account of modern principles of adult learning and must emphasize the motivational processes that are necessary to promote behavioural change.
- Be tailored to meet the requirements of patient groups with different risks of developing foot problems.

Education of patients, carers and health care providers is an essential component of an effective, multi-disciplinary team approach, but can be of only limited benefit unless the other components of the health care structure needed for diabetic foot care are adequately developed. These include effective systems and structures for screening, provision of chiropody and footwear, and prompt treatment when required.

ACKNOWLEDGEMENT

The author is very grateful to Dr Uwe Bott for much helpful discussion and advice during the preparation of this chapter.

REFERENCES

1. Boulton AJ. Why bother educating the multi-disciplinary team and the patient—the example of prevention of lower extremity amputation in diabetes. *Patient Educ Couns* 1995; **26**: 183–8.

2. Edmonds ME, Blundell MP, Morris ME, Maelor Thomas E, Cotton LT, Watkins PJ. Improved survival of the diabetic foot: the role of a specialized foot clinic. *Qu J. Med*, 1986; **232**: 763–71.

3. Falkenberg M. Metabolic control and amputations among diabetics in primary health care—a population-based intensified programme governed by patient education. *Scand J Prim Health Care* 1990; **8**: 25–9.

4. Kleinfeld H. Der "diabetische Fuß"—Senkung der Amputationsrate durch spezialisierte Versorgung in Diabetes-Fuß-Ambulanzen. *Münch Med Wochenschr* 1991; **133**: 711–15.

5. Larsson J, Apelqvist J, Agardh CD, Stenström A. Decreasing incidence of major amputation in diabetic patients: a consequence of a multidisciplinary foot care team approach. *Diabet Med* 1995; **12** :770–6

6. Malone JM, Snyder M, Anderson G, Bernhard VM, Holloway GA Jr, Bunt TJ. Prevention of amputation by diabetic education. *Am J Surg* 1989; 158: 520–3.

7. Litzelman DK, Slemenda CW, Langefeld CD, Hays LM, Welch MA, Bild DE, Ford ES, Vinicor F. Reduction of lower extremity clinical abnormalities in patients with non-insulin-dependent diabetes mellitus. A randomized, controlled trial. *Ann Intern Med* 1993; **119**: 36–41.

8. Barth R, Campbell LV, Allen S, Jupp JJ, Chisholm DJ. Intensive education improves knowledge, compliance, and foot problems in type 2 diabetes. *Diabet Med* 1991; **8**: 111–17.

9. Bloomgarden ZT, Karmally W, Metzger MJ, Brothers M, Nechemias C, Bookman J, Faierman D, Ginsberg-Fellner F, Rayfield E, Brown WV. Randomized, controlled trial of diabetic patient education: improved knowledge without improved metabolic status. *Diabet Care* 1987; **10**: 263–72.

10. Pieber TR, Holler A, Siebenhofer A et al. Evaluation of a structured teaching and treatment programme for type 2 diabetes in general practice in a rural area of Austria. *Diabet Med* 1995; **12**: 349–54.

11. Spraul M, Schönbach A, Mühlhauser I, Berger M. Amputationen und Mortalität bei älteren, insulinpflichtigen Patienten mit Typ 2 Diabetes. *Zentralbl Chir* 1999; **124**: 501–7.

12. Fletcher E, MacFarlane R, Jeffcoate WJ. Can foot ulcers be prevented by education? *Diabet Med* 1992; 9(suppl 2): S41–2 (abstr).

13. Grüßer M, Bott U, Ellermann P, Kronsbein K, Jörgens V. Evaluation of a structured treatment and teaching program for non-insulin-treated type II diabetic outpatients in Germany after the nationwide introduction of reimbursement policy for physicians. *Diabet Care* 1993; **16**: 1268–75.

14. Grüßer M, Hartmann P, Hoffstadt K, Spraul M, Jörgens V. Successful introduction of an annual health check for people with diabetes to detect diabetic complications. *Diabetologia* 1998; **41**(suppl 1): A250 (abstr).

15. Spraul M, Berger M, Huber HG. Prospective documentation of amputations in North Rhine. *Diabetologia* 1999; **42**(suppl 1): A304.

16. Crausaz FM, Clavel S, Liniger C, Albeanu A, Assal JP. Additional factors associated with plantar ulcers in diabetic neuropathy. *Diabetic Med* 1988; **5**: 771–5

17. Thomson FJ, Masson EA. Can elderly diabetic patients co-operate with routine foot care? *Age and Ageing* 1992; **21**: 333–7.

18. Macfarlane RM, Jeffcoate WJ. Factors contributing to the presentation of diabetic foot ulcers. *Diabet Med* 1997; **14**: 867–70.

19. WHO. Guidelines for education programmes. In Krans HMJ, Porta M, Keen H (eds), *Diabetes Care and Research in Europe: the St. Vincent Declaration Action*

Programme. Copenhagen: WHO, Regional Office for Europe, 1992; EUR/ICP/ CLR 055/3, 9–13.

20. Bott U, Schattenberg S, Mühlhauser I, Berger M. The diabetes care team: a holistic approach. *Diabet Rev Int* 1996; **5**: 12–14.

21. Maldonato A, Bloise D, Ceci M, Fraticelli E, Fallucca F. Diabetes mellitus: lessons from patient education. *Patient Educ Couns* 1995; **26**: 57–66.

10

Psychological and Behavioural Issues in Diabetic Neuropathic Foot Ulceration

LORETTA VILEIKYTE

University of Manchester, Manchester, UK

Although it is often stated that diabetic foot ulcers result from an interaction of physical and psychosocial/behavioural factors, the vast majority of studies into the pathogenesis of foot ulcers have focused solely on physical determinants of ulceration. This suggests either that psychosocial factors are not considered to be important or that we do not know how to approach them.

However, two studies from the Indianapolis group[1,2] have confirmed that certain foot care behaviours predict foot lesions and that their modification results in reduction in foot ulceration, thereby emphasizing the importance of behavioural factors. The fact that ulcer and amputation rates continue to rise[3,4], despite our attempts to control physical factors, should make us reappraise the importance of psychosocial variables.

In this chapter I will review previous reports of educational interventions for those patients at high ulcer risk, after which our earlier cross-sectional and prospective studies on psychosocial aspects will be summarized. Finally, results from the qualitative phase of our ongoing research into the psychological determinants of foot care behaviour and quality of life in diabetic neuropathic patients will be presented.

The Foot in Diabetes, 3rd edn. Edited by A. J. M. Boulton, H. Connor and P. R. Cavanagh.
© 2000 John Wiley & Sons, Ltd.

LIMITATIONS OF
FOOT CARE EDUCATION
STUDIES

In a recent systematic review covering the interventions for prevention and treatment of diabetic foot ulceration, Majid et al[5] found four randomized controlled trials[1,6,7,8] that evaluated the effects of foot care education on ulceration rates, and of these four studies only one[1] actually assessed foot care practice. The remaining studies assessed the direct relationship between information provision and reduction in ulceration, with the assumption that lower rates of ulceration imply better adherence to advice, and vice versa. However, this assumption may not be justified. To identify the role of preventative foot care behaviour in reducing ulcer rates, a behavioural assessment is essential. Moreover, in Litzelman's study[1] a system of reminders was introduced to tackle the non-intentional "non-compliance", simply assuming that patients forget to look after their feet because of the lack of symptoms. Non-adherence behaviours, however, fall broadly into two categories: non-intentional non-adherence occurs when the patient's intentions are thwarted by barriers such as forgetfulness or physical problems such as poor eye sight. Intentional or "intelligent non-compliance", from the patient's perspective, may be seen as a "common-sense" response to a lack of coherence between the patient's ideas and clinician's instructions[9].

The study of Malone et al[8] targeted patients with active foot problems, some of them unilateral amputees, whose perceptions of the health threat and their readiness to follow foot care advice may not be representative of the total high-risk population. Moreover, in order to motivate their patients, Malone and colleagues used fear arousal without previously assessing the levels of anxiety in subjects whose psychological distress might already have been high as a result of having a foot lesion, an approach that was probably unnecessary or even counterproductive. Inducing fear may lead to a destructive denial, especially in patients who are extremely threatened by their health situation and are already using denial to cope with excessive fear[10]. Furthermore, our qualitative studies[11] revealed that diabetic neuropathic patients have high levels of fear of amputation, and express hostility towards health care professionals who use a fear appeal to motivate them.

A major criticism of many educational interventions is that they employ general educational strategies, such as information provision, fear arousal or promotion of self-esteem, and are not grounded on preparatory research, and may not target the most important prerequisites for a particular behaviour in that particular population[12].

PSYCHOSOCIAL VARIABLES IN DIABETES SELF-MANAGEMENT

It is now well recognized that simple "knowledge transfer" approaches have been overemphasized in diabetes education. More recently, a number of studies have explored psychosocial factors related to diabetes self-management, mainly in relation to glycaemic control. In contrast to knowledge which is loosely, if at all, related to behaviour[13], social cognitive factors such as self-efficacy[14], social support[15], patients' beliefs and attitudes to diabetes[16,17] and internal locus of control[18] are rather stronger predictors of self-care behaviour.

In spite of this apparent recognition of the social-cognitive component of self-care behaviour in diabetes in general, to date no studies on the psychosocial constructs that might underpin preventative foot care behaviour have been reported, with the exception of a few anecdotal observations based on the common sense of clinical experts in the area.

PSYCHOLOGICAL ISSUES OF ULCERATION: CLINICIANS' VIEWS

In his classical paper on the psychology of peripheral insensitivity, Brand[19] wrote that: *"when sensation is lost, even intelligent people lose all sense of identity with their insensitive parts. An insensitive limb feels like a wooden block fastened to the body and is treated as such"*. Clinicians who treat diabetic feet have suggested that patients at high physical risk of developing ulcers exhibit strong negative emotions, such as fear, anger and depression, which may lead to "apparent carelessness" and "denial" of their situation[20]. Walsh et al[21] described a syndrome of "wilful self-neglect" occurring in patients with neuropathy, retinopathy and foot ulceration who exhibited a striking indifference to their condition. Thus, negative attitudes to feet, emotional upset and denial are commonly perceived by health care professionals to be important determinants of "non-compliance" in high risk diabetic neuropathic patients.

STUDIES OF PSYCHOSOCIAL FACTORS IN DIABETIC FOOT ULCERATION

We examined, cross-sectionally and prospectively, the role of those psychological variables considered by clinicians to be important determinants of foot ulceration in groups of patients with variable degrees of neuropathy[22]. Psychological assessment included a number of self-report scales. Thus, the Foot Health Questionnaire (FHQ) was specifically designed to assess patients' perceptions of the health status of their feet and the feelings diabetic patients have towards their feet[23]. The philosophy that guided the selection of items originated from Brand's observation[19] that peripheral neuropathy alters patients' attitudes towards their feet, leading to a neglect of their insensitive parts. This measure consists of a number of opposites, rated on a seven-point scale using semantic differential methodology that asks respondents to choose the point where their own views lie on the continuum of opposing views (e.g. my feet are: weak–strong; valuable–worthless). The Foot Problems Questionnaire (FPQ) covers the following areas: individuals' perception of the effectiveness of foot care advice (if I look after my feet, they will remain healthy); denial (when I have a foot ulcer, I tend to ignore it); fear of amputation (I am frightened of losing my leg). In addition, essential foot care knowledge and reported foot care practice regarding frequency of foot inspection, choice of footwear, barefoot walking, water temperature testing, methods of warming cold feet, care of callosities and toenails, and chiropody visits and reported foot care practice, were evaluated using a multiple-choice questionnaire.

The results of this study demonstrated that these high-risk patients are not ignorant of foot complications and have a good knowledge of essential foot care principles. Comparison of those patients with and those without an ulcer history at baseline showed that there was no difference in their levels of knowledge, but reported foot care practice was significantly better in those patients with previous ulceration as compared to those with no ulcer history. This suggests that behaviour does not change when health care professionals inform patients of their high risk of foot ulceration; it is the actual development of a foot ulcer that alters the behaviour. This finding may also apply to clinicians as well as to patients, because in a retrospective case–control study, del Aguila et al[24] found that clinicians provided more intensive education for those patients with a history of ulceration than for those with neuropathy or peripheral vascular disease but no history of ulceration. The cognitive processes involved in this behavioural change are not clear. We hypothesize that ulcer development alters patients' perception of the health threat, making it more real and giving rise to emotional responses that results in the behavioural change. Thus, patients' own judgement of the health status of their feet, as measured by the FHQ, might be an important catalyst in triggering this behavioural change. Indeed, in our study, patients with previous foot ulceration perceived their feet as significantly less healthy than those without ulcer history[22].

WHAT ABOUT DENIAL?

Denial is an abstract and highly complex psychological concept commonly applied to patients who: (a) do not accept their diagnosis; (b) minimize the implications of their illness; (c) delay seeking medical advice; (d) comply poorly with the treatment; or (e) appear unperturbed in the face of illness. Most commonly, denial has been used to describe a strategy or mechanism of defence, which serves to provide psychological protection against the perception of subjectively painful or distressing information.

In our study[22] we assessed several dimensions of denial—the extent to which the patients minimize the seriousness of having foot ulcers and delay seeking medical help. We did not find examples of extreme destructive denial in our group of high-risk patients. In fact, there was a significant negative correlation between fear of amputation and denial; patients with greater levels of fear were less likely to use denial as a means of coping with emotional upset and, indeed, were more likely to engage in preventative foot care. We hypothesize that fear has to be raised above a certain threshold before patients adopt denial rather than using preventative actions as a coping behaviour. It must be remembered that denial is a continuum of responses, ranging from biased defensive appraisal of personally relevant risk messages to a complete avoidance of anxiety-provoking thoughts to the extent that individuals will be convinced that they have not got a problem. Although overt denial was not documented in our study, defensiveness was not assessed and we speculate that those high-risk patients with no ulcer history may have employed defensive biases to appraise their risks, and this might have led them to minimize the health threat, resulting in the lack of preventative foot care.

Managing denial in the clinical situation can pose formidable problems and requires consideration of a number of issues:

- Is the patient's behaviour appropriately described as denial, or are there alternative explanations, such as ignorance, lack of understanding or a discrepancy in informed opinion, between the patient and the doctor?
- Is the patient's denial adaptive or maladaptive? In the short term, denial may be useful, as it protects the patient from being emotionally overwhelmed; if it is prolonged, it may impede adaptive coping.
- If judged to be maladaptive, how is such denial best tackled?

Confrontation, a strategy which can be attractive at first sight, may reduce compliance with treatment or may even precipitate a complete breakdown of the doctor–patient relationship. Addressing the issue of denial, Miller[25] suggested the following techniques: empathic listening, allowing patients to express personal views; reflection; summarizing; and discussion of behavioural alternatives.

Thus, clinical management of maladaptive denial poses a challenging problem which requires consideration of all factors pertaining to the patient, the nature of the illness, and the clinician. There is enough ambiguity in the entire picture of denial to suggest that the term should be made less invidious. The clinician–patient relationship would benefit from the avoidance of such terms, which may sometimes hinder attempts to discover the true reasons behind the maladaptive behaviour.

TESTING THE HEALTH BELIEFS MODEL

In order to explore the findings of our first study, we employed the modified Diabetes-specific Health Beliefs Questionnaire, which addresses perceived severity of vulnerability to foot complications and perceived benefits of, and barriers to, foot care, in the same group of high-risk patients[26]. Scores for perceived severity showed that foot complications rated as highly as other major complications of diabetes in all groups of high-risk patients, including those with and without ulcer history. Vulnerability scores were also similar for all major complications of diabetes in high-risk groups. Interestingly, however, patients with established neuropathy but no evidence of vascular complications perceived their vulnerability to vascular complications as being much greater than to foot ulceration, even though the results of the physical tests had been explained to them. This suggests that lay beliefs about vulnerability to vascular complications are strong, and this may have implications for educational interventions. In addition, high-risk patients, even those with previous ulceration, do not perceive their personal vulnerability to foot lesions as being any greater than that of an average diabetic patient, suggesting that appraisal of personal vulnerability is not a rational process. This observation is consistent with the literature indicating that vulnerability perceptions are not calmly reasoned beliefs; rather, they induce emotional distress, which can create barriers to preventative behaviour[27].

Weinstein[28] has documented an optimistic bias showing that most people perceive their individual risks to be lower than average. Croyle et al[29] describe ways in which individual representations of health threat can become distorted or less accessible following the receipt of positive information from screening tests. Their studies reveal a very consistent tendency in those identified as being at risk to play down the seriousness of the condition, to rate their own risk as being lower than it is, to perceive the test as unreliable and the health threat as relatively short-lived. The presence of these defensive biases and their role in shaping foot care behaviour require further investigation.

In our study, scores for perceived benefits of preventative foot care were universally and equally high in all patients studied; scores for barriers to wearing appropriate footwear were significantly higher than barriers to performing other aspects of foot care[26]. This could explain the frequent observation that only a minority of diabetic patients wear their prescribed footwear regularly. It is not surprising that one of the commonest precipitants of neuropathic foot ulcers is ill-fitting footwear.

The benefits of preventative behaviour are largely hypothetical, but the barriers are more real and comprise both psychological costs (e.g. unfashionable shoe style) and physical hindrances (e.g. restricted availability of appropriate footwear). Psychological barriers may vary as a function of the perceived health threat. For example, Breuer found that patients' perceptions of foot abnormalities affect their compliance with protective footwear[30].

However, when the physical and psychological variables were combined, the best independent predictors of ulceration were physical variables, such as past ulcer history, and quantitative sensory tests, such as vibration. Paradoxically, those reporting better foot care behaviour at baseline developed more ulcers during the first year of follow-up. This observation confirms the complex interaction between physical and behavioural factors in the genesis of foot ulceration, where the relative contributions of each varies along the continuum of severity of neuropathy. Thus, levels of foot care behaviour which might well be sufficient to prevent ulceration in patients with mild neuropathy are insufficient in those with more severe neuropathy. The challenge remains as to how to motivate those patients with milder neuropathy to adopt appropriate foot care practice.

Our studies have clearly indicated that patients' behaviour is not driven by the abstract designation of being "at risk", as defined by their clinicians; rather, behaviour is guided by patients' own perceptions of their risks. It follows that the content of patients' beliefs should be studied in a coherent way using an appropriate illness-focused model, an approach which can only succeed if there is close collaboration between clinicians and health psychologists.

STUDYING NEUROPATHY-SPECIFIC BELIEFS: A THEORETICAL PATIENT-CENTRED APPROACH

Increasing research evidence suggests that patients' own "common-sense" beliefs are fundamental in driving their illness-related behaviour[31,32]. These studies were guided by the self-regulatory model of behaviour described by Leventhal and colleagues[33], which proposes that individuals are active problem-solvers and construct their own representation of the health threat (e.g. neuropathy) derived from a number of sources, including their knowledge, experiences, beliefs and information from, for example, medical professionals.

In order to explore neuropathy-specific beliefs, we have used semi-structured interviews, conducted by health psychologists, in neuropathic patients (unpublished observations). The main themes emerging from these interviews suggest that patients have a distorted representation of neuropathy. They tend to conceptualize neuropathy as a circulatory problem and rely on symptoms when constructing their representation of neuropathy and monitoring its progress. Patients seem to link neuropathy directly with amputation; foot ulcers rarely feature in this pathway, unless previously experienced. These erroneous beliefs drive a fear emotion, specifically a fear of amputation. The second group of emotional responses includes anger and hostility, directed towards the health-care providers as a result of a perceived lack of clear explanation or perceived lack of compassion. This, in turn, leads to defensiveness and denial. Thus the doctor–patient interaction appears to be a powerful factor influencing initial appraisal of neuropathy, levels of emotional distress and adherence to preventative foot care.

These results of the qualitative phase of our research have informed the development of a Neuropathy Perception Inventory (NPI), which is currently undergoing validation. Hopefully the NPI will prove to be a useful tool that will enable us to assess individual needs of high-risk neuropathic patients in clinical practice and to identify determinants of behaviour and quality-of-life issues in further research studies.

At one time, the diabetic foot was regarded as the Cinderella of late diabetic complications, but this has changed in the last decade. It could now be stated that psychosocial problems are the Cinderella of diabetic foot research: I hope that this also will change in the near future.

REFERENCES

1. Litzelman DK, Slemenda CW, Langefeld CD, Hays LM, Welch MA, Bild DE et al. Reduction of lower extremity clinical abnormalities in patients with non-insulin dependent diabetes mellitus. *Ann Intern Med* 1993; **119**: 36–41.
2. Suico JG, Marriott DJ, Vinicor F, Litzelman DK. Behaviours predicting foot lesions in patients with non-insulin dependent diabetes mellitus. *J Gen Intern Med* 1998; **13**: 482–4.
3. Center for Disease Control, Atlanta, GA, USA. *Amputation Statistics*, October 1998.
4. Anonymous. An audit of amputations in rural health district. *Pract Diabet Int* 1997; **14**(6): 175–8.
5. Majid M, Cullum N, Fletcher A, O'Meara S, Sheldon T. Systematic review of interventions for the prevention and treatment of diabetic foot ulceration. Health Technology Assessment Report, in preparation.

6. Bloomgarden ZT, Karmally W, Metzger MJ, Brothers M, Nechemias C, Bookman J et al. Randomized, controlled trial of diabetic patient education: improved knowledge without improved metabolic status. *Diabet Care* 1987; **10**: 263–72.

7. Pieber TR, Holler A, Siebenhofer A, Brunner GA, Semlitsch B, Schattenberg S. Evaluation of a structured teaching and treatment programme for type 2 diabetes in general practice in a rural area of Austria. *Diabet Med* 1995; **12**: 349–54.

8. Malone JM, Snyder M, Anderson G, Bernhard VM, Holloway GA, Bunt TJ. Prevention of amputation by diabetic education. *Am J Surg* 1989; **158**: 520–4.

9. Weintraub M. Compliance in the elderly. *Clinics Geriat Med* 1990; **6**: 445–52.

10. Rubin RR, Peyrot M. Emotional responses to diagnosis. In Anderson BJ, Rubin RR (eds), *Practical Psychology for Diabetes Clinicians*. Alexandria: ADA Publications, 1996; 155–62.

11. Vileikyte L, Bundy CE, Tomenson B, Walsh T, Boulton AJM. Neuropathy-specific quality of life measure: construction of scales and preliminary tests of reliability and validity. *Diabetes* 1998; **47**: A44.

12. Kok G. Why are so many health promotion programs ineffective? *Health Promotion J Austral* 1993; **3**: 12–17.

13. Dunn SM. Rethinking the models and modes of diabetes education. *Patient Educ Couns* 1990; **16**: 281–6.

14. Kingery PM, Glasgow RE. Self-efficacy and outcome expectations in the self-regulation of non-insulin dependent diabetes mellitus. *Health Educ* 1989; **20**: 13–19.

15. Glasgow RE, Hampson SE, Strycker LA, Ruggiero L. Personal-model beliefs and social-environmental barriers related to diabetes self-management. *Diabet Care* 1997; **20**: 556–61.

16. Hampson SE, Glasgow RE, Toobert DJ. Personal models of diabetes and their relations to self-care activities. *Health Psychol* 1990; **9**: 632–46.

17. Bradley C, Gamsu DS, Moses JL, Knight G, Boulton AJM, Drury J et al. The use of diabetes-specific perceived control and health beliefs measures to predict treatment choice and efficacy in a feasibility study of continuous subcutaneous insulin infusion pumps. *Psychol Health* 1987; **1**: 133–46.

18. Peyrot M, Rubin RR. Structure and correlates of diabetes-specific locus of control. *Diabet Care* 1994; **17**: 994–1001.

19. Brand P. The diabetic foot. In Ellenberg M, Rifkin H (eds), *Diabetes Mellitus: Theory and Practice*, 3rd edn. New York: Med Exam Publishers, 1983; 824–49.

20. Foster A. Psychological aspects of treating the diabetic foot. *Pract Diabet* 1997; **14**: 56–8.

21. Walsh CH, Soler NG, Fitzgerald MG, Malins JM. Association of foot lesions with retinopathy in patients with newly diagnosed diabetes. *Lancet* 1975; **1**; 878–80.

22. Vileikyte L, Shaw JE, Carrington AL, Abbott CA, Kincey J, Boulton AJM. A prospective study of neuropathic and psychosocial factors in foot ulceration. *Diabet Med* 1996; **13**(suppl 7): S43.

23. Carrington AL, Mawdsley SKV, Morley M, Kincey J, Boulton AJM. Psychological status of diabetic people with or without lower limb disability. *Diabet Res Clin Pract* 1996; **32**: 19–26.

24. del Aguila MA, Reiber GE, Koepsell TD. How does provider and patient awareness of high-risk status for lower-extremity amputation influence foot-care practice? *Diabet Care* 1994; **17**: 1050–4.

25. Miller WR. Motivational interviewing. *Behav Psychother*, 1983; **11**: 147–72.

26. Vileikyte L, Shaw JE, Boulton AJM. Diabetic foot: patients' perceptions of risks and barriers to foot care may be the final determinants of ulceration. *Diabetes* 1997; **46**(suppl 1): 147A.
27. Cameron LD. Screening for cancer: illness perceptions and illness worry. In Petrie KJ & Weinman JA (eds), *Perceptions of Health and Illness*. Amsterdam, Netherlands: Harwood Academic, 1997; 291–322.
28. Weinstein N. Unrealistic optimism about illness susceptibility: conclusions from a community-wide sample. *J Behav Med* 1987; **10**: 481–500.
29. Croyle RT, Yi-Chun Sun, Hart M Processing risk information: defensive biases in health-related judgements and memory. In Petrie KJ, Weinman JA (eds), *Perceptions of Health and Illness*. Amsterdam, Netherlands: Harwood Academic, 1997; 267–90.
30. Breuer U. Diabetic patient's compliance with bespoke footwear after healing of neuropathic foot ulcers. *Diabetes Metabol* 1994; **20**: 415–19.
31. Petrie KJ, Weinman J, Sharpe N, Buckley J. Role of patients' view of their illness in predicting return to work and functioning after myocardial infarction: longitudinal study. *Br Med J* 1996; **312**: 1191–4.
32. Hampson SE, Glasgow RE, Zeiss AM. Personal models of osteoarthritis and their relation to self-management activities and quality of life. *J Behav Med* 1994; **17**: 143–58.
33. Leventhal H, Meyer D, Nerenz D. The common representation of illness danger. In Rachman S (ed.), *Medical Psychology*, vol. 2. New York: Pergamon, 1980.

11

Footwear for the High-risk Patient

ERNST CHANTELAU

Heinrich Heine Universität, Düsseldorf, Germany

Half of all amputations in diabetic patients are preceded by injury from footwear[1], but such damage is rarely seen in non-diabetic people. Footwear can be particularly harmful to the feet of diabetic subjects when protective sensation is lost. In addition, foot deformity[2] aggravates this deleterious impact of footwear (Figure 11.1). Both conditions put diabetic feet at high risk of injuries from pressure and shear stresses, caused by mismatch between footwear and foot. While healthy feet are protected by pain sensation, which prevents or limits exposure to harmful pressure forces, insensate diabetic feet will allow the exposure to continue until tissue is damaged. In diabetic feet, such damage occurs predominantly at the forefoot (Figure 11.2), where most footwear-related pressure stress occurs[3].

The National Institute of Diabetes and Digestive and Kidney Diseases (NIDDK) and the US Department of Health and Human Services have issued a *Guide to Preventing Diabetic Foot Problems*[4], with a summarized differentiation between low-risk and high-risk diabetic feet (Table 11.1). According to this document, patients with high-risk feet should be given special footwear, namely depth-inlay (stock) shoes with stock or customized inserts (insoles), or custom-moulded shoes with inserts. However, the report gives little other information about the type of footwear which is needed, stating only that it "should relieve areas of excessive pressure, reduce shock and shear, and accommodate, stabilize and support deformities", and that "shoes should be long enough and have

The Foot in Diabetes, 3rd edn. Edited by A. J. M. Boulton, H. Connor and P. R. Cavanagh.
© 2000 John Wiley & Sons, Ltd.

Plantar aspect of the foot

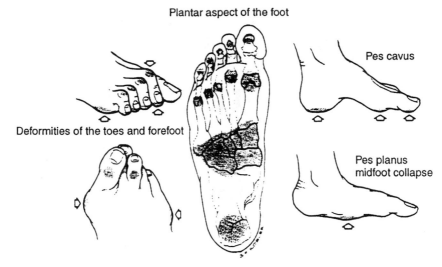

Shaded areas and arrows indicate primary regions 'at risk' for developing ulcers

Figure 11.1 The "at-risk" diabetic foot. Illustration by G. Kogler, reproduced with permission from reference 2

room in the toe area and over the instep"[4]. This chapter will describe the evidence-base for the use of diabetic footwear and how such products should be constructed.

Footwear for high-risk diabetic feet, "diabetic" footwear, needs to be much more sophisticated than normal footwear to match the requirements of extremely vulnerable feet. Moreover, it must meet the requirements of elderly people, since many patients with high-risk diabetic feet are elderly and often handicapped by co-morbidity.

RECENT STUDIES ON PLANTAR PRESSURE REDUCTION BY FOOTWEAR

With the widespread application of the in-shoe dynamic plantar pressure measurement, which was first described as early as 1975[5], there have been many papers on peak plantar pressure (PPP) in relation to various pressure-reducing materials and shoe design (Table 11.2). Although the methodology of this surrogate parameter is not yet standardized in respect of the equivalence of the various systems on the market (e.g. accuracy and precision of the measurements, temperature dependency of the pressure transducers), or to the measurement procedure (e.g. measurement at a fixed or habitual walking speed or stride length), or the reporting of the data (as absolute values in percentage bodyweight,

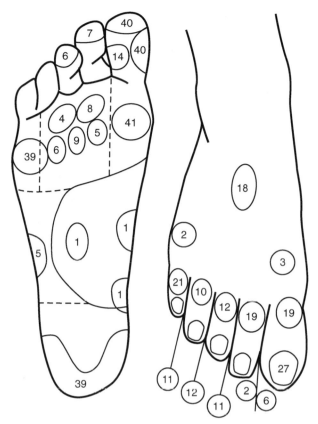

Figure 11.2 Localization of 439 diabetic foot ulcers. Reproduced by permission of *Prosthetics and Orthotics International*, from reference 3

kPa, g or N per cm², or as intra-individual changes from reference values), the data do allow some preliminary conclusions to be drawn. Firstly, human PPP measurements confirm earlier data obtained by mechanical materials testing[13,18,19], which show that some materials are

Table 11.1 Factors and markers of low-risk versus high-risk diabetic feet

Low-risk foot	High-risk foot
All of the following: Intact protective sensation Pedal pulses present No severe deformity No prior foot ulcer No amputation	One or more of the following: Loss of protective sensation Absent pedal pulses Severe foot deformity History of foot ulcer or pre-ulcerative callus Prior amputation Limited foot joint mobility

After reference 4.

Table 11.2 Peak plantar pressure (PPP) reduction during walking

Reference	Sole design or materials	Subjects (H*, D*)	By comparison with:	PPP reduction at metatarsal heads
6	PPT*, Berkelast, PZ*, MCR* 7 mm	H	Barefoot walking	0–40% depending on material
6	Jogging shoe	?	Oxford leather-soled shoe	30%
7	Ordinary shoes, not specified	H, D	Barefoot walking	30% (H) 35% (D)
8	Custom-moulded PZ +MCR insoles 10 mm	D	Barefoot walking	50%
9	Ordinary shoes, from leather or rubber	H	Barefoot walking	50%
10	Running shoes, leather-soled Oxford shoes	H, D	Barefoot walking	<10% (Oxford shoes), 30% (running shoes)
11	Extra-depth shoe +stock insole	D	Oxford canvas shoes	12%
12	Stock shoes + PZ/ urethane insoles 4 mm	D	Stock shoes, no insoles	5–20%
13	PPT 2–13 mm	D	Barefoot walking	21–29%
14	Alcapy/PPT 3 mm	D	Barefoot walking	<10%
15	Oxford shoe leather-soled, running shoe, extra-depth shoe ±cork/PPT custom inlay		Barefoot walking	0% leather-soled shoe, 35% running shoe, 0% cork, 35% PPT
16	Rocker bottom	Amputated D	Normal shoes	25%
17	Rocker bottom, various heights	?	Normal shoes	40–55%
11	Total contact cast + rocker	D	Oxford canvas shoes	84%
14	Semi-rocker bottom	D	Barefoot walking	<10%

*Abbreviations: H=healthy subjects; D=diabetic subjects; PPT=open cell urethane foam; PZ=plastazote (polyethylene foam); MCR=microcellular rubber.

better than others in terms of shock absorption and durability. Hence, technical characteristics like hardness, thickness, elasticity and durability appear to be predictive of a material's performance when used in footwear, and need not be confirmed by human studies. Secondly, load distribution by total plantar contact orthoses has been proved to reduce PPP substantially, for example in a total contact cast with a high rocker bottom[11,16,17]. Thus, the two established principles of reducing PPP, namely shock absorption and load distribution, that had been reported qualitatively[20,21], have now been confirmed quantitatively, rendering them useful for footwear design.

RECENT STUDIES ON THE CLINICAL EFFECTIVENESS OF PLANTAR PRESSURE REDUCTION BY "DIABETIC" FOOTWEAR

Only a few studies have so far been published on footwear-related PPP reduction and clinical endpoints, i.e. protection from foot lesions (Table 11.3). However, these studies suffer from methodological shortcomings. Most of them rely on patient-reported data as to the timing and the nature of the endpoints (erythema, blister, ulcer). How can neuropathic patients accurately recall such an event? Not every footwear-induced injury might have been due to the footwear under study (as there can be no certainty that patients wore only the study footwear). Neither is it possible to be sure that all injuries were due to an elevated PPP. Finally, the patients' risk category (Table 11.4), callosities and quality of foot care must be taken into account, as they are strong confounders of the desired clinical outcomes. Nevertheless, the three cohort studies[8,23,24] and one randomized trial[22] in undeformed feet, and one short-term randomized trial in severely deformed feet[16] suggest that prolonged reduction of PPP during walking reduces the rate of foot lesions, including ulcer relapses.

Table 11.3 Clinical effectiveness of PPP reduction in diabetic patients

Reference	Shoe design	PPP reduction	Outcome	Follow-up
8	Tovey-style[20] custom-moulded shoes with PZ+MCR insoles	50% vs barefoot walking	Minus 50% ulcer relapses*	2 years
22	Tovey-style[20] stock shoes with semi-rocker bottom	?	Minus 50% ulcer relapses	1 year
16	Rocker bottom, custom-moulded insole	25% vs normal shoes	Minus >50% skin lesions	1 month
23	Tovey-style[20] stock shoes, viscoelastic insole and outsole	30% vs barefoot walking	Minus >50% ulcer relapses*	1 year
24	Tovey-style[20] stock shoes, viscoelastic insole, semi-rocker bottom	30% vs barefoot walking	Minus 50% ulcer relapses*	1 year

*Depending on wearing time >8 hours/day.
Abbreviations: see Table 11.2.

Table 11.4   Updated footwear recommendation by risk category

Risk category	Protective footwear
0 Protective sensation intact	Shoes of proper style and fit
1 Loss of protective sensation	Shock-absorbing stock insoles extra-depth stock shoes
2 Loss of protective sensation and high plantar pressure, or callosities, or history of ulcer	Custom-moulded, shock-absorbing insoles, extra-depth stock shoes
3 Loss of protective sensation and history of ulcer, and severe foot or toe deformation ± limited joint mobility	Custom-moulded, extra-depth shoes and insoles, rigid rocker outsole and accommodative modifications
4 Neuropathic fracture, healed	Custom-moulded, rigid total plantar contact orthoses, extra-depth shoes, rocker outsole

Based on reference 26.

STOCK VS CUSTOM-MOULDED BESPOKE "DIABETIC" SHOES

Custom-moulded "diabetic" footwear was shown to be clinically effective in diabetic feet without major deformities[8], and in deformed feet with forefoot amputation[16]. Stock "diabetic" footwear was clinically effective in diabetic feet without major deformities[22–24], but not in deformed feet[23]. While several studies on stock "diabetic" footwear have included technical details of the footwear[22–24,25], comparable reports on custom-moulded bespoke footwear are rare[8,16]. Hence, the production of custom-moulded "diabetic" footwear is still mostly empirical, and not scientifically based. The prescription of stock or custom-moulded footwear will depend on the risk category of the patient (Table 11.4).

ASSESSMENT OF FORCES FROM THE SHOE UPPER

Shear forces, as well as pressure forces, may be exerted by the shoe upper, and especially by a toe-cap. Schröer[27] used an experimental metal toe-cap of variable diameter inside a shoe model to assess these effects. Interdigital pressure was measured between the fourth and fifth toes. High-risk patients with limited joint mobility displayed increased interdigital pressure in a toe-cap which fitted well to the forefoot diameter. Narrowing the toe-cap, as well as bending the forefoot (to simulate the push-off phase of the gait cycle), further increased interdigital pressure. A soft, way-giving, upper significantly attenuated toe compression when compared with a rigid toe-cap. Healthy controls displayed substantially less interdigital pressure under all study conditions[27]. Thus, toe-caps must be avoided in "diabetic" footwear (Figure 11.3), in order to protect high-risk toes from injuries[20,28].

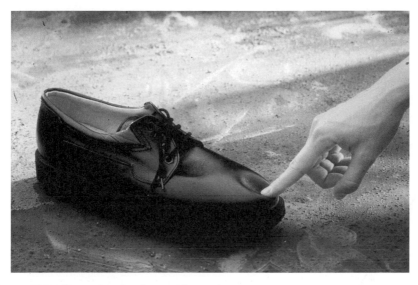

Figure 11.3   Example of a shoe without toe cap

LASTS FOR "DIABETIC" STOCK FOOTWEAR

While customized footwear is manufactured over individualized lasts (made from plaster models of each foot), stock shoes are made over standardized lasts. It is not known whether the normal standard lasts used by the footwear industry are appropriate for "diabetic" footwear, such as extra-depth shoes which can accommodate inlays. Normal standard lasts are tabulated according to the shoe-number (English or French system) in length and width. To assess whether the dimensions used for normal footwear would fit diabetic feet, 1112 feet of 568 diabetic patients with peripheral neuropathy were investigated (excluding feet with severe deformities like Charcot fracture, amputation or hallux valgus). Length and width, as well as the shoe-number (French system), were obtained automatically using a rectangular device (WMS-measuring apparatus, kindly provided by Professor K. Mattil, PFI, Pirmasens, Germany). The patient data were compared with standard footwear size tables (Fagus GmbH, Alfeld, Germany). Seventy-six per cent of all diabetic feet were broader than the size-related width 7 (equal to English width G), which is the most prevalent width in normal footwear, and 62% were even larger than the next, extra-large, width 8 (equal to English width H)[29]. Thus, stock shoes for diabetic high-risk feet require special lasts, and must not be made over the standard lasts used for normal footwear.

Table 11.5   Evidence-based items of "diabetic" footwear design

Item	Definition by study data
Width	Larger than "extra large" of the standard shoe size system[29]
"Way-giving" shoe upper	Reduces toe compression[27]
Toe-cap	Increases toe compression[27], causes toe ulcers[28]
Shock-absorbing insole	Reduction of PPP by >30%, vs barefoot walking, lowers incidence of foot lesions[8,16,24]; insoles must have 7–12 mm thickness (PPT) to give desired effect[13], and hardness 15–25 °Shore[18]*
Depth of anterior part	Must allow for forefoot plus appropriately thick (approx 10 mm[13]) insole
Total plantar contact	Custom-moulded rigid insole, to accommodate severely deformed foot (Charcot fractures); requires rocker-bottom[16,17] to prevent shear stress at foot–shoe interface
Rocker-bottom	Reduces PPP at metatarsal heads, depending on height of the rocker[17], affects postural stability and gait[31]
Outsole	Rubber-made outsoles (running shoes) reduce PPP, as compared to leather-made Oxford-style shoes[6,10,15]

*°Shore is a measure of hardness.

In summary, recent data have provided better evidence on which the manufacture of "diabetic" footwear for the high-risk patient should now be based (Table 11.5). However, many old[30] and new issues remain on the agenda. These include potential adverse effects of different types of "diabetic" footwear, e.g. on gait acceleration, climbing stairs and postural stability[31], and potential beneficial effects of plantar cushioning on neuropathic foot pain.

"DIABETIC" FOOTWEAR, A MEDICAL PRODUCT ON PRESCRIPTION

"Diabetic" footwear is, by definition, a medical product, as it differs in terms of major construction items, shape and purpose from normal footwear. Patients with loss of protective sensation in their feet are unable to judge for themselves whether or not a particular shoe is suitable for them. Hence, "diabetic" footwear must be prescribed and controlled by professionals who are experienced in this field. This is what the NIDDK document rightly requires and, most importantly, it also requires that reimbursement by medical insurance be conditional on the suitability of the footwear being approved by the prescribing physician[4]. However doctors are often not prepared to do this[32]. More guidance on the appropriateness of the "diabetic" footwear on the market is therefore necessary. Help may come from European Community (EC) legislation. The EC Medical Product Directive 93/42 requires that only medical products which fulfil certain technical safety standards may be distributed within the EC. "Diabetic"

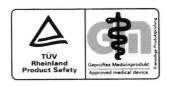

Figure 11.4 Stamp of approval, according to European Community Directive 93/42 on Medical Products (see text)

footwear belongs to Class 1, the lowest class of medical products. Medical products may optionally be certified as an "Approved Medical Device" upon proof of their clinical effectiveness (Figure 11.4). To date, at least one brand of "diabetic" stock shoes (Thanner GmbH, Höchstädt, Germany) has applied for and received this certificate. However, no custom-moulded bespoke footwear has so far been approved for this certificate; bespoke shoe-making for high-risk diabetic feet continues to be haphazard.

Footwear for the high-risk diabetic foot is intended to prevent, but not to heal, foot lesions. To quote Tovey[20], "it must be emphasized that all ulcers must be healed first by bed rest or non-weightbearing, and that protective footwear will not heal ulcers". This is because foot lesions can be prevented by a significant reduction in harmful pressures, but abolition of pressure is needed to heal an established lesion. Thus, strategies and devices for treatment must differ from those for prevention. The footwear required for prevention will depend on the patient's risk category, as described in Table 11.4. The availability of good "diabetic" footwear will continue to increase, making it possible to prescribe approved stock "diabetic footwear" more readily and at an earlier stage. In this way many first "lesions" will be prevented.

OUTLOOK

Continuous quality control is urgently required; it will increase the acceptance of "diabetic" footwear by medical professionals and by patients alike. As a consequence, the clinical benefits of this very important preventative tool will hopefully become more popular. As long as there are insufficient technical data to predict the clinical outcome of a particular footwear design, controlled clinical trials will remain the gold standard for the evaluation of "diabetic" footwear, where clinical efficiency must be proved in every single case. The many variables that should be considered when planning trials of footwear must include measurement of the daily duration of ambulation (usually the number of hours out of bed) and the length of time that the footwear is worn each day (ideally by using in-built, step-on sensors). An example from a recent study[24] is shown in Figure 11.5.

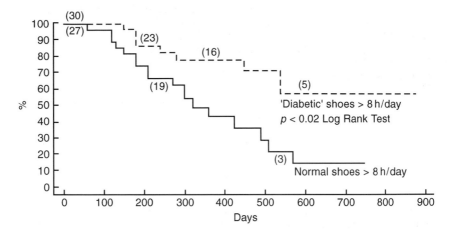

Figure 11.5 Percentage of patients free of foot ulcer relapses over time, whether wearing normal shoes or "diabetic" shoes for more than 8 hours/day. Kaplan–Meier analysis; numbers of patients under observation in parentheses. Reproduced by permission of Urban & Vogel GmbH, Munich, from reference 24

Randomized prospective studies that compare different types of stock "diabetic" footwear with normal shoes, with measurement of shock absorption vs load distribution, would be needed to provide the most sceptical of medical statisticians with the ultimate proof of efficacy. However, not every high-risk patient may wish to be randomized into the control group, as the disadvantages of normal footwear for high-risk patients are already indisputable.

REFERENCES

1. Reiber GE.   Who is at risk of limb loss and what to do about it? *J Rehabil Res Dev* 1994; **31**: 357–62.
2. Boulton AJM, Gries FA, Jervell JA.   Guidelines for the diagnosis and out-patient management of diabetic peripheral neuropathy. *Diabet Med* 1998; **15**: 508–14.
3. Larsen K, Holstein P, Deckert T.   Limb salvage in diabetics with foot ulcers. *Prosthet Orthot Int* 1989; **13**: 100–3.
4. National Institute of Diabetes and Digestive and Kidney Diseases and US Department of Health and Human Services.   *Feet Can Last a Lifetime. A Health Care Provider's Guide to Preventing Diabetes Foot Problems*. Bethesda, MD, 1997.
5. Stokes IA, Faris IB, Hutton WC.   The neuropathic ulcer and loads on the foot in diabetic patients. *Acta Orthop Scand* 1975; **46**: 839–47.
6. Schaff PS, Siebert WE.   Ulcusprophylaxe am diabetischen Fuss. *Orthopädie-Schuhtechnik* 1988; **June**: 16–23.
7. Sarnow MR, Veves A, Giurini JM, Rosenblum BI, Chrzan JS, Habershaw GM.   In-shoe foot pressure measurements in diabetic patients with at-risk feet and in healthy subjects. *Diabet Care* 1994; **17**: 1002–6.

8. Chantelau E, Haage P: An audit of cushioned diabetic footwear: relation to patient compliance. *Diabet Med* 1994; **11**: 114–16.
9. Nyska M, McCabe C, Linge K, Laing P, Klenerman L. Effect of the shoe on plantar foot pressures. *Acta Orthop Scand* 1995; **66**: 53–6.
10. Perry JE, Ulbrecht JS, Derr JA, Cavanagh PR. The use of running shoes to reduce plantar pressures in patients who have diabetes. *J Bone Joint Surg* 1995; **77**A: 1819–28.
11. Lavery LA, Vela SA, Lavery DC, Quebedeaux TL. Reducing dynamic foot pressures in high risk diabetic subjects with foot ulcerations. *Diabet Care* 1996; **19**: 818–21.
12. Lavery LA, Vela SA, Fleischli JG, Armstrong DG, Lavery DC. Reducing plantar pressure in the neuropathic foot. *Diabet Care* 1997; **20**: 1706–10.
13. Lemmon D, Shiang TY, Hashmi A, Ulbrecht JS, Cavanagh PR. The effect of insoles in therapeutic footwear—a finite element approach. *J. Biomechanics* 1997; **30**: 615–20.
14. Uccioli L, Toffolo M, Volpe A, et al. Efficacy of different shoes and insoles in reducing plantar pressures in diabetic neuropathic patients [abstract]. *Diabetologia* 1997; **40** Suppl. 1: A 489.
15. Kästenbauer T, Sokol G, Auinger M, Irsigler K. Running shoes for relief of plantar pressure in diabetic patients. *Diabet Med* 1998; **15**: 518–22.
16. Mueller MJ, Strube MJ, Allen BT. Therapeutic footwear can reduce plantar pressures in patients with diabetes and transmetatarsal amputation. *Diabet Care* 1997; **20**: 637–41.
17. Cavanagh PR, Ulbrecht JS, Zanine W, Welling RL, Leschinsky D, van Schie C. A method for the investigation of the effects of outsole modifications in therapeutic footwear. *Foot Ankle Int* 1996; **17**: 706–8.
18. Patil KM, Babu TS, Oommen PK, Srinivasan H. Foot pressure measurement in leprosy and footwear designs. *Ind J Leprosy* 1986; **58**: 357–66.
19. Brodsky JW, Kourosh S, Stills M, Mooney V. Objective evaluation of insert material for diabetic and athletic footwear. *Foot Ankle Int* 1988; **6**: 26–33.
20. Tovey FI. The manufacture of diabetic footwear. *Diabet Med* 1984; **1**: 69–71.
21. Brand PW. The diabetic foot. In Ellenberg M, Rifkin H (eds), *Diabetes Mellitus. Theory and Practice*. 3rd edn. New Hyde Park, NY: Medical Examination Publishing Co, 1983: 829–49.
22. Uccioli L, Faglia E, Monticone G, Favales F, Durola L, Aldeghi A, Quarantiello A, Calia P, Menzinger G. Manufactured shoes in the prevention of diabetic foot ulcers. *Diabet Care* 1995; **18**: 1376–8.
23. Baumann R. Industriell gefertigte Spezialschuhe für den diabetischen Fuss. *Diab Stoffw* 1996; **5**: 107–12.
24. Striesow F. Konfektionierte Spezialschuhe zur Ulkusrezidivprophylaxe beim diabetischen Fusssyndrom. *Med Klin* 1998; **93**: 695–700.
25. Reiber GE, Smith DG, Boone DA, et al. Design and testing of the DVA/Seattle footwear system for diabetic patients with foot insensitivity. *J Rehabil Res Dev* 1997; **34**: 1–8.
26. Sims DS, Cavanagh PR, Ulbrecht JS. Risk factors in the diabetic foot: recognition and management. *Phys Ther* 1988; **68**: 1887–902.
27. Schröer O. A toe-box in the shoe increases interdigital pressure—a risk for the diabetic foot. *Med Orthop Technik* 1999; **19**: 58–61.
28. Samata A, Burden AC, Sharma A, Jones GR. A comparison between "LSB" shoes and "space" shoes in diabetic foot ulceration. *Pract Diabet Int* 1989; **6**: 26.

29. Chantelau E, Gede A. Diabetic feet are broader than normal footwear [abstract]. *Diabetologia* 1999; **42**(suppl 1): A311.
30. Ulbrecht JS, Perry J, Hewitt FG, Cavanagh PR. Controversies in footwear for the diabetic foot at risk. In Kominsky SJ (ed.), *Medical and Surgical Management of the Diabetic Foot*. St. Louis, MO: Mosby–Year Book, 1994; 441–53.
31. Fleischli JG, Vela SA, Lavery LA, Lavery DC. Postural instability in devices to facilitate healing in diabetic foot ulceration [astract]. *Diabetes* 1997; **46**(suppl.1): 148A.
32. Sugarman JR, Reiber GE, Baumgardner G, Prela CM, Lowery J. Use of the therapeutic footwear benefits among diabetic Medicare beneficiaries in three states, 1995. *Diabet Care* 1998: **21**: 777–81.

12

The Rational Use of Antimicrobial Agents in Diabetic Foot Infection

GREGORY M. CAPUTO

The Milton S. Hershey Medical Center, Hershey, PA, USA

GENERAL CONSIDERATIONS

Foot infections are the most common cause of admission to hospital in patients with diabetes, and infection is a precursor to amputation in many cases[1–5]. Antibiotics are, of course, important tools in the management of infection, but their inappropriate use has important and far-reaching consequences. First, there are worrisome epidemiological trends in the patterns of resistance to antimicrobial agents among pathogenic bacteria. Gram-positive cocci, such as *Staphylococcus aureus* and the enteroccus, have developed resistance to several commonly employed agents. Gram-negative bacilli have likewise become increasingly resistant to standard drugs. Misuse of antibiotics is believed to have contributed significantly to increased antimicrobial resistance. Second, potentially serious side reactions, such as colitis due to *Clostridium difficile*, take a costly human toll. Anaphylaxis, renal and haematological toxicity are other serious complications that are minimized by the judicious use of antibiotics. Third, a mistaken focus on antibiotics as the only required measure in the management of diabetic foot infection may diminish the perceived importance of other critical factors, such as surgical debridement, drainage and pressure relief. Last, the inappropriate use of antibiotics leads to unnecessary financial costs. The newer broad-spectrum regimens are all more expensive than older, more narrow-spectrum agents, and the latter

The Foot in Diabetes, 3rd edn. Edited by A. J. M. Boulton, H. Connor and P. R. Cavanagh.
© 2000 John Wiley & Sons, Ltd.

are more appropriate in some circumstances, such as non-limb-threatening cellulitis. All of these factors support the commonly-heard plea to be more rational in the prescription of antibiotic agents. This chapter examines the evidence that is available to help clinicians achieve this goal.

There are several general questions that should be answered in the rational approach to antibiotic selection. First is the question of whether or not infection is present. There remains some controversy over whether all colonized foot ulcers are infected, but most authors have suggested that the absence of inflammatory findings implies the absence of infection[6-8]. Second, the severity of infection should be carefully assessed by careful bedside inspection and palpation. Gently exploring the wound with a surgical probe and debridement of necrotic tissue should be part of the comprehensive initial examination. Third, an assessment of the likely microbiological aetiology of infection is critical in choosing appropriate empiric agents. This depends on the severity and extent of infection and whether recent treatment with antibiotics may have altered the local flora. Fourth, an analysis of host factors that may impact on toxicity should be undertaken. For example, neurotoxicity is more likely with imipenem if the patient has known neurological disease. Prior drug allergy should be carefully explored. Pre-existing renal disease may make nephrotoxicity more likely with aminoglycosides, which should generally be avoided in the diabetic patient. Last, the antimicrobial spectrum, pharmacodynamic properties, and cost of specific agents are major factors that help the clinician select a regimen tailored to the specific needs of the individual patient.

THE UNCOMPLICATED NEUROPATHIC ULCER

Like most wounds, virtually all foot ulcers are colonized with a variety of bacterial flora. The open lesion is an ideal micro-environment for the growth of bacteria, and swabs of uninflamed lesions commonly produce growth of staphylococci, streptococci and Gram-negative bacilli. This poses a dilemma for the clinician, since a common response to a positive culture result is to treat with antibiotics. The knowledge that diabetic foot infections can be limb and even life-threatening heightens the clinician's inclination towards antibiotic treatment. However, there is no clearly convincing evidence that the micro-organisms recovered from cultures of uninflamed diabetic foot ulcers require treatment with antibiotics. In fact, there is some evidence that attention to careful wound management without antibiotics can lead to healing of neuropathic ulcers. Chantelau and colleagues' study[9], for example, which included patients with and without cellulitis, demonstrated that patients with neuropathic ulcers healed at similar rates whether or not they received antibiotics.

The diagnosis of an infected ulcer is thus not made in the microbiology laboratory but at the bedside, supported by the presence of inflammatory signs and/or drainage. This can only be accomplished with a meticulous bedside examination of the wound in full lighting and with close inspection for subtle signs of erythema, induration or drainage. In the absence of such findings, however, an ulcer can be classified as uninfected or uncomplicated.

The management of the uncomplicated ulcer demands careful debridement of all devitalized tissue (repeatedly if necessary), the application of appropriate dressings, and pressure relief at the ulcer site. A fully enclosed total contact cast is frequently used to manage uncomplicated ulcers. A plain film is performed routinely at the time the ulcer is first documented in order to assess bony integrity and to detect radio-opaque foreign bodies.

As noted, the use of antibiotics to treat uninflamed ulcers remains somewhat controversial, but the approach at our centre is to withhold antibiotics unless inflammation is noted. Avoiding the routine culture of clearly uninflamed ulcers will help to avoid inappropriate use of antibiotics, with the attendant risks enumerated above. Close follow-up is required, however, since these ulcers may subsequently become infected, and occult osteomyelitis may be present even if the initial plain radiograph is normal[10]. A repeat radiograph 2–3 weeks after the first film is recommended. If there is any doubt about underlying osteomyelitis on plain radiograph, a radio-labelled leukocyte scan can be performed.

In summary, ulcers without apparent inflammation should be managed with careful wound care and pressure relief; there is no clear evidence that cultures or antibiotics are required.

MILD CELLULITIS

Soft tissue infection may be categorized as either limb-threatening or non-limb-threatening (mild) cellulitis. Non-limb-threatening infection is defined as having less than 2 cm of cellulitis, a non-full thickness ulcer, no evidence of ischaemia or deep-seated infection, and a patient with good metabolic control, adequate home support and a high likelihood of adherence to medical advice and close follow-up[3]. Non-limb-threatening infection is usually caused by Gram-positive cocci—typically *S. aureus* and/or *Streptococcus* spp.[3,11,12]. Antibiotic-resistant strains of these micro-organisms (e.g. methicillin-resistant *Staphylococcus aureus*; MRSA) may be recovered, but most often the antibiotic-susceptible strains are implicated in mild cellulitis[11]. In hospitalized patients with diabetic foot cellulitis, however, MRSA and enterococci are becoming more prevalent[13].

Because the microbiological aetiology of non-limb-threatening cellulitis is reasonably predictable, it is not clear whether cultures are important to the patient's management in every case. If a culture is taken, the most reliable

Table 12.1   Recommended empiric antibiotics for non-limb-threatening
diabetic foot cellulitis. Use any one of these as a single agent

- First-generation cephalosporin (e.g. cephalexin)
- Clindamycin
- Dicloxacillin
- Amoxicillin–clavulanate

specimens are obtained by curettage (with a curette or scalpel) of the base of
the ulcer after preparing with antiseptic solution. Needle aspiration is a
technique that produces reliable microbiological information but should be
reserved for the patient with a fluctuant area. A superficial swab of the
lesion is considered unreliable in detecting the pathogen because of the
presence of colonizing flora, although culture (by swab) of frankly purulent
drainage may be helpful.

Recommended empiric oral antibiotics for mild cellulitis include a first-
generation cephalosporin, such as cephalexin or cefadroxil (Table 12.1).
Later-generation cephalosporins (e.g. cefuroxime or cefixime) are not
indicated—their spectrum of activity is not appropriate and they are
unduly expensive. Oral clindamycin is a useful alternative in patients that
cannot tolerate β-lactam agents[11]. Dicloxacillin has suitable antimicrobial
coverage. Amoxicillin/clavulanate is an oral agent that includes coverage
for all of the most commonly recovered micro-organisms and is a
reasonable agent for non-limb threatening cellulitis. Amoxicillin alone,
however, is not recommended, since its spectrum is too limited, having no
anti-staphylococcal activity.

In general, the use of a fluoroquinolone as a single agent is not
recommended, particularly since ciprofloxacin has suboptimal Gram-
positive activity. However, there are several studies that do confirm the
efficacy of fluoroquinolones in diabetic foot infections[14–16]. The activity of
levofloxacin against Gram-positive micro-organisms is significantly better
than ciprofloxacin, but it has not been studied specifically in diabetic foot
infections. The newer fluoroquinolone agent, trovafloxacin, may ultimately
prove useful as an alternative for patients who cannot tolerate β-lactam
agents or clindamycin, since its Gram-positive activity is excellent, but
published studies are currently lacking. The recommended duration of
therapy for non-limb-threatening infection is 7–14 days.

With careful follow-up, most patients with mild cellulitis can be treated
as outpatients. In addition to appropriate antibiotics, debridement of
devitalized tissue, pressure relief at the ulcer site, and assurance of
adequate arterial flow are measures that are critical for healing. Patients
must be seen frequently and follow-up plain radiographs to detect
osteomyelitis are recommended, as noted above for patients with
uncomplicated ulcers.

LIMB-THREATENING SOFT-TISSUE INFECTION

This is a dreaded lower extremity complication of diabetes with a high risk of associated amputation[1-5]. Those soft tissue infections not meeting the criteria listed above are classified as limb-threatening[3]. Extensive cellulitis may be found in association with necrotizing fasciitis, localized abscess, septicaemia and/or underlying osteomyelitis. The finding of crepitance suggests soft tissue gas and necrosis; fluctuance indicates undrained suppuration. The extent of the infection may not be readily apparent until the wound is carefully explored. Indeed, surgical exploration frequently detects extensive soft tissue and/or bone involvement in the face of rather subtle superficial findings. Fever may not be present, even in life-threatening sepsis; its presence is often associated with deep tissue collections or distant, metastatic infection.

Most cases of limb-threatening infection have a polymicrobial aetiology. Gram-positive cocci (e.g. *S. aureus* and streptococci), strict anaerobes (e.g. *Bacteroides fragilis*) and facultative Gram-negative bacilli (e.g. *Escherichia coli*) are usually isolated in mixed cultures[3,12]. Deep tissue and/or bone cultures should be taken at the time of surgical exploration and debridement. Specimens should be submitted for both aerobic and anaerobic culture.

The patient with limb-threatening infection should be hospitalized immediately. A multidisciplinary approach to management is recommended. Surgical consultation is integral to the management of the patient with limb-threatening cellulitis. Consultation with diabetologists or infectious disease specialists should be considered as needed. If there is any doubt about the adequacy of arterial flow, a vascular surgeon should be consulted. A plain radiograph is performed to detect soft tissue gas, foreign bodies and bony abnormalities. Soft tissue gas indicates necrotizing infection that requires immediate exploration and drainage. A deep specimen for culture should be taken at the time of the initial debridement and drainage.

The role of the surgeon in the management of limb-threatening infections cannot be overemphasized. The focus in the care of such patients is often directed towards the correct antibiotic regimen, and the proper choice of antibiotic is clearly important. However, antibiotics are usually insufficient for complete cure; devitalized and necrotic tissue is frequently present in cases of limb-threatening infection and debridement is thus required. The wound must be explored and sites of loculated purulence must be drained. There is evidence that aggressive treatment of limb-threatening infection, using a combined medical–surgical approach using early debridement and drainage, can limit the need for above-ankle amputation[2]. Lastly, the adequacy of the arterial circulation is of prime importance in the successful management of such infections, and an experienced vascular surgeon should be consulted immediately if there is any doubt about ischaemia in a patient with limb-threatening infection.

There are several reasonable empiric intravenous antibiotic regimens for limb-threatening infection[17,14,22]. However, there are surprisingly few prospective, randomized trials of different antibiotic regimens in this common infection[11,14,18,19]. In a recent study by Lipsky et al[14], two broad-spectrum parenteral-to-oral regimens were found comparable in efficacy and cost. One-hundred and-eight patients hospitalized with diabetic foot infection were randomized to either intravenous ofloxacin followed by oral ofloxacin, or ampicillin–sulbactam followed by amoxicillin–clavulanate. Rates of adverse affects were likewise similar in the two groups. In a study by Grayson et al[18], ampicillin–sulbactam was found to be as effective as imipenem–cilistatin for the initial empiric and subsequent definitive treatment of limb-threatening infection. Improvement at 5 days occurred in 94% and 98% in the ampicillin–sulbactam and imipenem–cilistatin groups, respectively, and cure rates were also similar (81% and 85%, respectively). The authors found that, even if the infecting micro-organisms were resistant to the empiric regimen, a comprehensive approach that included modification of the regimen, wound care, and appropriate debridement of devitalized tissue allowed for cure in 10/16 cases of infection with resistant organisms. Patients with life-threatening infection were excluded from their study. This study was particularly important, since it showed that the broadest-spectrum agent is not necessary for empiric therapy of limb-threatening infection as long as careful modification of the regimen is undertaken if needed.

The recommended regimens for limb-threatening infection are listed in Table 12.2. If the patient does not respond promptly, the regimen should be expanded to cover pathogens for which the empiric regimen is not active. However, expansion of the spectrum is not recommended if the patient is improving on the initial empiric regimen, since the isolates recovered may include colonizing flora as well as pathogens. This will prevent unnecessarily broad coverage and decrease the selective pressure towards

Table 12.2 Selected empiric intravenous antibiotic regimens for limb-threatening diabetic foot infections. The regimen should be modified depending upon the patient's clinical progress and the results of cultures. The potential for particularly resistant pathogens (e.g. methicillin-resistant *Staphylococcus aureus*) should be considered, based on patient history and local epidemiological factors

- β-lactam–β-lactamase inhibitor, used as a single agent (e.g. ampicillin–sulbactam, ticarcillin–clavulanate, or piperacillin–tazobactam)
- Clindamycin plus a fluoroquinolone (e.g. ciprofloxacin)
- Clindamycin plus a late-generation cephalosporin (e.g. ceftazadime)
- For life-threatening infection, consider vancomycin plus imipenem–cilistatin

the development of resistant strains. Likewise, if the patient is improving, the regimen can be modified to a narrower spectrum if indicated by the culture results.

OSTEOMYELITIS

The diagnosis and management of pedal osteomyelitis is perhaps the most controversial topic related to diabetic foot infection[10,20]. There are a wide variety of diagnostic tests available for diagnosis, and each has strengths and disadvantages[21,22]. For example, plain radiographs are insensitive early in the course of osteomyelitis; nuclear scans lack optimum specificity; and magnetic resonance imaging is expensive and its role is not fully defined in diagnosis and management. In our programme we use a combination of the bedside "probe-to-bone" test and serial plain radiographs in the initial evaluation of patients with possible osteomyelitis. The "probe-to-bone" test has been shown to have a high positive predictive value for osteomyelitis[22]. Indium-labelled leukocyte scans, or rarely, magnetic resonance imaging are reserved for patients in whom the diagnosis remains in significant doubt.

The combination of surgical removal of all infected bone coupled with prolonged intravenous antibiotics has long been the standard approach to the management of pedal osteomyelitis in the diabetic patient. However, there are no prospective, randomized trials to define the optimal approach. Several papers have challenged the conventional wisdom that surgical removal of infected bone and prolonged intravenous antibiotics are required for cure, but selection of appropriate patients for medical treatment only has not been carefully established[16,23,24]. One recent study that used decision analysis techniques came to the conclusion that non-invasive testing added little (except expense) to the management of possible pedal osteomyelitis in diabetic patients[25]. Based on their analysis, Eckman et al[25] recommended a 10 week course of antibiotics following surgical debridement for patients without systemic toxicity. Eckman's study did not consider the use of "probe-to-bone testing", however. In our programme, we perform an initial plain film and "probe-to-bone" test. If either is positive and the patient is clinically stable without necrotizing infection or other reasons for hospitalization, we usually recommend a 4–6 week course of oral or intravenous antibiotics based on a deep culture specimen. We are particularly likely to recommend this approach if bony destruction is limited or absent on plain radiograph. If there is progressive bony destruction or clinical deterioration, surgical removal of infected bone is then considered. Obviously, the recommendation must be individualized for each patient.

SUMMARY

The appropriate use of antimicrobial agents is a critical factor in treating foot infection in the diabetic patient. Antibiotic misuse has the potential to lead to clinical failure, widespread antimicrobial resistance, unnecessary complications, and increasing costs. Antibiotics should be reserved for obviously inflamed ulcers. For mild infection, a limited-spectrum oral agent is the most appropriate choice. In limb-threatening cases, a broad-spectrum regimen should be used empirically and then modified, based on the patient's clinical course and the results of appropriately taken cultures. The management of osteomyelitis remains controversial, but selected patients may be cured with prolonged antibiotic regimens without surgery.

REFERENCES

1. Criado E, DeStefano AA, Keagy BA, Upchurch GR, Johnson G. The course of severe foot infection in patients with diabetes. *Surg Gynecol Obstet* 1992; **175**: 135.
2. Tan JS, Firedman NM, Hazelton-Miller C, Flanagan JP, File TM. Can aggressive treatment of diabetic foot infections reduce the need for above-ankle amputations? *Clin Infect Dis* 1996; **23**: 286–91.
3. Gibbons GW, Eliopoulos GM. Infection of the diabetic foot. In Kozak GP, Hoar CS Jr, Rowbotham RL, et al (eds), *Management of Diabetic Foot Problems*. Philadelphia: W.B. Saunders, 1984; 97–102.
4. Mills JL, Beckett WC, Taylor SM. The diabetic foot: consequences of delayed treatment and referral. *South Med J* 1991; **84**: 974.
5. Eneroth M, Apelqvist J, Stenstrom A. Clinical characteristics and outcome in 223 diabetic patients with deep foot infections. *Foot Ankle Int* 1997; **18**: 716–22.
6. Lipsky BA, Pecoraro RE, Wheat LJ. The diabetic foot: soft tissue and bone infection. *Infect Dis Clin N Am* 1990; **3**: 409.
7. Caputo GM, Cavanagh PR, Ulbrecht JS, Gibbons GW, Karchmer AW. Assessment and management of foot disease in patients with diabetes. *N Engl J Med* 1994; **331**: 854–60.
8. Van der Meer JWM, Koopman PP, Lutterman JA. Antibiotic therapy in diabetic foot infection. *Diabet Medicine* 1996: **13**: S48–51.
9. Chantelau E, Tanudjaja T, Altenhofer F, Ersanli Z, Lacigova S, Metzger C. Antibiotic treatment for uncomplicated forefoot ulcers in diabetes: a controlled trial. *Diabet Med* 1996; **13**: 156–9.
10. Newman LG, Waller J, Palestro CJ et al. Unsuspected osteomyelitis in diabetic foot ulcers: diagnosing and monitoring by leukocyte scanning with indium, In 111 oxyquinolone. *J Am Med Assoc* 1991; **266**: 1246–51.
11. Lipsky BA, Pecoraro RE, Larson SA, Hanley ME, Ahroni JH. Outpatient management of uncomplicated lower-extremity infections in diabetic patients. *Arch Intern Med* 1990; **150**: 790–7.
12. Wheat LJ, Allen SD, Henry M et al. Diabetic foot infections: bacteriologic analysis. *Arch Intern Med* 1986; **146**: 1935–40.
13. Goldstein EJC, Citron DM, Nesbit CA. Diabetic foot infections: bacteriology and activity of 10 oral antimicrobial agents against bacteria isolated from consecutive cases. *Diabet Care* 1996; **19**: 638–41.

14. Lipsky BA, Baker PD, Landon GC, Fernau R. Antibiotic therapy for diabetic foot infections: a comparison of two parenteral-to-oral regimens. *Clin Infect Dis* 1997; **24**: 643–8.
15. Gentry LO. Review of quinolones in treatment of infections of the skin and skin structure. *J.Antimicrob Chemother* 1991; **28**(suppl C): 97–110.
16. Peterson LR, Lissack LM, Canter MLT, Fasching CE, Clabots C, Gerding DN. Therapy of lower extremity infections with ciprofloxacin in patients with diabetes, peripheral vascular disease, or both. *Am J Med* 1989; **86**: 801–8.
17. Karchmer AW, Gibbons GW. Foot infections in diabetes: evaluation and management. *Curr Clin Top Infect Dis* 1994; **14**: 1–22.
18. Grayson ML, Gibbons GW, Habershaw GM et al. Use of ampicillin/sulbactam versus imipenem/cilistatin in the treatment of limb-threatening foot infections in diabetic patients. *Clin Infect Dis* 1994; **18**: 683–93.
19. Hughes CE, Johnson CC, Bamberger DM et al. Treatment and long term follow-up of foot infections in patients with diabetes or ischemia: a randomized, prospective, double-blind comparison of cefoxitin and ceftizoxime. *Clin Ther* 1987; **10**(suppl A0): 36–49.
20. Lipsky BA. Osteomyelitis of the foot in diabetic patients. *Clin Infect Dis* 1997; **25**: 1318–36.
21. Longmaid HE, Kruskal JB. Imaging infections in diabetic patients. *Infect Dis Clin N Am* 1995; **9**: 163–82.
22. Grayson ML, Balogh K, Levin E et al. Probing to bone in infected pedal ulcers: a clinical sign in underlying osteomyelitis in diabetic patients. *J Am Med Assoc.* 1995; **273**: 721.
23. Venkatesan P, Lawn S, Macfarlane RM, Fletcher EM, Finch RG, Jeffcoate WJ. Conservative management of osteomyelitis in the feet of diabetic patients. *Diabet Med* 1996; **14**: 487–90.
24. Bamberger DM, Daus GP, Gerding DN. Osteomyelitis in the feet of diabetic patients. *Am J Med* 1987; **83**: 653–60.
25. Eckman MH, Greenfield S, Mackey WC, Wong JB, Kaplan S, Sullivan L, Dukjes K, Paulker SG. Foot infection in diabetic patients: decision and cost-effectiveness analysis. *J Am Med Assoc* 1995; **273**: 712–20.

13

Use of Dressings: Is there an Evidence Base?

NICKY CULLUM, MARIAM MAJID, SUSAN O'MEARA
and TREVOR SHELDON
University of York, York, UK

The promotion of a local wound environment conducive to healing through the judicious use of wound dressings is seen as an essential component of diabetic foot ulcer treatment. There is uncertainty as to the best means of achieving this, leading to keen debate. A variety of wound dressings is used on diabetic foot ulcers, although none is marketed specifically for this indication. However, what is the research evidence?

When setting out to summarize the evidence for or against any health care intervention, it is essential to review all the original research that is relevant to the question and appropriate in research design[1]. Pioneering work by health researchers in the 1980s and 1990s has shown us the dangers of not using systematic, rigorous methods to summarize the research evidence on the effectiveness of a health care intervention. In 1992 Antman and colleagues[2] showed that over the years, "experts"—authors of textbooks and review articles on the treatment of myocardial infarction—had consistently failed to recommend effective treatments that had been shown in trials to save lives. The same "experts" had continued to recommend harmful treatments long after the evidence had accumulated against them. Thus, unless we go out of our way to minimize biases and mistakes when undertaking overviews of research, we run a great risk of peddling misinformation. Rigorous overviews of this nature have been termed "systematic reviews" to distinguish them from the more

The Foot in Diabetes, 3rd edn. Edited by A. J. M. Boulton, H. Connor and P. R. Cavanagh.
© 2000 John Wiley & Sons, Ltd.

commonplace, haphazard reviews, which were often biased in that they reflected only the studies with which the reviewer agreed, or was aware of[3].

Systematic reviews generally follow the following process[4]:

- Formulation of the problem—in this case: *which wound dressings are the most effective for healing diabetic foot ulcers?*
- Location and selection of studies.
- Critical appraisal of studies.
- Collection of data from the original studies.
- Analysis and presentation of results.
- Interpretation of results.
- Ongoing improvement and updating.

This chapter reports the findings of a systematic review undertaken to summarize the available evidence on wound dressings for diabetic foot ulcers. This review is one of a series of systematic reviews on interventions for chronic wounds conducted by a larger team, including the authors, and funded by the UK NHS Health Technology Assessment Programme.

REVIEW QUESTION

How effective are different wound dressings in promoting the healing of diabetic foot ulcers?

REVIEW METHODS

Location and Selection of Studies

In order to minimize bias, systematic reviewers make *a priori* decisions about the types of study eligible for inclusion in a review. The study eligibility criteria for this review are summarized in Table 13.1. Evaluations were included if they were randomized controlled trials (RCTs)[†] or, in the absence of RCTs, controlled clinical trials with a contemporaneous control, which evaluated the effectiveness of wound dressings for diabetic foot ulcers. RCTs provide the most reliable evidence as to the effectiveness of health care interventions, and non-randomized trials often misjudge treatment effects[5,6]. Trials were eligible irrespective of whether they had been published, as publication is associated with a bias towards studies

---

[†]A randomized trial is one where the allocation of patients to one of two or more alternative treatments (e.g. experimental treatment and control) is by some random method, such as a computer-generated random sequence of treatments. This mechanism of allocation ensures that the play of chance alone determines the treatment received, and if the study is large enough the treatment groups should be similar in all other respects.

Table 13.1   Study eligibility criteria

- Randomized controlled trials and controlled trials of dressings for healing diabetic foot ulcers
- Published or unpublished
- Written in any language
- Measured foot ulcer healing by some objective and valid measure, such as proportion of total ulcers healed; rate of reduction in original wound area; time to ulcer healing

Table 13.2   Databases searched

Cochrane Controlled Trials Register/CENTRAL
MEDLINE
EMBASE
CINAHL
ISI Science Citation Index (on BIDS)
BIOSIS (on Silver Platter)
British Diabetic Association Database
CISCOM (Complementary Medicine Database of the RCCM)
Conference Proceedings (on BIDS)
Database of Abstracts of Reviews of Effectiveness (DARE)
Dissertation Abstracts
Royal College of Nursing Database (CD-ROM)
CRIB (Current Research in Britain)
DHSS-Data
SIGLE
Healthstar (1992-Dec 1996)
UK National Research Register
Amed

which identify a statistically significant finding; thus, a review which includes only published studies may only cover a biased subset of the total research[7]. Trials which included patients with wounds of various aetiologies, including a subgroup of patients with diabetic foot ulcers, were included if results were presented for the diabetic foot ulcer patients separately.

Eighteen electronic databases were searched for RCTs (see Table 13.2) and the reference lists of all primary papers and review articles identified were examined for additional studies. The proceedings of 12 conferences were hand-searched and, where relevant studies were identified in abstract form, the authors were contacted to obtain full study details. A number of wound dressing manufacturers were contacted and asked to provide details of relevant studies. Finally, five specialist wound care journals were systematically hand-searched until the end of 1997.

The series of systematic reviews which we have conducted of interventions in chronic wound care has benefited from the ongoing support of an advisory panel of specialists in various aspects of wound care, including diabetic foot ulcers. The panel helped to identify relevant research and to ensure that the review reflected the current issues.

The decision on whether any study should be included or excluded from the review was made independently by two reviewers (MM and SOM), and disagreements were resolved by discussion.

Critical Appraisal of Studies

After a decision to include a study had been made, each study included in this review was individually peer-reviewed as part of the review process. The methodological quality of each study was assessed by the two reviewers independently and any disagreement on quality resolved by discussion (see Table 13.3 for results of Methodological Quality Assessment).

Collection of Data from the Original Studies

Relevant details were extracted from each original study by the primary reviewer (MM) onto a standardized, pre-prepared data extraction form for the following variables:

- Inclusion/exclusion criteria applied in the study.
- Study setting.
- Description of the main interventions and comparison/control interventions evaluated in the study; description of any co-interventions; numbers of patients in each group; duration of treatment; duration of follow-up.
- Summary of the baseline characteristics of the patients in each group for important variables, e.g. age, gender, size of ulcers, stage of ulcers, duration of diabetes, type of diabetes, type of foot ulcer (ischaemic, neuropathic, mixed).
- Summary of results for important outcomes, e.g. ulcers healed, time to healing, percentage of patients followed up, reasons for withdrawal.

Analysis of Results

The results are largely presented as a narrative review. There was little opportunity for meta-analysis (pooling of individual, similar trials to derive an overall estimate of effect), as most studies identified were unique or unreplicated comparisons of interventions. Pooling was undertaken where appropriate and where studies were not heterogeneous, using the Peto fixed effects model[8], and summary results presented as an overall odds ratio* with 95% confidence intervals.

---

*The odds ratio (OR) refers to the odds of patients in the experimental group experiencing the outcome—in this review usually ulcer healing—divided by the odds of patients in the control group experiencing the same outcome. An OR > 1 for an outcome of ulcer healing in a trial of two ulcer dressings indicates that more ulcers healed in the experimental dressing group than the control group. An OR < 1 indicates that the experimental dressing is less effective than the comparison dressing.

Table 13.3 Quality of studies included

Reference	Sample size (no. of arms)	Concealment of allocation?	A priori sample size calculation described?	Baseline comparability of groups described?	Inclusion/ exclusion criteria described?	Adequate follow-up period?	Withdrawals and patients lost to follow-up reported?	Intention-to-treat analysis?
9	19 (2)	Yes	No	Yes	Yes	No	Yes	Yes
10	30 (2)	No	No	Yes	Yes	No	Yes	No
11	29 (2)	No	No	Yes	Yes	No	Yes	No
12	18 (2)	Unclear	No	Yes	No	No	Yes	No
13	40 (2)	No	Yes	Yes	No	Yes	Numbers but no reasons	No
14	75 (2) unequal randomization	No	No	Yes	Yes	No	Yes	Yes
15	40 (2)	No	No	Yes	No	No	No	No
16	(i) 82 (2) (ii) 99 (2)	No	No	No	Yes	No	No	No
17	100 (2)	No	Yes	For some variables but not ulcer area	Yes	No	No	No
18	41 (2)	Yes	No	Described as "similar" but data not presented	Yes	No	Yes	No
19	44 (2)	No	No	Yes	Yes	No	Yes	No

Statistical heterogeneity was assessed by χ^2 test and, where this was significant, pooling was not undertaken[4].

RESULTS OF THE REVIEW

Eleven studies met the inclusion criteria for the review and two of these were unpublished; nine studies evaluated wound dressings and two evaluated debriding agents. Two studies compared alginate dressings with a hydrocellular dressing[9,10]; the remainder were unique comparisons: hydrogel vs dry gauze plus antiseptics[11]; polymeric membrane dressing vs wet–dry saline gauze[12]; polyurethane gel dressing vs hydrocellular dressing[13]; collagen–alginate dressing vs saline-soaked gauze[14]; dimethyl-sulphoxide (DMSO) vs standard treatment[15]; glycyl–histidine–lysine–copper complex vs vehicle[16]; topical phenytoin vs dry occlusive dressing[17]; cadexomer iodine dressing vs standard treatment[18]; zinc oxide tape vs hydrocolloid[19].

Alginate Dressings vs a Hydrocellular Dressing

Two RCTs compared different alginate dressings with the hydrocellular dressing Allevyn[9,10]. In a small unpublished study, Baker[9] compared the calcium–alginate dressing (Sorbsan) with Allevyn in 19 patients with neuropathic foot ulcers; whilst Foster et al[10] compared calcium–sodium alginate (Kaltostat) with Allevyn in 30 patients. The two studies were sufficiently similar to pool them statistically (Figure 13.1). Overall there was no significant difference in healing between ulcers treated with the alginate dressing and those treated with the hydrocellular dressing (pooled OR 0.41;

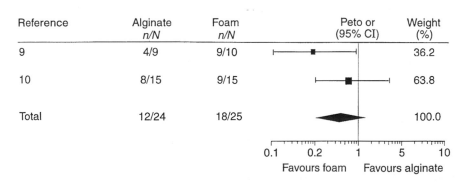

Figure 13.1   Two randomized controlled trials comparing alginate dressings with foam dressings for the treatment of diabetic foot ulcers. Pooled using a fixed effects model. Outcome: ulcers completely healed (different follow-up periods)

95% CI 0.13–1.28). However, both studies together involved only 49 patients, and so this test lacks sufficient power to detect clinically important differences as statistically significant.

DMSO vs Standard Treatment

Studies in animal models have suggested that dimethylsulphoxide (DMSO) aids healing by increasing tissue oxygen saturation and local vasodilation, decreased thrombocyte aggregation and increased oxygen diffusion to the tissue[20,21]. In a single study, DMSO (500 ml 25% solution of DMSO in normal saline) applied topically plus standard treatment (debridement, dry dressings, soft shoes and treatment of cellulitis with antibiotics) was compared with standard treatment alone in 40 hospitalized diabetic patients with chronic neuropathic foot ulceration[15]. The patients were treated for 20 weeks, and in that time 14/20 (70%) of the ulcers in the DMSO group completely healed, compared with 2/20 (10%) in the standard treatment group—a difference that is statistically significant (OR 11.44; 95% CI 3.28–39.92).

Glycyl-L-histidine-L-lysine–Copper (GHK–Cu) Gel

The peptide complex glycyl-L-histidine-L-lysine–copper (Iamin Gel) is thought to be a modulator of wound healing and has been reported to be a potent chemo-attractant for cells essential to the healing process.

Mulder and colleagues[16] reported two multicentre studies comparing Iamin Gel with vehicle gel in patients with chronic neuropathic ulcers. In the first trial, following debridement of their foot ulcers, patients in one group received 2% Iamin Gel, and those in the other group received vehicle, for 8 weeks. Significantly more plantar foot ulcers healed in patients who received Iamin Gel than in patients who received vehicle (median percentage closure of ulcers, 98.5% and 60.8%, respectively, $p<0.05$). The infection rate was also significantly lower in the Iamin Gel group (7% vs 34%). In the second trial, patients were initially treated with vehicle alone for 4 weeks, then one group had 2% Iamin Gel and the other 4% Iamin Gel for an additional 8 weeks. The mean percentage ulcer closure was 40% for the lower concentration of Iamin and 68% for the higher concentration—it is noteworthy, however, that data were only analysed for the subgroup of patients who had plantar ulcers (80% of the total).

Topical Phenytoin vs Dry Oclusive Dressing

In a single controlled clinical trial where patients were matched for key variables and not randomized, following debridement the ulcers of 50 patients with type 2 diabetes were treated with phenytoin powder "in a thin, uniform layer" covered with a dry dressing, and 50 with the dry dressing alone[17]. Patients were treated for 35 days, at which point the mean percentage reduction in baseline ulcer area in the phenytoin-treated group was $90 \pm 3.9\%$ compared with $50 \pm 4.4\%$ in the control group ($p < 0.005$). Importantly, baseline ulcer area data was not presented for this trial.

Adhesive Zinc Oxide Tape vs Hydrocolloid Dressings

Apelqvist et al[19] compared a zinc oxide tape (MeZinc) with an occlusive hydrocolloid (DuoDerm) in 44 diabetic patients with necrotic foot ulcers. Zinc oxide tape was more effective in completely eradicating or reducing by more than 50% the area of necrotic tissue (OR 4.44; 95% CI 1.34–14.70). However, reduction of necrotic tissue is a surrogate outcome measure that has never been shown to accurately predict the rate of ulcer healing (ulcer healing was not measured in this study).

DISCUSSION

No significant differences in outcome were identified in any of the other trials identified (all 11 studies are summarized in Table 13.4). However, because of the small size of the studies, this should be interpreted as insufficient evidence of effect, rather than evidence of no effect. In common with so much of research in wound care, sample sizes in these trials were extremely small (mean 56) and this has two important consequences:

- There is a very high probability of type 2 errors, i.e. failure to detect a clinically important effect of a dressing as statistically significant where it exists. Thus, we can generally conclude that "there is insufficient evidence of an effect", but rarely can we categorically state "there is no difference in effectiveness" between alternative dressings.
- There is a high probability that randomization of small numbers of patients will not succeed in evenly distributing known and unknown prognostic factors between treatment groups. Thus, the estimates of effect may be biased. This is particularly relevant for important variables such as baseline ulcer size. The direction in which an imbalance in baseline ulcer size biases the results depends on the way in which the outcome is measured. If healing is reported as percentage change in baseline ulcer area, a treatment group with smaller ulcers at baseline will have an advantage. Conversely, if healing is reported as rate of change of area in cm^2, a group with larger ulcers will appear to

Table 13.4 Study details

Reference (study type)	Sample and Setting	Intervention	Baseline Characteristics	Results
9 (UK, RCT)	19 people with clean neuropathic ulcers on weightbearing areas of the foot. Palpable foot pulses, no claudication or rest pain 10 males, 9 females Setting: outpatients	I_1, hydrocellular dressing (Allevyn) (n=10); I_2, calcium alginate dressing (Sorbsan) (n=9) Duration of treatment up to 12 weeks	Mean age (years): I_1, 58.9 SD 18.5; I_2, 54.1 SD 15.8 Mean ulcer duration (days): I_1, 19.8 SD 21.9; I_2, 26.3 SD 49.2 Mean ulcer area (cm^2): I_1, 0.89 SD 0.62; I_2, 0.82 SD 0.73 History of previous ulceration: no previous ulceration: I_1, 3; I_2, 4: 1 episode: I_1, 2; I_2, 3: 2 episodes: I_1, 2; I_2, 0: not known: I_1, 3; I_2, 2	Ulcers healed at 12 weeks: I_1, 9/10 (90%); I_2, 4/9 (44%) (OR 0.14, 95% CI 0.02, 0.89) Median time to healing (days): I_1, 28; I_2, >84 Withdrawals: I_1, 1; I_2, 2 (1 from each group due to poor compliance; 1 from I_2 as lack of exudate meant alginate contraindicated)
10 (UK, RCT)	30 patients over 18 years with clean foot ulceration 20 males, 0 females Setting: outpatient clinic	I_1, hydrocellular dressing (Allevyn) (n=15); I_2, calcium–sodium alginate dressing (Kaltostat) (n=15) Duration of treatment: up to 8 weeks	Mean age (years): I_1, 61; I_2, 70 IDDM/DDM: I_1, 6/9; I_2, 4/11 Mean area (mm^2): I_1, 88; I_2, 79 Mean duration (days): I_1, 107; I_2, 170 Aetiology (ischaemia/neuro): I_1, 6/9; I_2, 4/11 Depth (superficial/deep): I_1, 12/3; I_2, 13/2	Ulcers healed at 8 weeks: I_1, 9/15 (60%); I_2, 8/15 (53%) (OR 0.77, 95% CI 0.19, 3.18) Withdrawals: I_1, 0; I_2, 4 (1 due to pain, 3 due to blockage of drainage)
11 (Belgium, RCT)	29 diabetic patients who have had previous amputation of toe/s 13 males, 16 females Setting: unclear	I_1, ulcers cleansed with cleanser made up of saline and 0.8% acetic acid and moist hydrogel (Elastogel) (65% glycerine/ 17.5% water/17.5% polyacrylamide) dressing applied (n=15); I_2, ulcers cleansed with chlorhexidine (0.05%) and dressed with Betadine cream and dry gauze dressing twice/day (n=14) Duration of treatment: 3 months	Mean age (years): I_1, 62.6; I_2, 65.3 Neuropathy: I_1, 9/15 (60%); I_2, 9/14 (64%) Infection present before trial: I_1, 1/15 (7%); I_1, 1/14 (7%) Completely mobile: I_1, 12/15 (80%); I_2, 11/14 (79%)	Complete healing at 3 months: I_1, 7/15 (47%); I_2, 5/14 (36%); (OR 1.55, 95% CI 0.36, 6.61) Withdrawals: I_2, 2 due to death

(Continued)

Table 13.4 *(Cont.)*

Reference (study type)	Sample and Setting	Intervention	Baseline Characteristics	Results
12 (USA, RCT)	18 diabetic patients with partial- or full-thickness foot ulcers free from hard eschar 17 males, 1 female Setting: outpatients	I$_1$, polymeric membrane dressing (n=11); I$_2$, standard treatment (wet to dry saline gauze) (n=7) Duration of treatment: 6 months or until ulcer healed	Male/female: I$_1$, 11/0; I$_2$, 6/1 Mean age (years) ± SE: I$_1$, 59 ± 5; I$_2$, 51 ± 4 Mean ulcer area ± SE (cm^2): I$_1$, 2.67 ± 1.2; I$_2$, 1.81 ± 0.75 Mean ulcer duration ± SE (weeks): I$_1$, 25 ± 7; I$_2$, 28 ± 6 Mean glycated haemoglobin ± SE (%): I$_1$, 8.4 ± 0.9; I$_2$, 9.5 ± 1.1	Ulcers completely healed at 2 months: I$_1$, 3/11 (27%); I$_2$, 0/7 (OR 6.39, 95% CI 0.54, 75.62) Baseline area at 2 months (%): I$_1$, 35 ± 16%; I$_2$, 105 ± 26% (OR −70.00; 95% CI −91.46, −48.54) NB: data for 2 months only presented, as 5 patients crossed over from I$_2$ to I$_1$ Withdrawals: 2 patients in each group progressed to Wagner Stage III ulceration and were excluded from final analysis
13 (Germany, RCT)	40 diabetic outpatients with superficial neuropathic ulcers of 1–5 cm diameter; no signs of osteomyelitis 32 males, 8 females, aged 18–80 years Setting: diabetic outpatients	I$_1$, hydroactive polyurethane gel dressing (Cutinova Hydro) plus standard treatment of wound cleansing, pressure relief, wound debridement, infection control (n=20); I$_2$, hydrocellular dressing (Allevyn) plus standard treatment (n=20) Duration of treatment: 16 weeks or until healing	Male/female: I$_1$, 15/5; I$_2$, 17/3 Mean age (years) ± SD: I$_1$, 58.9 ± 11.6; I$_2$, 53.2 ± 14.6 Mean duration of ulcer ± SD (days): I$_1$, 162.37 ± 325.55; I$_2$, 165.00 ± 318.68 Mean area of ulcer (mm^2): I$_1$, 205.09; I$_2$, 207.83 Systemic antibiotics—Yes/No: I$_1$, 14/6; I$_2$, 15/5 Recurrence of ulcer—Yes/No: I$_1$, 15/5; I$_2$, 15/5	Mean time to healing ± SD (days): I$_1$, 25.19 ± 23.53; I$_2$, 20.43 ± 14.74; (OR 4.76; 95% CI −7.4, 16.93) Wound area at 4 weeks ± SD (mm^2): I$_1$, 32.32 ± 54.21; I$_2$, 33.46 ± 75.22 (OR −1.09; 95% CI −41.7, 39.5) Withdrawals: I$_1$, 2; I$_2$, 4
14 (USA, RCT)	75 diabetic patients with foot ulcers of at least 1 cm^2 diameter after initial debridement. All subjects were over 21 years with adequate nutritional intake, as indicated by serum albumin > 2.5 g/dl; all also had adequate blood flow to extremities 54 males, 21 females Setting: outpatients	I$_1$, collagen–alginate topical wound dressing (Fibracol) and limited weightbearing (n=50); I$_2$, Saline-soaked gauze and limited weightbearing (n=25) Duration of treatment: 8 weeks or until ulcer healed	Male/female (range): I$_1$, 59 (30–81); I$_2$, 60 (33–79) Mean area of ulcer ± SE (cm^2): I$_1$, 2.2 ± 0.5; I$_2$, 3.3 ± 0.8 Mean duration diabetes (years) (range): I$_1$, 19 (4–47); I$_2$, 17 (2–25) Mean ulcer duration ± SE (days): I$_1$, 153 ± 83; I$_2$, 241 ± 131 Ulcers at Wagner ulcer stage—I/II/III (%): I$_1$, 9/70/11; I$_2$, 6/88/6	Ulcers completely healed: I$_1$, 24/44 (54.4%); I$_2$, 9/17 (52.9%) (OR 1.07; 95% CI 0.35, 3.25) Mean time to complete healing ± SD (days): I$_1$, 43.4 ± 19.8; I$_2$, 40.6 ± 21.00 Mean reduction in area ± SD (%): I$_1$, 80.6 ± 0.1; I$_2$, 61.1 ± 0.3 Withdrawals: I$_1$, 6/50; I$_2$, 8/25

Table 13.4 (*Cont.*)

Study	Patients/Setting	Treatment	Baseline characteristics	Outcomes
15 (Israel, RCT)	40 diabetic (NIDDM and IDDM) patients with chronic perforating ulcers for 7–36 months, 22 males and 18 females aged 46–78 years. All had nephropathy; PVD in 20 patients; all had neuropathy. Setting: hospital 3–5 days, then treated as outpatients	I_1, local application of DMSO (500 ml 25% DMSO in saline) for 20 mins tid. Plus standard treatment (debridement, dry dressings, treatment of cellulitis with antibiotics, soft shoes). When ulcers infected, 80 mg gentamycin added to the solution. If no healing by 6th week, conc of DMSO increased to 50% ($n=20$); I_2, standard treatment ($n=20$)	Mean duration diabetes (years): I_1, 14; I_2, 15.5. Presence of PVD: I_1, 14/20 (70%); I_2, 12/20 (60%). Duration of ulcer (months): I_1, 16; I_2, 14	Complete ulcer healing: I_1, 14/20 (70%); I_2, 2/20 (10%) (OR 11.44; 95% CI 3.28, 39.93). The authors report that DMSO had analgesic properties in patients with PVD. The 50% solution caused irritation of skin and burning sensation
16 (USA, RCT)	181 diabetic outpatients with neuropathic full-thickness ulcers. Systolic toe pressure >40 mmHg, aged 21–90 years. Min ulcer area 25 mm²; max ulcer area 2700 mm². Excluded patients with osteomyelitis, gangrene, Wilson's disease, venous stasis. Patients stratified by ulcer location (plantar vs other). Plantar group divided into large ulcers (>100 mm²) and small (<100 mm²). Setting: outpatient clinics (multi-centre study)	Duration of treatment: 20 weeks. Trial 1 immediate treatment I_1, lamin gel for 8 weeks ($n=40$; 28 plantar ulcers); I_2, vehicle gel for 8 weeks ($n=42$, 32 plantar ulcers). Trial 2 treatment delayed for 4 weeks: I_1, 2% lamin gel for additional 8 weeks ($n=49$, plantar 39); I_2, 4% lamin gel for additional 8 weeks ($n=50$, plantar 42). All patients received sharp debridement before commencement of treatment and regular cleansing, daily dressing changes, metered dosing of gel, standardized pressure-relieving footwear, patient education. Infection treated with systemic antibiotics	Average age: 60 years. Mean duration diabetes: 15 years. Type 1 diabetes, 44 patients; type 2 diabetes, 137. No significant differences between groups reported at baseline	Median ulcer closure (%) (100% closure=complete healing). All plantar ulcers: I_1, 98.5%; I_2, 60.8% ($p<0.05$). Small plantar ulcers: I_1, 98.5% I_2, 98.5%. Large plantar ulcers: I_1, 89.2%; I_2, −10.4% ($p<0.01$). Trial 1: patients with >98% closure. All plantar ulcers: I_1, 54%; I_2, 31%. Large plantar ulcers: I_1, 43%; I_2, 6% ($p<0.05$). Small plantar ulcers: I_1, 64%; I_2, 56%. Infection rates (%): I_1, 7%; I_2, 34% ($p<0.05$). Withdrawals: 4, but unclear which group/s. Trial 2: delayed lamin treatment. Median closure (%): I_1, 40%; I_2, 68.2%. Mean closure ± SEM (%): I_1, 31.1 ± 10.1%; I_2, 33.9 ± 12.9%

(Continued)

Table 13.4 *(Cont.)*

Reference (study type)	Sample and Setting	Intervention	Baseline Characteristics	Results
17 (India; not randomized trial, but controlled trial with matching of patients and controls for "key" variables)	100 NIDDM patients with foot ulcers, class I and II (Meggitt classification). Aged 40–80 years. Setting: inpatients	I_1, daily topical phenytoin powder in thin layer with sterile dry dressing (n=50); I_2 dry sterile occlusive dressing (n=50). All ulcers debrided and cleansed with saline. Systemic antibiotics used where infection, as per culture and sensitivity. Duration of treatment: 35 days	Male/female: I_1, 27/23; I_2, 27/23. Groups reported to be well-matched for age, sex, duration of ulcer and initial area, but data not presented.	Mean time to complete healing (days): I_1, 21; I_2; 45 ($p<0.05$) Mean reduction in ulcer area at 35 days ± SD (%): I_1, 90 ± 3.9; I_2, 50 ± 4.4 ($p<0.005$) Excess granulation tissue was observed in 18 phenytoin-treated patients
18 (Sweden, RCT)	41 diabetic outpatients with deep exuding ulcers on the foot (Wagner grade I or II). Ulcer area >1 cm², and systolic toe pressure >30 mmHg, or systolic ankle pressure >80 mmHg. All patients Caucasian and aged over 40 years. Setting: outpatients	I_1, cadexomer iodine applied topically, changed once per day during 1st week, and every 1–3 days thereafter (n=22); I_2 standard treatment (gentamicin if infected, enzymic debridement if necrotic; dry saline gauze during exudation; paraffin gauze thereafter) All patients were given appropriate footwear and antibiotics for infection. Ulcers cleansed with saline Duration of treatment: 12 weeks	Not given, but described as "similar"	Ulcers completely healed: I_1, 5/17 (29%); I_2, 2/18 (11%) (OR 3.04; 95% CI 0.59, 15.56) Ulcers requiring surgical revision: I_1, 3/17 (18%); I_2, 5/18 (28%) Withdrawals: 2 due to violation of inclusion criteria (ulcers too large and too deep); 2 due to hospitalization for cardiac problems; 1 non-compliant No adverse events reported

Table 13.4 (*Cont.*)

19 (Sweden, RCT)	44 diabetic outpatients with necrotic foot ulcers (superficial and full-thickness skin ulcer below ankle; systolic toe pressure >45 mmHg; ulcers 1–25 cm² with >50% of area covered with dry/wet necrotic tissue) largest ulcer chosen where multiple ulcers present; Setting: outpatients	I_1, adhesive zinc oxide tape (MeZinc) (*n*=22); I_2, occlusive hydrocolloid dressing (DuoDerm) (*n*=22) Duration of treatment: 5 weeks	Mean age ±SD (years): I_1, 63±13; I_2, 62±18 Treated with insulin: I_1, 17/22; I_2, 18/22 Mean duration of diabetes ±SD (years): I_1, 22±15; I_2, 19±12 Mean ulcer area (range) (cm²): I_1, 2.2 (1–10.5); I_2, (0.9–19.2) Dry/wet necrotic ulcer: I_1, 15/7; I_2, 16/6	Reduction of baseline necrotic area 50–100%: I_1, 14/21 (67% of ulcers); I_2, 6/21 (29% of ulcers) (OR 4.44; 95% CI 1.34, 14.70) Reduction of necrotic area 25–50%: I_1, 1/22 (5%), I_2, 2/22 (9%) Treatment failures (increase in necrosis of >50% area): I_1, 4; I_2, 5 Withdrawals: treatment stopped in 8/9 patients above due to increase in area of necrosis by >100%, associated with pain and oedema Adverse events commonly seen in both groups: maceration of skin

Key: I_1, treatment group 1; I_2, treatment group 2; RCT, randomized controlled trial; SD, standard deviation; neuro, neuropathic; OR, odds ratio; CI, confidence interval; SE, standard error; SEM, standard error of the mean; PVD, peripheral vascular disease; DMSO, dimethylsulphoxide; tid, 3 times/day; An OR whose 95% CI includes 1 indicates no significant difference between the effects of the two treatments.

do better, as the absolute area of healing will be larger but the percentage change smaller.

Future trials of dressings for diabetic foot ulcers, therefore, need to address and avoid these methodological deficiencies. In addition, the role of co-interventions, such as wound debridement and weightbearing measures, as well as wound dressings, should be explored. Studies should also be of sufficient duration to capture a high proportion of ulcers which heal completely, analysis should be on an intention-to-treat basis[6], ideally including all participants in the final analysis, and reasons for withdrawal should be clearly documented. Trialists might also consider incorporating an economic analysis in order to answer questions of cost-effectiveness.

CONCLUDING REMARKS

There should be three important consequences of completing a systematic review in health care:

1. Clinical decisions can be better informed by the research evidence, even if this evidence is inconclusive.
2. A research agenda can be defined which aims to fill the important gaps in the research evidence.
3. The review should be kept up-to-date, to incorporate the results of new research as it becomes available.

The Cochrane Collaboration is an international network of thousands of individuals keen to undertake, maintain and disseminate systematic reviews of health care interventions[22]. These systematic reviews are undertaken in all clinical areas, and made available on CD-ROM and the Internet:

(http://www.update-software.com/ccweb/cochrane/cdsr.htm)

Reviews of interventions to prevent and treat diabetic foot ulceration are undertaken by international collaborators within the Cochrane Wounds Group (whose editorial base is at the University of York), and the Group is always keen to recruit new reviewers. We would also particularly like to hear about ongoing and unpublished trials in wound care so that we can ensure their early inclusion in systematic reviews.

ACKNOWLEDGEMENTS

This review was funded by the Health Technology Assessment Programme of the UK National Health Service Research and Development Programme. We are very grateful to Julie Glanville, Information Service Manager of the

NHS Centre for Reviews and Dissemination, University of York, who designed and executed the literature search.

REFERENCES

1. NHS Centre for Reviews and Dissemination (CRD). *Undertaking Systematic Reviews of Research on Effectiveness: CRD Guidelines for Those Carrying out or Commissioning Reviews.* CRD Report 4. NHS Centre for Reviews and Dissemination, York YO10 5DQ, UK, 1996.
2. Antman EM, Lau J, Kupelnick B, Mosteller F, Chalmers TC. A comparison of results of meta-analyses of randomized control trials and recommendations of clinical experts. Treatments for myocardial infarction. *J Am Med Assoc* 1992; **268**: 240–8.
3. Chalmers I, Altman DG. *Systematic Reviews.* London: British Journal of Medicine Publishing Group, 1995.
4. Mulrow CD, Oxman AD (eds). Cochrane Collaboration Handbook [updated September 1997]. In *The Cochrane Library* [database on disk and CD-ROM]. The Cochrane Collaboration, Oxford: Update Software, 1994; issue 4.
5. Sacks HS, Chalmers TC, Smith H Jr. Sensitivity and specificity of clinical trials. Randomized vs historical controls. *Arch Intern Med* 1983; **143**: 753–5.
6. Pocock SJ. *Clinical Trials: a Practical Approach.* Chichester: Wiley, 1983.
7. Dickersin K, Min YI. Publication bias: the problem that won't go away. *Ann NY Acad Sci* 1993; **703**: 135–48.
8. Laird NM, Mosteller F. Some statistical methods for combining experimental results. *Int J Tech Assess in Health Care* 1990; **6**: 5–30.
9. Baker N. Allevyn vs Sorbsan in the treatment of diabetic foot ulcers. Unpublished study, conducted at the Diabetes Resource Centre, Royal South Hants Hospital, Southampton, UK.
10. Foster A, Greenhill M, Edmonds M. Comparing two dressings in the treatment of diabetic foot ulcers. *J Wound Care* 1994; **3**: 224–8.
11. Vandeputte J, Gryson L. Diabetic foot infection controlled by immunomodulating hydrogel containing 65% glycerine—presentation of a clinical trial. Unpublished study, conducted at St. Josef Clinic, Ostend, Belgium.
12. Blackman J, Senseng D, Quinn L et al. Clinical evaluation of a semipermeable polymeric membrane dressing for the treatment of chronic diabetic foot ulcer. *Diabet Care* 1994; **17**: 322–5.
13. Clever H, Dreyer M. Comparing two wound dressings for the treatment of neuropathic diabetic foot ulcers. *Proceedings of the 5th European Conference on Advances in Wound Management.* London: Macmillan, 1996.
14. Donaghue VM, Chrzan JS, Rosenblum BI. A clinical evaluation of a collagen-alginate topical wound dressing (FIBRACOL) in the management of diabetic foot ulcers. *Adv Wound Care* 1998; **11**: 114–19.
15. Lishner M, Lang R, Kedar I, Ravid M. Treatment of diabetic perforating ulcers (malperforant) with local dimethylsulfoxide. *J Am Geriat Soc* 1985; **33**: 41–3.
16. Mulder G, Patt L, Sanders L, Rosenstock J, Altman MI, Hanley ME, Duncan GW. Enhanced healing of ulcers in patients with diabetes by topical treatment with glycl-L-histidyl-L-lysyl:copper. *Wound Rep Reg* 1994; **2**: 259–69.
17. Muthukumarasamy M, Sivakumar G, Manoharan G. Topical phenytoin in diabetic foot ulcers. *Diabet Care* 1991; **14**: 909–11.

18. Apelqvist J, Tennvall R.   Cavity foot ulcers in diabetic patients: a comparative study of cadexomer iodine ointment and standard treatment. An economic analysis alongside a clinical trial. *Acta Derm Venereol* 1996; **76**: 231–5.
19. Apelqvist J, Larsson J, Stenstrom A.   Topical treatment of necrotic foot ulcers in diabetic patients: a comparative trial of Duoderm and MeZinc. *Br J Dermatol* 1990; **123**: 787–92.
20. Page D, Kovacs J, Klevans L.   DMSO inhibits platelet aggregation in partially obstructed canine coronary vessels. *Fed Proc* 1982; **41**: 1530.
21. Finney J, Urshel H, Belle G.   Protection of the ischemic heart with DMSO alone or DMSO with hydrogen peroxide. *Ann NY Acad Sci* 1967; **141**: 231.
22. Chalmers I. The Cochrane Collaboration: preparing, maintaining, and disseminating systematic reviews of the effects of health care. *Ann NY Acad Sci* 1993; **703**: 156–65.

14

New Treatments for Diabetic Foot Ulcers
(a) Growth Factors

VINCENT FALANGA

Boston University School of Medicine, Roger Williams Medical Center, Providence, RI, USA

Over the past several decades, the discovery of growth factors has led to much hope and speculation about the use of these potent peptides in the treatment of difficult-to-heal wounds, particularly chronic wounds. *In vitro* experiments showed that growth factors were very effective in regulating cell proliferation, chemotaxis, and extracellular matrix formation. Animal experiments confirmed the notion that growth factors could accelerate wound repair, although most such experiments dealt with wounds created by acute injury. However, it was not until later, when further advances in recombinant technology made it possible to obtain large amounts of purified growth factors, that these agents could be tested in human clinical trials. Over the last 10–15 years, a large number of trials have been performed to evaluate the safety and effectiveness of growth factors in the healing of chronic wounds due to pressure (decubitus ulcers), diabetic neuropathy, and venous insufficiency[1]. Platelet-derived growth factor (PDGF) is now approved for topical treatment of diabetic neuropathic ulcers[2]. In this brief discussion, I will review growth factors, their mode of action, and the experience from clinical trials, with particular emphasis on the use of PDGF in diabetic foot ulcers. The discussion will end with the provision of a perspective on the future of growth factors in chronic wounds, including diabetic foot ulcers.

The Foot in Diabetes, 3rd edn. Edited by A. J. M. Boulton, H. Connor and P. R. Cavanagh.
© 2000 John Wiley & Sons, Ltd.

GENERAL ASPECTS OF GROWTH FACTORS

Although more easily conceptualized by the division into three distinct phases (inflammation, fibroplasia, and maturation), the process of wound repair is characterized by a series of complex cellular and molecular events with a great degree of overlap and interdependence[3]. Growth factors play fundamental roles in this process, by stimulating chemotaxis and cellular proliferation, by providing signalling among cells of the same and different types, by controlling extracellular matrix formation and angiogenesis, by regulating the process of contraction, and by re-establishing tissue integrity. As soon as blood vessels are disrupted, platelets enter the wound in great numbers and release several growth factors, including platelet-derived growth factor (PDGF) and transforming growth factor-$\beta 1$ (TGF-$\beta 1$). These and other growth factors are chemotactic for a number of cell types critical to the repair process, such as macrophages, fibroblasts, and endothelial cells. Later, during the proliferative phase of wound repair, several growth factors, including vascular endothelial growth factor (VEGF), fibroblast growth factors (FGFs) and PDGF and TGF-β isoforms, provide a potent stimulus for angiogenesis and for fibroblasts to synthesize key extracellular components (i.e. collagens, proteoglycans, fibronectin, elastin). During the later stages of wound repair, growth factors are important in tissue remodelling, aided by the action of matrix-degrading metalloproteinases (MMPs). It is likely, however, that the action of growth factors does not end with wound closure and tissue remodelling, but that they are key players in the maintenance of tissue integrity and in cell-to-cell communication.

Growth factors are multifunctional peptides that are extremely potent *in vitro*, often in the picogram (10^{-12} M) range[4]. Table 14a.1 shows a list of growth factors, some of them grouped into families, which have been tested for the treatment of chronic wounds. This list is not meant to be inclusive, and many more clinical studies have been performed than suggested by the number of published results. The nomenclature used to define growth factors tends to be confusing to the clinician for a number of reasons. First of all, the names of growth factors have more to do with the circumstances in which they were identified than with their specific effects on cells. Thus, fibroblast growth factors (FGFs) are very potent angiogenic factors, and transforming growth factor-βs (TGF-βs) are not transforming to cells and actually appear to be important in preventing cancer. Also, the term "growth factor" is generally used in a broad sense, to indicate substances which increase cell proliferation, mitogenic activity, and extracellular matrix formation. The actual category in which such substances are placed often depends on the context in which they were discovered. For example, the chances are that the same substance identified by a biochemist, an

Table 14a.1 Partial list of growth factors used to accelerate the repair of chronic wounds in humans

Factor	Cell or tissue of origin	Selected target cells or tissue	Selected stimulatory (S) or inhibitory (I) actions	Clinical trials
EGF	Macrophages, monocytes	Epithelium, endothelial cells	S: proliferation of keratinocytes, fibroblasts, and endothelial cells S: keratinocyte migration	Venous ulcers
FGF	Monocytes, macrophages, endothelial cells	Endothelium, fibroblasts, keratinocytes	S: proliferation of endothelial cells, keratinocytes, and fibroblasts S: chemotaxis, ECM	Diabetic ulcers, venous ulcers, pressure ulcers
GMCSF	Macrophages, fibroblasts, endothelial cells	Haematopoietic, inflammatory cells, neutrophils, fibroblasts	S: chemotaxis of endothelial cells, inflammatory cells S: keratinocyte proliferation, activation of neutrophils	Venous and arterial ulcers
HGH	Pituitary gland	Hepatocytes, bone, fibroblasts	S: IGF-1 production	Venous ulcers
IL-1	Lymphocytes, macrophages, keratinocytes	Monocytes, neutrophils, fibroblasts, keratinocytes	S: monocytes, neutrophils S: macrophage chemotaxis	Pressure ulcers
PDGF	Platelets, macrophages, neutrophils, smooth muscle cells	Fibroblasts, smooth muscle cells	S: proliferation of smooth muscle cells and fibroblasts S: chemotaxis S: ECM, contraction	Diabetic ulcers, pressure ulcers
TGF-β	Platelets, bone, most cell types	Fibroblasts, endothelial cells, keratinocytes, lymphocytes, monocytes	S: ECM, fibroblast activity S: chemotaxis I: proliferation of keratinocytes, endothelial cells	Venous ulcers, pressure ulcers

Abbreviations: EGF=epidermal growth factor; FGF=fibroblast growth factor, GMCSF=granulocyte-macrophage colony-stimulating factor; HGH=human growth hormone; IL-1=interleukin-1; IGF-1=insulin growth factor-1; PDGF=platelet-derived growth factor; TGF-β=transforming growth factor-β.

immunologist, and a haematologist would be called a growth factor, an interleukin, and a colony stimulating factor, respectively.

Growth factors work by binding to specific cell surface receptors and can target cells in a number of recognized ways or "modes". Release of these substances into the blood stream allows them to get to distant targets (endocrine mode). From the cell of origin, growth factors can diffuse over short distances to affect other cells (juxtacrine mode), and to influence neighbouring cells (paracrine mode). Growth factors can also act on the cell in which they are produced (autocrine mode). These different modes are all likely to be operative during tissue repair[1,4].

After binding to receptors, growth factors can have a profound influence on cell proliferation, chemotactic activity, and extracellular matrix synthesis. Interestingly, not all of these actions are stimulatory and not for all cell types. For example, transforming growth factor-βs (TGF-βs) are potent inhibitors of keratinocyte and endothelial cell proliferation. However, these same agents are a potent stimulus for the deposition of collagen and other extracellular matrix proteins. Harvesting the inhibitory activities of growth factors has great therapeutic potential, e.g. using antibodies to TGF-βs to decrease scarring.

MODE OF ACTION OF GROWTH FACTORS

Much of the progress made in the last 10 years in the basic science aspects of growth factors has been in identifying and cloning their specific cellular receptors and in elucidating the complex signalling pathways leading from receptor binding to a biological response (reviewed in reference 5). Tyrosine kinase receptors are membrane-spanning molecules with kinase activity (ability to phosphorylate or add phosphate groups) on the cytoplasmic domain. The kinase activity is activated upon binding of the growth factor (ligand). Almost 60 tyrosine kinases have been described, and they have been grouped in 14 families. Dimerization of several tyrosine kinase molecules is brought about by ligand binding (i.e. PDGF). After activation, the receptor can add phosphate groups to certain downstream targets or, by virtue of its phosphotyrosine residues, can bring other molecules into the signalling complex. There are other ways to transmit the initial signals. For example, the downstream target phosphorylated by the insulin receptor tyrosine kinase is a small protein called insulin receptor substrate-1 (IRS-1). Some receptors, i.e. those for interferons, do not have intrinsic tyrosine kinase activity. They instead recruit molecules possessing this ability to phosphorylate. The intracellular domain of these receptors is associated with a protein kinase family of the Janus family (JAKs) which, once autophosphorylated, recruits signal transducers and activators or transcription (STATs).

Receptors of the TGF-β superfamily of molecules have intrinsic serine/threonine kinase activity[6]. TGF-β binds to a class II receptor, which is a constitutively active kinase. Binding results in recruitment of a Type I receptor, which is phosphorylated and can activate downstream targets, such as SMADs proteins, which can move to the nucleus and interact with transcription factors. More than 10 SMADs proteins have been identified, with some causing activation (Smad 4) and others donwnregulating the signalling (Smad 6 and Smad 7).

Once tyrosine kinase activation and initial targeting occurs, further signals are generally transmitted by the Ras–Raf–MAP kinase pathway and the phospholipase C-γ-activated second messenger system[7]. These systems work in a cascade-like manner, and often involve a series of phosphoryla-tions, from one molecule to another. There is a Ras pathway, consisting of Rac and Rho proteins and cycling between GTP-associated (active) and GDP-associated (inactive) states. Another prominent system for downstream activation is the MAP (mitogen-activated protein kinase) pathway. Ras and Raf molecules are involved here, with Raf phosphorylating a MAP kinase kinase (MAPKK) or Mek (MAPK/Erk) kinase.

GROWTH FACTORS IN HUMAN ACUTE WOUNDS

The greatest potential of growth factors is to accelerate the healing of chronic wounds. Still, there are situations where accelerating the healing of acute wounds would be highly desirable and perhaps cost-effective. Moreover, acute wounds are in general less complex than chronic wounds, and allow investigators to develop "proof of principle" for certain parameters, such as dose of growth factors, development of optimal vehicle and delivery system, and other important variables. Split-thickness donor sites are in many ways the ideal acute wound for testing growth factors in humans. These wounds are easily made in a reproducible way, generally on the thighs. They offer a side-to-side comparison for testing products, are shallow, and normally heal within 7–10 days, which is a reasonable time period for testing effectiveness in acute wounds. Importantly, there is great value in accelerating the healing of split-thickness graft donor sites, for this would allow clinicians to re-harvest skin more quickly in burns patients.

There have been four studies of graft donor sites treated with growth factors. These have been reviewed in more detail elsewhere[1]. Topically applied EGF, bFGF, IL-1β and HGH have been tested. bFGF was found not to accelerate the healing of these acute wounds. The magnitude of the positive effect of growth factors in healing donor sites was generally not very dramatic. However, the results of these studies do show that growth factors can accelerate human healing when applied topically.

GROWTH FACTORS IN HUMAN CHRONIC WOUNDS

It is not possible to describe in detail all the trials that have been reported with growth factors and chronic wounds. Table 14a.2 is a partial list; it must be recognized that the results of unsuccessful trials are generally not published. As shown in Table 14a.2, a number of growth factors have been tested in more than one type of chronic wound. Although the results were not statistically significant in most of these studies, overall wounds treated with the growth factor seemed to do better than those treated with the placebo. All of the studies listed in Table 14a.2 were done with topically applied growth factors, except for GMCSF; this peptide was injected into the skin surrounding the

Table 14a.2   Double-blind, placebo-controlled trials of growth factors and chronic wounds

Growth factor	Reference	Target wound type (No. of subjects)	Dose of Growth Factor	Results
EGF	8	Venous (44)	10 μg/ml, twice daily	N.S.
HGH	9	Venous (37)	1 IU/cm^2 per week	N.S.
GMCSF	10	Venous+arterial (25)	400 μg, injected once around the wound	N.S.
TGF-β2	11	Venous (36)	2.5 μg/cm^2, three times per week	N.S.
PDGF-BB	12	Pressure (20)	1, 10 and 100 μg/ml, daily	N.S.
PDGF-BB	13	Pressure (45)	1 and 3 μg/ml, daily	N.S.
PDGF-BB	14	Diabetic (118)	2.2 μg/cm^2, daily	$p=0.01$
PDGF-BB	15	Diabetic (382)	30 and 100 μg/g, daily	$p=0.007$ for 100 μg dose
bFGF	16	Diabetic (17)	0.25 to 0.75 μg/cm^2, daily	N.S.
bFGF	17	Pressure (50)	1, 5 and 10 μg/cm^2	N.S.
IL-1β	18	Pressure (25)	0.01, 0.1 and 1 μg/cm^2, daily	N.S.

Abbreviations: EGF=epidermal growth factor; HGH=human growth hormone; GMCSF=granulocyte-macrophage colony-stimulating factor; TGF-β2=transforming growth factor-β2; PDGF-BB=platelet-derived growth factor BB; bFGF=basic fibroblast growth factor; IL-1β=interleukin-1β; N.S.=statistically non-significant.

wound[10]. Particularly promising results were obtained with PDGF[12] and FGF[17] in pressure (decubitus) ulcers, EGF[8] and TGF-β2[11] in venous ulcers, and PDGF in diabetic ulcers[14]. The results obtained in the treatment of diabetic ulcers with PDGF have been confirmed in larger trials[2,15] and will be described in more detail in the next section. Predictably, specific growth factors may be more effective in certain types of wounds. For example, growth factors capable of stimulating extracellular matrix formation and angiogenesis (i.e. PDGF and FGFs) are more likely to be useful in deep wounds, such as pressure ulcers. EGF was promising in venous ulcers[8], where failure of re-epithelialization is the major clinical problem[19].

One must be careful in evaluating the published literature on the use of growth factors in chronic wounds, such as the information in Table 14a.2, in which, apart from the PDGF trials in diabetic ulcers, the rest were pilot studies consisting of a small number of patients, sometimes from a single centre. However, it is highly likely that large, multicentre studies were performed with most of the growth factors shown in Tables 14a.1 and 14a.2, but that the results were not satisfactory and were not published.

This discussion has dealt exclusively with purified or recombinant growth factors. There has been a considerable amount of information on the use of autologous platelet preparations for accelerating the healing of chronic wounds, including diabetic ulcers[20,21]. The results have been promising, and the approach is based on the principle that more than one growth factor is needed for accelerating wound repair and that platelets are a rich source of growth factor peptides. However, these studies have been small, and it remains unclear whether autologous platelet releasate preparations are reliably active.

PDGF AND DIABETIC FOOT ULCERS

The only growth factor that has more convincingly been shown to stimulate healing of chronic wounds and which is approved for use in diabetic neuropathic ulcers by the Food and Drug Administration (FDA) and the European Medicines Evaluation Agency (EMEA) is PDGF-BB (becaplermin). In a Phase II clinical trial, Steed and colleagues tested the effect of a recombinant human PDGF-BB (rhPDGF-BB) gel preparation in the treatment of neuropathic diabetic ulcers of at least 8 weeks' duration[14]. A total of 118 patients were randomized to receive either rhPDGF-BB gel or placebo gel until complete wound closure or 20 weeks, whichever came first. The gel preparation was spread over the wound, and covered with a non-adherent saline-soaked gauze dressing. This primary dressing was held in place with roll gauze. Dressings were changed twice daily, 12 hours apart, but the study or placebo gel preparation were applied only once daily. The study was randomized, double-blind, and placebo-controlled, and patients were enrolled from 10 centres. There were no differences in the patients receiving the study drug or the placebo, except that patients treated with rhPDGF-BB were on average 5 years older ($p=0.02$). By approximately 6 weeks of therapy, differences emerged between the active and placebo group. Throughout the 20 weeks of the study, 29 (48%) of 61 patients treated with rhPDGF-BB achieved complete wound closure, compared to 14 (25%) of the 57 patients in the placebo group ($p=0.01$). Wounds also healed more quickly in the rhPDGF-BB group, by about 30–40 days ($p=0.01$). No statistically significant differences were present in the rate of ulcer recurrences between the two groups, the mean time for recurrence being 8.5 weeks. The rhPDGF-BB gel preparation proved to be safe.

A very interesting relationship between wound debridement and the effect of rhPDGF-BB emerged in the trial just described and published by Steed et al[14]. Surgical debridement, with removal of the callus around the ulcer, was performed at the beginning of the study and throughout the trial, as required. However, there were differences in the rate of wound debridement, depending on the study site. In general, a lower rate of healing was observed in those centres performing less frequent debridement[22]. It appears that there may have been a synergistic effect of aggressive surgical debridement and the use of rhPDGF-BB. The reasons behind this interesting observation are not clear. At higher debridement rates in the placebo group, there was no definite relationship between the healing rate and the frequency of debridement. An attractive hypothesis is that debridement removes tissue containing cells that are no longer responsive to the action of growth factors.

The effectiveness of rhPDGF-BB in the treatment of diabetic neuropathic ulcers have been confirmed in an additional and larger study, although a higher dose of the peptide (100 μg/g) were required for optimal efficacy[15]. This was a multicentre double-blind placebo-controlled Phase III trial of 382 patients. Ulcers were treated once daily with either 30 or 100 μg/g of rhPDGF-bb or placebo gel. As in the previous study, dressings were changed twice daily, and consisted of saline-soaked gauze. Compared to placebo gel, rhPDGF-BB in a dose of 100 μg/g increased the incidence of complete wound closure by 43% (p=0.007) and decreased the time to complete healing by 32% (86 vs. 127 days; p=0.013). It remains unclear why the lower dose of rhPDGF-BB did not prove as effective in this larger follow-up study. However, the safety of the rhPDGF-BB preparation remains established[23].

PERSPECTIVE ON GROWTH FACTOR THERAPY OF DIABETIC ULCERS

Substantial progress has been made with regard to growth factors in the treatment of chronic wounds. It appears that no serious safety issues have arisen; systemic absorption appears to be minimal, and no untoward local effects have been reported. These peptides have not caused cancer at the site of application, they have not been absorbed in substantial amounts and caused fibrosis, and they have not worsened diabetic retinopathy. Of course, much still remains to be done. It may very well be that the delivery systems used in these clinical trials were ineffective and did not allow the peptides to reach their target cells and tissues. Another reason, probably related to the first, is that the micro-environment of these chronic wounds is very hostile to proteins, and that breakdown of peptides by proteases is very likely. The success of PDGF in diabetic ulcers may be due to the persistence of biological activity of the peptide in the wound micro-environment[24]. A possible third reason is that the resident cells in chronic wounds have been altered by the pathogenic mechanisms responsible for the wounds in the first place. There is indeed evidence that fibroblasts from chronic wounds, including diabetic ulcers, are not able to respond to certain growth factors[25]. Removal of tissue from around the wound, as has been advocated for the use of PDGF in diabetic ulcers[22], may remove these unresponsive cells and allow peptides to function as they should.

There are, of course, other ways to deliver growth factors to wounds. Gene therapy may be ideal for wounds, because peptides would only be needed for a short period of time. Bioengineered skin products and skin substitutes represent another very exciting development and a major advance in the treatment of chronic wounds. Some of these agents supply matrix materials alone, while others contain living cells that are probably able to adjust to the wound micro-environment and provide growth factors and other substances that may be lacking in chronic wounds[26,27]. We still do not know whether the transplanted cells survive in the wound, but we think that they remain there long enough to stimulate and accelerate wound healing. These bioengineered products may well provide growth factors in the right concentration and in the right sequence, something that has proved difficult to achieve with the topical application of recombinant growth factors. It is also likely that these bioengineered skin products will be engineered to deliver certain growth factors in large quantities, e.g. PDGF[28]. This type of delivery may render growth factor therapy more effective.

REFERENCES

1. Robson MC.   Exogenous growth factor application effect on human wound healing. *Progress Dermatol* 1996; **30**: 1–7.
2. Dahn MS.   The role of growth factors in wound management of diabetic foot ulcers. *Fed Pract* 1998; **July**: 14–19.
3. Lawrence TW.   Physiology of the acute wound. In Granick MS, Long CD, Ramasastry SS (eds), *Clinics in Plastic Surgery. Wound Healing: State of the Art.* Philadelphia: WB Saunders, 1998; 321–40.
4. Falanga V.   Growth factors and wound healing. *Dermatol Clin* 1993; **11**: 667–75.
5. Twyman RM.   *Advanced Molecular Biology. Signal Transduction.* New York: Springer-Verlag, 1998; 425–42.
6. Barford D.   Molecular mechanisms of the protein serine threonine phosphatases. *Trends Biochem Sci* 1996; **21**: 407–12.
7. Robinson MJ, Cobb MH.   Mitogen-activated kinase pathways. *Curr Opin Cell Biol* 1997; **9**: 180–6.
8. Falanga V, Eaglstein WH, Bucalo B, Katz MH, Harris B, Carson P.   Topical use of human recombinant epidermal growth factor (h-EGF) in venous ulcers. *J Dermatol Surg Oncol* 1992; **18**: 604–6.
9. Rasmussen LH, Karlsmark T, Avnstrorp C, Peters K, Jorgensen M, Jensen LT. Topical human growth hormone treatment of chronic leg ulcers. *Phlebology* 1991; **6**: 23–30.
10. da Costa RM, Jesus FM, Aniceto C, Mendes M.   Double-blind randomized placebo-controlled trial of the use of granulocyte-macrophage colony-stimulating factor in chronic leg ulcers. *Am J Surg* 1997; **173**: 165–8.
11. Robson MC, Phillips LG, Cooper DM, Lyle WG, Robson LE, Odom L et al.   The safety and effect of transforming growth factor-B2 for the treatment of venous stasis ulcers. *Wound Repair Regen* 1995; **3**: 157–67.
12. Robson MC, Phillips LG, Thomason A, Altrock BW, Pence PC, Heggers JP et al.   Recombinant human platelet-derived growth factor-BB for the treatment of chronic pressure ulcers. *Ann Plast Surg* 1992; **29**: 193–201.

13. Mustoe TA, Cutler NR, Allman RM, Goode P, Deuel TF, Pruse JA et al.   Phase II study to evaluate recombinant PDGF-BB in the treatment of pressure sores. *Arch Surg* 1994; **129**: 213–19.

14. Steed DL and the Diabetic Ulcer Study Group.   Clinical evaluation of recombinant human platelet-derived growth factor for the treatment of lower extremity diabetic ulcers. *J Vasc Surg* 1995; **21**: 71–81.

15. Wiemann TJ, Smiell JM, Su Y.   Efficacy and safety of a topical gel formulation of recombinant human platelet-derived growth factor-BB (becaplermin) in patients with chronic neuropathic diabetic ulcers. A phase III randomized placebo-controlled double-blind study. *Diabet Care* 1998; **21**: 822–7.

16. Richard JL, Parer-Richard C, Daures JP, Clouet S, Vannereau D, Bringer J, Rodier M, Jacob C, Comte-Bardonnet M.   Effect of topical basic fibroblast growth factor on the healing of chronic diabetic neuropathic ulcer of the foot. A pilot, randomized, double-blind, placebo-controlled study. *Diabet Care* 1995; **18**: 64–9.

17. Robson MC, Phillips LG, Lawrence WT, Bishop JB, Youngerman JS, Hayward PG et al.   The safety and effect of topically applied recombinant basic fibroblast growth factor on healing of chronic pressure sores. *Ann Surg* 1992; **216**: 401–8.

18. Robson MC, Abdullah A, Burns BF, Phillips LG, Garrison L, Cowan W et al.   Safety and effect of topical recombinant human interleukin-1B in the management of pressure sores. *Wound Repair Regen* 1994; **2**: 177–81.

19. Falanga V, Grinnell F, Gilchrest B, Maddox YT, Moshell A.   Experimental approaches to chronic wounds. *Wound Repair Regen* 1995; **3**: 132–40.

20. Knighton DR, Ciresi KF, Fiegel VD, Schumerth S, Butler E, Cerra F.   Stimulation of repair of chronic, non-healing, cutaneous ulcers using platelet-derived wound healing formula. *Surg Gynecol Obstr* 1990; **170**: 56–60.

21. Steed DL, Goslen JB, Holloway GA, Malone JM, Bunt TJ, Webster MW.   Randomized prospective double-blind trial in healing chronic diabetic foot ulcers. CT-102-activated platelet supernatant, topical vs placebo. *Diabet Care* 1992; **15**: 1598–604.

22. Steed DL, Donohoe D, Webster MW, Lindsley L.   Effect of extensive debridement and treatment on the healing of diabetic foot ulcers. Diabetic Ulcer Study Group. *J Am Coll Surg* 1996; **183**: 61–4.

23. Smiell JM.   Clinical safety of becaplermin (rhPDGF-BB) gel. Becaplermin Studies Group. *Am J Surg* 1998; **176**: 68–73S.

24. Castronuovo JJ Jr, Ghobrial I, Giusti AM, Rudolph S, Smiell JM.   Effects of chronic wound fluid on the structure and biological activity of becaplermin (rhPDGF-BB) and becaplermin gel. *Am J Surg* 1998; **176**: 61–7S.

25. Hasan A, Murata H, Falabella A, Ochoa S, Zhou L, Badiavas E, Falanga V.   Dermal fibroblasts from venous ulcers are unresponsive to the action of transforming growth factor-β 1. *J Dermatol Sci* 1997; **16**: 59–66.

26. Falanga V, Margolis D, Alvarez O, Auletta M, Maggiacomo F, Altman M et al.   Healing of venous ulcers and lack of clinical rejection with an allogeneic cultured human skin equivalent. *Arch Dermatol* 1998; **134**: 293–300.

27. Gentzkow GD, Iwasaki SD, Hershon KS, Mengel M, Prendergast JJ, Ricotta JJ, Steed DP, Lipkin S.   Use of Dermagraft, a cultured human dermis, to treat diabetic foot ulcers. *Diabet Care* 1996; **19**: 350–4.

28. Eming SA, Medalie DA, Tompkins RG, Yarmush ML, Morgan JR.   Genetically modified human keratinocytes overexpressing PDGF-A enhance the performance of a composite skin graft. *Human Gene Ther* 1998; **9**: 529–39.

14

New Treatments for Diabetic Foot Ulcers
(b) Dermagraft and Granulocyte-colony Stimulating Factor (GCSF)

MICHAEL E. EDMONDS

King's College Hospital, London, UK

The diabetic foot remains a major problem, with often considerable difficulties in healing ulcers and controlling infection. Recently, two new therapies have been explored; these comprise Dermagraft to treat neuropathic ulceration and granulocyte-colony stimulating factor to treat infection.

DERMAGRAFT

Dermagraft is a bioengineered human dermis designed to replace a patient's own damaged or destroyed dermis. It consists of neonatal dermal fibroblasts cultured *in vitro* on bio-absorbable mesh to produce a living metabolically active tissue containing the normal dermal matrix proteins and cytokines.

Dermagraft is manufactured through the process of tissue engineering, the science of growing living human tissues for transplantation. Human fibroblast cells established from newborn foreskins are cultivated on a three-dimensional polyglactin scaffold. As fibroblasts proliferate within the scaffold, they secrete human dermal collagen, fibronectin, glycosaminoglycans, growth factors and other proteins embedding themselves in a

---

The Foot in Diabetes, 3rd edn. Edited by A. J. M. Boulton, H. Connor and P. R. Cavanagh.

self-produced dermal matrix. This results in a metabolically active dermal tissue with the structure of a papillary dermis of newborn skin. A single donor foreskin provides sufficient cell seed to produce 250 000 square feet of finished Dermagraft tissue. Maternal blood samples and cultured cells are tested throughout the manufacturing process to ensure that Dermagraft is free from known pathogenic agents, including HIV, human T-cell lymphotropic virus (HTLV), herpes simplex virus (HSV), cytomegalovirus (CMV) and hepatitis viruses.

After manufacture, Dermagraft is stored at $-70°C$. Since it is designed to be a living tissue, remaining viable and giving growth factors and matrix proteins into the wound bed after implantation, the metabolic activity of the product is assessed, pre- and post-cryroprecipitation, by measurement of specific levels of collagens and other matrix proteins. Dermagraft is then shipped on dry ice to clinical sites. Prior to implantation, the product is thawed, rinsed three times with sterile saline, cut to the wound size and placed into the wound bed. The fibroblasts, evenly dispersed throughout the tissue, remain metabolically active after implantation and deliver a variety of growth factors which are key to neovascularization, epithelial migration and differentiation and integration of the implant into the patient's wound bed. Thus, Dermagraft rebuilds a healthy dermal base over which the patient's epidermis can migrate and close the wound. No sutures are required but dressings are needed to ensure the dermal implant remains in place.

Clinical experience has included pilot and pivotal studies. The pilot study evaluated healing over a 12 week period in 50 patients with full-thickness neuropathic plantar and heel ulcers, greater than 1 cm² in size[1]. Patients were randomized into four groups (three different dosage regimes of Dermagraft and one control group). Ulcers treated with the highest dose of Dermagraft (one piece applied weekly for 8 weeks) healed significantly more often than those treated with conventional wound closure methods; 50% of the Dermagraft-treated ulcers healed completely compared with only 8% of the control ulcers ($p=0.03$). Also, after a mean of 14 months of follow-up (range 11–22 months) there were no recurrences in the Dermagraft-healed ulcers.

In the pivotal study, 281 patients with similar foot ulcers were enrolled into a multicentre, randomized controlled study to evaluate wound closure at 12 weeks, with a follow-up at 32 weeks[2]. At 12 weeks, 50.8% of the Dermagraft group experienced complete wound closure, compared with 31.7% in controls ($p=0.006$). Furthermore, at week 32, Dermagraft patients still had a statistically significant higher number of healed ulcers, 58% compared with 42% in controls ($p=0.04$).

However, at the time of a planned interim analysis, there was evidence that some patients had received product of low metabolic activity at the time of implantation and that these patients had significantly poorer healing results. A complete analysis of all *in vitro* and clinical data at the conclusion of the study showed that the metabolic activity of Dermagraft must lie within a definite therapeutic range to ensure that the tissue is sufficiently active after implantation to affect wound healing. The total evaluable Dermagraft group, which included many patients who had not received metabolically active Dermagraft at their early doses, had a higher rate of healing than the control group, 38.5% vs 31.7%, but the difference did not reach statistical significance. However, when evaluable patients who received Dermagraft with metabolic activity within the therapeutic range were analysed, 50.8% had experienced complete wound closure compared with 31.7% in controls ($p=0.006$). Furthermore, at week 32, Dermagraft patients still had a statistically significant higher number of healed ulcers, 58% compared with 42% in controls ($p=0.04$).

These data illustrate the importance of implanting Dermagraft within the appropriate metabolic range and the commercial manufacturing system is now designed to produce Dermagraft within this defined therapeutic range. Indeed, in a supplemental study to the pivotal trial, a further 50 patients were treated with Dermagraft and again showed an ulcer healing rate at 12 weeks above 50%. Preliminary uncontrolled studies at King's College Hospital, London, have shown similar results; 10 patients with "hard-to-heal" neuropathic plantar ulcers of a mean duration of 40 ± 29 months have been treated and seven healed within 32 weeks.

Thus, tissue engineering offers the ability to replace the damaged or destroyed dermis of a patient suffering from a full-thickness ulcer with a manufactured living dermal implant. Hitherto, Dermagraft has been used in the indolent plantar neuropathic ulcer to kick-start persistent lesions that are reluctant to heal. However, it may also be useful in the recently formed neuropathic ulcer and also in the neuro-ischaemic ulcer, and further studies are awaited with these types of ulcers.

Using clinical data obtained from the pivotal study and projecting costs for a cohort of 100 patients over 52 weeks in the British health care system, a cost-effective analysis developed by the York Health Economics Consortium, has shown that Dermagraft is cost-saving to the health care system[3]. It is estimated that the cost of healing ulcers using conventional therapy per year is £4327. However, when Dermagraft is used, more ulcers are healed and healed significantly faster. The cost to achieve such healing is lower at £3475 per healed ulcer per year, resulting in an £852 saving per healed ulcer when using Dermagraft.

Dermagraft is a very safe treatment and more than 1000 pieces of Dermagraft have been implanted with no immune rejection observed. Clinical experience has shown no significant difference between Dermagraft and control groups with respect to incidence of infection, cellulitis or osteomyelitis. However, Dermagraft should not be used if infection is present in the wound.

At present, Dermagraft presents a new and exciting treatment for the indolent plantar neuropathic ulcer that has failed to respond to conventional treatment.

GRANULOCYTE-COLONY STIMULATING FACTOR (GCSF)

Foot infection is common in patients with diabetes mellitus. The incidence and severity of such infections is greater in people with diabetes than in the non-diabetic population. The higher risk may be related to abnormalities in host defence mechanisms, including defects in neutrophil function[4,5]. Effective neutrophil antimicrobial action depends on the generation of several oxygen-derived free radicals. These toxic metabolites, (e.g. superoxide anion) are formed during the respiratory (or oxidative) burst that is activated after chemotaxis and phagocytosis. Deficiencies in neutrophil chemotaxis, phagocytosis, superoxide production, respiratory burst activity, and intracellular killing have been described in association with diabetes.

Granulocyte-colony stimulating factor (GCSF) is an endogenous haemopoietic growth factor that induces terminal differentiation and release of neutrophils from the bone marrow. The recombinant form is used widely to treat chemotherapy-induced neutropenia. Endogenous GCSF concentrations rise during bacterial sepsis in both neutropenic[6] and non-neutropenic states[7]; these findings suggest that GCSF may have a central role in the neutrophil response to infection[8]. In addition, GCSF improves function in both normal and dysfunctional neutrophils[9].

Since diabetes represents an immunocompromised state secondary to neutrophil dysfunction, we investigated the effect of systemic recombinant human GCSF (filgrastim) treatment in diabetic patients with foot infection. The aims of the study were to assess the effects of the GCSF on the clinical response and to measure the generation of neutrophil superoxide in patients and healthy controls[10].

Patients received either GCSF or a similar volume of placebo (saline solution). GCSF or placebo was administered as a daily subcutaneous injection for 7 days. Glycaemic control was optimized with insulin in all participants, by means of a continuous intravenous infusion or a multiple-dose regimen. Primary study objectives were time to resolution of infection (cellulitis), intravenous antibiotics requirements, and time to hospital discharge. Secondary objectives were the need for surgery, effects of GCSF on the generation of neutrophil superoxide, and the time taken for pathogens to be eliminated from the wound.

Forty diabetic patients with foot infections were enrolled in a double-blind placebo-controlled study. On admission, patients were randomly assigned to GCSF therapy (n=20) or placebo (n=20) for 7 days. There were no significant differences between the groups in clinical or demographic characteristics on entry to the study. Both groups received similar antibiotic and insulin treatment. Neutrophils from the peripheral blood were stimulated with opsonized zymosan, and superoxide production was measured by a spectrophotometric assay based on reduction of ferricyto-chrome *c*. The maximum skin temperature within the area of cellulitis was recorded with an infra-red thermometer. These readings were compared with those taken from the corresponding site on the non-infected foot. Any decisions about surgical debridement or amputation were based on clinical signs, including the presence of non-viable tissue, the development of gangrene, abscess formation, and lack of improvement despite optimum antimicrobial therapy.

GCSF therapy was asociated with earlier eradication of pathogens from infected ulcers [median 4 (range 2–10) vs 8 (2–79) days in the placebo group; $p=0.02$], quicker resolution of cellulitis [7 (5–20) vs 12 (5–93) days; $p=0.03$], shorter hospital stay [10 (7–31) vs 17.5 (9–100) days; $p=0.02$], shorter duration of intravenous antibiotic treatment [8.5 (5–30) vs 14.5 (8–63) days; $p=0.02$].There was a significant reduction in the temperature difference between the infected and non-infected foot by day 7 in the GCSF-treated group; by contrast, in the placebo group the reduction was not significant. No GCSF-treated patient needed surgery, compared with four in the placebo group. Four patients had ulcers healed at day 7 in the GCSF group, compared with none in the placebo group ($p=0.09$). After 7 days' treatment, neutrophil superoxide production was higher in the GCSF group than in the placebo group [16.1 (4.2–24.2) vs 7.3 (2.1–11.5) nmol per 10^6 neutrophils in 30 minutes; $p<0.0001$]. GCSF therapy was generally well tolerated. Patients who received GCSF therapy had significantly earlier eradication of bacterial pathogens from wound swabs, quicker resolution of cellulitis, shorter hospital stays, and shorter duration of intravenous antibiotic treatment than placebo recipients. Metabolic control did not differ significantly between the groups.

GCSF therapy was associated with the development of leukocytosis, due almost entirely to an increase in neutrophil count. Total white-cell and neutrophil counts increased significantly after two doses of GCSF, and the increases were maintained until day 7. There were also significant increases in lymphocyte and monocyte populations in patients receiving GCSF. All cell counts returned to near-baseline values within 48 hours of the end of treatment.

CONCLUSION

This study showed that in diabetic patients with foot infection, GCSF treatment significantly accelerated resolution of cellulitis, shortened hospital stay, and decreased antibiotic requirements. Thus, GCSF may be an important adjunct to conventional therapy. Clinical improvements with GCSF were supported by a significant decrease in foot temperature difference, and a shorter time to negative wound culture.

REFERENCES

1. Gentzkow G, Iwasaki S, Hershon K, Mengel M, Prendergast J, Ricotta J, Steed D, Lipkin S. Use of Dermagraft, a cultured human dermis, to treat diabetic foot ulcer. *Diabet Care* 1996; **19**: 350–4.
2. Naughton G, Mansbridge J, Gentzkow G. A metabolically active human dermal replacement for the treatment of diabetic foot ulcers. *Artifical Organs* 1997; **21**: 1203–10.
3. York Health Economics Consortium. Evaluation of the cost-effectiveness of Dermagraft in the treatment of diabetic foot ulcers in the UK. University of York, 1997.
4. Sato N, Shimizu H, Shimomura Y, Mori M, Kobayashi I. Myeloperoxidase activity and generation of active oxygen species in leukocytes from poorly controlled diabetic patients. *Diabet Care* 1992; **15**: 1050–2.
5 Marphoffer W, Stein M, Maeser E, Frederlin K. Impairment of polymorpho-nuclear leukocyte function and metabolic control of diabetes. *Diabet Care* 1992; **15**: 256–60.
6. Cebon J, Layton JE, Maher D, Morstyn G. Endogenous haemopoietic growth factors in neutropenia and infection. *Br J Haematol* 1994; **86**: 265–74.
7. Selig C, Nothdurft W. Cytokines and progenitor cells of granulocytopoiesis in peripheral blood of patients with bacterial infections. *Infect Immun* 1995; **63**: 104–9.
8. Dale DC, Liles WC, Summer WR, Nelson S. Granulocyte colony stimulating factor (GCSF): role and relationships in infectious diseases. *J Infect Dis* 1995; **172**: 1061–75.
9. Roilides E, Walsh TJ, Pizzo PA, Rubin M. Granulocyte colony stimulating factor enhances the phagocytic and bactericidal activity of normal and defective neutrophils. *J Infect Dis* 1991; **163**: 579–83.
10. Gough A, Clapperton M, Tolando N, Foster AVM, Philpott-Howard J, Edmonds ME. Randomised placebo-controlled trial of granulocyte-colony stimulating factor in diabetic foot infection. *Lancet* 1997; **350**: 855–9.

14

New Treatments for Diabetic Foot Ulcers
(c) Larval Therapy

STEPHEN THOMAS

Princess of Wales Hospital, Bridgend, UK

HISTORY

In the treatment of infected or necrotic areas on the diabetic foot, as with most types of chronic wounds, it is axiomatic that before the process of healing can begin, the affected areas must be thoroughly cleansed of all devitalized tissue. If surgical intervention is not an option, most practitioners use hydrogels to promote autolytic debridement[1] or resort to the use of other agents of questionable value. These include preparations containing povidone iodine and other lotions and potions containing sodium hypochlorite. Enzymatic debriding agents such as those containing streptodornase and streptokinase have also been used, although results of clinical trials involving these preparations have been disappointing.

Within the last few years, an alternative approach has been described that involves the use of sterile maggots, larvae of the common greenbottle, to effect wound debridement. This is not a new technique but a revival of a procedure that was widely used in the first half of the century as a treatment for osteomyelitis and soft tissue infections.

An early reference to the ability of maggots to cleanse wounds and prevent infection was made by Larrey, a military surgeon to Napoleon, who reported that when these creatures accidentally developed in wounds sustained in battle, they prevented the development of infection and accelerated the process of wound healing[2].

The Foot in Diabetes, 3rd edn. Edited by A. J. M. Boulton, H. Connor and P. R. Cavanagh.
© 2000 John Wiley & Sons, Ltd.

During the First World War, Baer, an American orthopaedic surgeon, also observed the cleansing action of maggots in extensive traumatic injuries. Some 10 years later, when Clinical Professor of Orthopaedic Surgery at the Johns Hopkins Medical School, he remembered this experience and began to use maggots to treat cases of intractable osteomyelitis. He found that the wounds of many of his patients, which had failed to respond to all other therapies, healed within 6 weeks with the continued application of the larvae[3]. As a result of Baer's work, the clinical use of maggots became commonplace in the USA during the 1930s[4] and remained so for about a decade until the development of antibiotics offered an easier and more aesthetically acceptable form of treatment for serious wound infections.

In recent years, however, multiresistant strains of bacteria such as *Staphylococcus aureus* (MRSA) have evolved. The clinical problems caused by these organisms, combined with a general recognition that conventional debriding agents are of limited efficacy in the management of problem or potentially limb-threatening wounds such as those on the diabetic foot, have caused some practitioners to revert to the use of maggots, often with impressive results.

The revival of larval therapy began in the USA in 1983 when Sherman et al[5] used maggots for treating pressure ulcers in persons who had suffered spinal cord injuries. This was followed by further reports of the use of larval therapy in podiatry[6] and recurrent venous ulceration[7].

In the UK, sterile larvae under the brand name of LarvE are produced in the Biosurgical Research Unit in South Wales[8]. Over a 4 year period, about 10 000 containers of sterile larvae have been supplied by this unit to about 700 centres, mainly in the UK, but also in Sweden, Germany and Belgium. A significant proportion of these larvae has been used in the treatment of wounds associated with diabetes. These vary in size from small neuropathic ulcers to more serious infected wounds involving one or more toes[9,10] as well as wounds such as leg ulcers and pressure sores[8,9,11–13].

A particularly graphic account of the use of larvae in the management of diabetic patients with extensive ulceration of the feet was published by Rayman et al[14]. These initial reports of the value of larval therapy are now being tested in randomized controlled trials to compare larvae with conventional treatments in the management of different types of necrotic wounds.

Treatment times vary according to the severity of the wound and the number of larvae applied. A small wound may only require one application lasting 3 days, but for more extensive wounds containing large amounts of necrotic tissue additional treatments may be required. Experience suggests that the continued application of larvae to a chronic or indolent wound following complete debridement will help to prevent further infection and may actually promote healing. Although larvae are generally applied to cleanse wounds in order to promote healing, they have also been used to improve the quality of life for terminally ill patients, for whom healing is not a realistic option. In such situations it has been reported that they may eliminate odour and reduce wound-related pain. One paper describes how larvae used in this way removed extensive amounts of necrotic tissue, including the toes, from a terminally ill gentleman with diabetes[15].

FLIES USED IN LARVAL THERAPY

The maggots used clinically are the larvae of *Lucilia sericata* a member of the family Calliphoridae, also classified as higher Diptera (Muscamorpha)[16]. The adult insects are a metallic coppery green colour, hence the common name, "greenbottles". They are facultative parasites, able to develop both on carrion and live hosts. In some animals such as sheep, greenbottle larvae produce serious wounds—a condition known as sheep-strike—but in human hosts the larval enzymes appear able only to attack dead or necrotic tissue.

The life cycle of the insect involves four stages; the egg, the larval form, the pupa (in its puparium) and the adult. Adult flies lay their eggs directly onto a food source and these hatch within about 18–24 hours, according to temperature, into larvae 1–2 mm long. These larvae immediately begin to feed using a combination of mouth hooks and proteolytic secretions and excretions. If conditions are favourable, the larvae grow rapidly, moulting twice before reaching maturity. The full-grown larvae, some 8–10 mm long, stop feeding and search for a dry place to pupate and complete the life cycle with the emergence of a new adult fly.

Sterile larvae for clinical use are collected in the laboratory from eggs the outer surface of which have treated to remove the very high numbers of bacteria that are normally present. The absence of micro-organisms on these newly hatched larvae is subsequently confirmed by a sterility test.

MODE OF ACTION OF STERILE LARVAE

Maggots remove dead tissue by means of complex mechanisms which involve both physical activity and the production of a broad spectrum of powerful enzymes that break down dead tissue to a semi-liquid form, which is then ingested by the larvae. Young et al[17] showed that the range of molecules secreted by larvae is complex and dynamic, changing quite dramatically over a short time frame of a few days. The majority of these agents belong to the serine class of proteases and some are developmentally regulated.

In order to maximize the efficiency of their extra-corporeal digestive process, larvae tend to congregate into groups, feeding in the head-down position, concentrating initially on small defects or holes in the tissue.

In human wounds it is believed that the enzymes produced by *Lucilia sericata* are inactivated by enzyme inhibitors in healthy tissue which are not present in necrotic tissue or slough. Some evidence for this hypothesis comes from the observation that if a significant quantity of larval enzymes are allowed to escape from the area of the wound and spread onto the surrounding skin, they can cause severe excoriation, eventually penetrating right through the keratinized epidermal layer. Once the enzymes breach the epidermis, however, no further damage occurs[9]. It is therefore assumed that the enzymes are inactivated at this point by proteolytic enzyme inhibitors in the dermis.

The mechanisms by which larvae prevent or combat infection are also complex. Pavillard, in 1957[18], demonstrated that secretions of larvae of the black blowfly contained an antibiotic agent that, when partially purified and injected into mice, protected them from the lethal effects of intraperitoneal injection with a suspension of Type 1 pneumococci. It has been shown in studies conducted in the author's laboratory that actively feeding larvae produce a marked increase in the pH of their local environment, which is sufficient to prevent the growth of some pathogenic Gram-positive bacteria. Furthermore, it has been shown that other bacteria which are not susceptible to pH changes within the wound are ingested by feeding larvae and killed as they pass through the insects' gut[19].

The early literature contained numerous references to the fact that maggots appeared to stimulate the production of granulation tissue[3,20,21], and this effect has also been noted in more modern studies. There are a number of possible explanations for this observed effect. Prete[22] demonstrated the existence of intrinsic fibroblast growth-stimulating factors in the haemolymph and alimentary secretions of maggots which may have some stimulatory effects *in vivo*. It may also be that the presence of the larvae, or their metabolites, stimulates cytokine production by macrophage cells which initiate or potentiate the inflammatory response within the wound and thus enhance the ability of the body to resist the development of infection and initiate healing.

LARVAE: METHOD OF USE

Various techniques have been described for retaining larvae in a wound[7,12]. In the main these rely upon the use of a piece of sterile net anchored to a suitable substrate applied to the area surrounding the wound to form a simple enclosure. A simple absorbent pad completes the dressing system. The adhesive substrate, which may consist of a hydrocolloid dressing, a zinc paste bandage or some other suitable alternative, fulfils three important functions. It provides a sound base for the net, protects the skin from the potent proteolytic enzymes produced by the larvae, and prevents any tickling sensation caused by the larvae wandering over the intact skin surrounding the area of the wound. If larvae are applied to or between the toes, it is prudent to protect the areas between the adjacent toes with small amount of alginate fibre to absorb any excess secretions.

The outer absorbent dressing can be changed as often as required and, because the net is partially transparent, the activity of the larvae can be determined without removing the primary dressing. As a rule of thumb, about 10 larvae/cm^2 should be introduced into a small wound (a circular wound 35 mm in diameter has an approximate area of 10 cm^2 and could therefore be treated with about 100 larvae). The fully grown larvae are generally removed from the wound after 2–3 days.

Studies have shown that larvae are unaffected by the concurrent administration of systemic antibiotics[23] but residues of hydrogel dressings within the wound may have an adverse effect upon their development[24]. Unpublished studies have shown that larvae appear to be unaffected by X-rays and therefore do not need to be removed if a patient requires such an investigation.

CONCLUSIONS

Larvae are living chemical factories that produce a complex mixture of biologically active molecules, many of which have yet to be fully characterized. Long-term clinical experience with maggots in wounds has been extremely positive and the wealth of recorded observations concerning the ability of these creatures to debride wounds and stimulate healing are gradually beginning to be substantiated by structured clinical investigations. It has also been shown that the use of larvae produces a wound bed that is very suitable for grafting.

Whilst some patients find the use of larvae unacceptable, generally there is much less resistance to this form of treatment than might have been expected. Some medical and nursing staff initially find the idea distasteful or consider that it represents an outmoded or unacceptable form of therapy, but once they have seen the benefits of larval therapy at first hand many become enthusiastic converts.

Although larval therapy has been used for all types of chronic wounds, the technique is of particular value in the treatment of the diabetic foot. The larvae are frequently able to remove all traces of necrotic tissue and eliminate wound infections in a fraction of the time taken by conventional therapies. The procedure may often be carried out in the patient's own home, thus reducing or eliminating the need for hospitalization, with important implications for overall treatment costs.

At the present time larval therapy is regarded by some as a treatment of "last resort". For this reason it is only offered to patients when all other options have been exhausted and when some form of amputation is considered inevitable. If the technique were to be applied at an earlier stage, it might prevent relatively small isolated areas of infection extending to threaten a foot or even an entire limb.

REFERENCES

1. Thomas S. *Wound Management and Dressings*. London: Pharmaceutical Press, 1990.
2. Livingstone SK, Prince LH. The treatment of chronic osteomyelitis with special reference to the use of the maggot active principle. *J Am Med Assoc* 1932; **98**: 1143–9.
3. Baer WS. The treatment of chronic osteomyelitis with the maggot (larva of the blowfly). *J Bone Joint Surg* 1931; **13**: 438–75.
4. Robinson W. Progress of maggot therapy in the United States and Canada in the treatment of suppurative diseases. *Am J Surg* 1935; **29**: 67–71.
5. Sherman RA, Wyle F, Vulpe M. Maggot therapy for treating pressure ulcers in spinal cord injury patients. *J Spinal Cord Med* 1995; **18**: 71–4.
6. Stoddard SR, Sherman RM, Mason BE, Pelsang DJ. Maggot debridement therapy. *J Am Podiat Med Assoc* 1995; **85**: 218–20.
7. Sherman RA, Tran JM-T, Sullivan R. Maggot therapy for venous stasis ulcers. *Arch Dermatol* 1996; **132**: 254–6.
8. Thomas S, Jones M, Andrews A. The use of fly larvae in the treatment of wounds. *Nursing Standard* 1997; **12**: 54–9.
9. Thomas S, Jones M, Shutler S, Jones S. Using larvae in modern wound management. *J Wound Care* 1996; **5**: 60–9.
10. Mumcuoglu KY, Lipo M, Ioffe-Uspensky I, Miller J, Galun R. Maggot therapy for gangrene and osteomyelitis. *Harefuah* 1997; **132**: 323–5, 382.
11. Thomas S. A wriggling remedy. *Chem Ind* 1998; **17**: 665–712.
12. Thomas S, Jones M, Andrews M. The use of larval therapy in wound management. *J Wound Care* 1998; **7**: 521–4.
13. Thomas S, Jones M, Shutler S, Andrews A. Wound care. All you need to know about . . . maggots. *Nursing Times* 1996; **92**: 63–6, 68, 70 *passim*.
14. Rayman A, Stansfield G, Woolard T, Mackie A, Rayman G. Use of larvae in the treatment of the diabetic necrotic foot. *Diabet Foot* 1998; **1**: 7–13.
15. Evans H. A treatment of last resort. *Nursing Times* 1997; **93**.
16 Crosskey RW. Introduction to the Diptera. In Lane RP, Crosskey RW (eds), *Medical Insects and Arachnids*. London: Chapman & Hall, 1995.
17. Young AR, Mesusen NT, Bowles VM. Characterisation of ES products involved in wound initiation by *Lucilia cuprina* larvae. *Int J Parasitol* 1996; **26**: 245–52.
18. Pavillard ER, Wright EA. An antibiotic from maggots. *Nature* 1957; **180**: 916–17.
19. Robinson W, Norwood VH. Destruction of pyogenic bacteria in the alimentary tract of surgical maggots implanted in infected wounds. *J Lab Clin Med* 1934;**19**: 581–6.

20. Fine A, Alexander H. Maggot therapy—technique and clinical application. *J Bone Joint Surg* 1934; **16**: 572–82.
21. Buchman J, Blair JE. Maggots and their use in the treatment of chronic osteomyelitis. *Surg Gynecol Obstet* 1932; **55**: 177–90.
22. Prete P. Growth effects of *Phaenicia sericata* larval extracts on fibroblasts: mechanism for wound healing by maggot therapy. *Life Sci* 1997; **60**: 505–10.
23. Sherman RA, Wyle FA, Thrupp L. Effects of seven antibiotics on the growth and development of *Phaenicia sericata* (Diptera: Calliphoridae) larvae. *J Med Entomol* 1995; **32**: 646–9.
24. Thomas S, Andrews A. The effect of hydrogel dressings upon the growth of larvae of *Lucilia sericata*. *J Wound Care* 1999; **8**: 75–7.

15

The Role of Radiology in the Assessment and Treatment of the Diabetic Foot

JOHN F. DYET, DUNCAN F. ETTLES and
ANTHONY A. NICHOLSON
Hull and East Yorkshire Hospitals NHS Trust, Hull, UK

Radiology has an important role in the diagnosis of the underlying bony abnormalities encountered in the diabetic foot. Whilst plain film radiography will demonstrate the basic bone pathology, newer modalities such as magnetic resonance imaging (MRI) add a further dimension by being able to detect dynamic changes. The interventional radiologist is able to use endovascular techniques to improve the blood supply to the diabetic foot, which is often affected by ischaemia.

PATHOGENESIS

Radiological manifestations in diabetic foot disease result from a combination of neuropathy, infection and vascular disease, all of which are present to a greater or lesser extent in diabetic foot problems. The disease affects all parts of the diabetic foot, including skin, soft tissues, muscles, blood vessels and bones. It is the neuropathy which is the foundation upon which the other aspects of the diabetic foot are superimposed.

The severity of the bone disease in the absence of osteomyelitis is due to the neuropathy[1]. It is generally believed that loss of sensation allows repeated minor trauma. The patient continues to weight bear, so leading to

---

The Foot in Diabetes, 3rd edn. Edited by A. J. M. Boulton, H. Connor and P. R. Cavanagh.
© 2000 John Wiley & Sons, Ltd.

progressive joint destruction. This is accelerated by sympathetic denervation of small blood vessels causing hyperaemia, which in turn causes increased osteoclastic activity with bone resorption, thus weakening the bone structure[2].

Atheromatous vascular disease is approximately four times more common in diabetic patients than in the non-diabetic population[3] and the pattern of vascular disease is also different. In non-diabetic patients, disease in the femoral and popliteal arteries is most common, followed by disease in the aorto-iliac segment. In patients with diabetes, multiple stenoses and occlusions in the popliteal and tibial arteries occur most frequently, with relative sparing of the vessels around the ankle and foot[4,5]. Another characteristic of diabetic vascular disease is Mönckeberg's medial calcification, which is found in the intermediate-sized vessels and is thought to be caused by autonomic denervation. The affected artery has been likened to a lead pipe which is non-compressible (Figure 15.1).

DIABETIC OSTEOPATHY AND NEUROARTHOPATHY

"Diabetic osteopathy" is the term commonly used to describe the bone changes in the neuropathic foot that are usually associated with joint destruction (neuro-arthropathy). Bone changes associated with primary neuro-arthropathy are most common in the phalanges and metatarsals, although the tarsal bones and ankles may also be involved. Whilst it is the older age group (60+) who are most commonly affected, the younger patient is not immune[6].

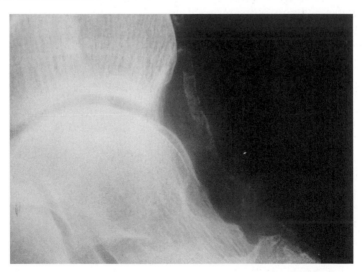

Figure 15.1   Calcification in the anterior tibial artery at the ankle

The early radiographic signs are those of soft tissue swelling with joint effusion. This may be followed by mild subluxation and peri-articular fractures (Figure 15.2a). As the process worsens, subluxation and frank osteoclastic destruction predominate (Figure 15.2b). Attempts at healing with periosteal new bone formation may cause the bones to have a sclerotic appearance (Figure 15.3). Eventually the peri-articular surfaces become completely resorbed due to excessive osteoclastic activity, and the resulting appearance has been described variously as a pencil-like deformity, sucked candy, and wax running down a burnt candle (Figures 15.2b and 15.3). Resorptive changes predominate in the metatarsals and phalanges, whereas in the tarsal bones and ankle the changes are mainly destructive. The destruction causes a deranged and unstable joint (Figures 15.3 and 15.4). Synonyms for the process include neuro-osteoarthropathy and Charcot joint[7].

INFECTION

Soft tissue infection is always a possibility where ulceration and fissuring are found in the diabetic foot. Direct spread of infection to the adjacent bone (Figure 15.5) and/or joint may occur, leading to osteomyelitis and septic

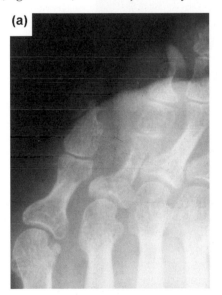
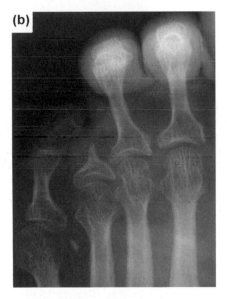

Figure 15.2 Bony changes as a result of diabetic neuroarthopathy. (a) There are fractures at both ends of the shaft of the proximal phalanx of the fourth toe. There is partial erosion of the distal phalanges of the fourth and fifth toes. (b) The middle and distal phalanges of the fourth toe have been amputated. The proximal phalanx now shows the classical "sucked candy" appearance

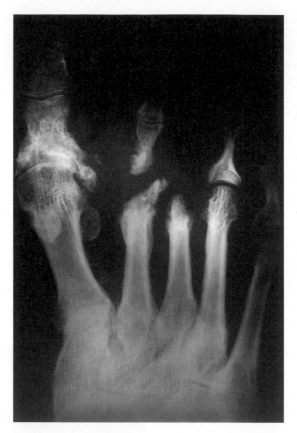

Figure 15.3 Diabetic neuroarthopathy. There is destruction of most of the phalanges. The heads of the second and third metatarsals are also destroyed. The upper ends of their shafts are sclerotic, and the appearance on the second metatarsal is like wax running down a candle. The first metatarsophalangeal joint is disorganized (the so-called Charcot joint)

arthritis. Plain film radiography is poor at differentiating between neuropathic changes and neuropathy plus osteomyelitis. Both processes cause bone resorption with cartilage and joint destruction. The presence of infection may lead to more abundant periosteal reaction and also more marked soft tissue swelling[8]. Other factors that may help in diagnosis are the fact that changes may be localized to one site and an adjacent soft tissue ulcer may be visible (Figure 15.6).

Because of the difficulty of diagnosing osteomyelitis on plain film radiography, other techniques have been employed. Bone scintigraphy, using the isotope ^{99m}Tc-MDP, has been useful in helping to differentiate the early changes of osteomyelitis from uncomplicated neuropathic changes[9].

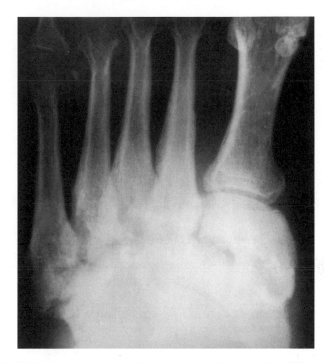

Figure 15.4 Diabetic neuroarthopathy involving the second to fifth tarso-metatarsal joints

However, in their article, Yuh et al[2] found that due to lack of spatial resolution and the coexistent neuropathy, scintigraphy proved less than reliable. In their series of 29 patients in whom pathological specimens had been obtained, only MRI accurately diagnosed the presence or absence of infection in all cases. Scintigraphy proved to give a high false-positive rate for the presence of infection. The MRI studies showed a normal bone marrow signal in the absence of infection but a high signal intensity in osteomyelitis (Figure 15.7). However, studies with leucocyte scans using indium (^{111}In oxyquinoline) were also shown to be superior to bone scintigraphy and radiology, with a sensitivity of 89%[10].

MAGNETIC RESONANCE IMAGING

Early and accurate diagnosis of infection or neuropathy is the key to successful management of the diabetic foot. In addition, it is essential that developing angiopathy be treated early in order to avoid ischaemia. This requires high quality imaging of the arterial supply to the leg and foot. Spin echo MRI combined with 2D time-of-flight sequences can

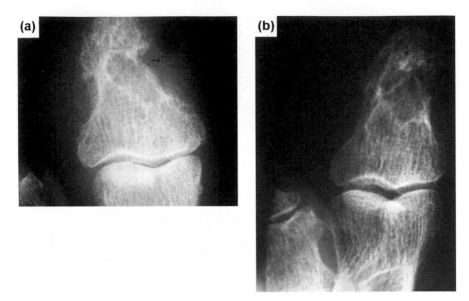

Figure 15.5 Infection in diabetic neuropathy. (a) A soft tissue ulcer can be seen and there is erosion of the adjacent bone. There is no periosteal reaction. (b) One month later, the erosion is much more extensive, suggesting infection, but there is still no periosteal reaction

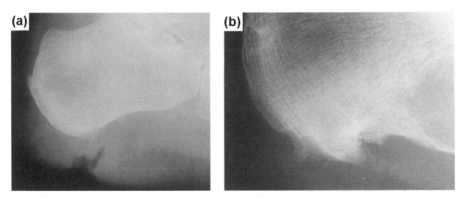

Figure 15.6 Infection in diabetic neuropathy. (a) There is an obvious soft tissue ulcer but the underlying bone is not obviously infected. (b) The ulcer has now healed but marked periosteal thickening of the underlying bone indicates that it was infected

provide all this information. The time-of-flight sequences look at blood flow rather than blood vessels. Thus, blood flowing in both arteries and veins is imaged. Because this would be confusing, a system of saturation bands is used in order that the blood returning to the heart (i.e. venous

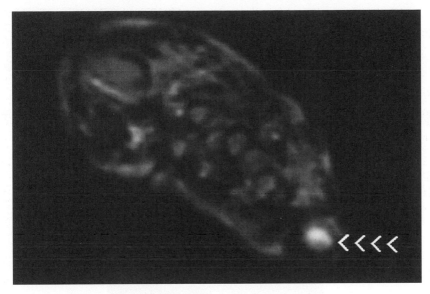

Figure 15.7 Magnetic resonance imaging in infection. A transverse image taken through the heads of the metatarsals. The head of the fifth metatarsal gives a very high-intensity signal, indicating infection

blood) is presaturated, such that on exposure to the radiofrequency pulses, no return signal is produced. As discussed above, distinguishing osteomyelitis and neuro-arthropathy frequently presents a clinical and radiological challenge in diabetic patients. In osteomyelitis, signal intensity changes in the bone marrow (low signal on T1- and high signal on T2-weighted images (Figure 15.7), associated occasionally with cortical lesions and often with soft tissue abnormalities. Decreased signal in bone, regardless of pulse sequence or no signal change, is the characteristic of chronic neuro-arthropathy. However, patients with acutely evolving neuropathy can have signal intensity changes in the marrow, which can be a source of diagnostic error. The use of contrast agents such as gadolinium dimeglumine has not been shown to be helpful in distinguishing between osteomyelitis and neuro-arthropathy[11]. Although the later stages of osteomyelitis may produce a soft tissue mass, this is not seen in the first week. Similarly, cortical changes can take 7–10 days to become visible on plain radiographs, and although seen earlier by MRI, do not help acutely. Despite this potential pitfall, the diagnostic sensitivity, specificity and accuracy of MRI has been shown to be 88%, 100% and 95% respectively[12]. This compares with plain radiography (22%, 94% and 70%), technetium bone scanning (50%, 50% and 50%) and labelled white cell studies (33%, 60% and 58%) from the same study. In addition, MRI accurately delineates

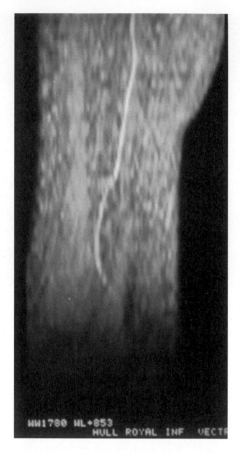

Figure 15.8 Magnetic resonance (MR) angiography. Time-of-flight MR images showing a distal peroneal artery that was not visible on digital subtraction angiography

the limits of the infection, reducing the incidence of recurrent infection post surgery. This makes MRI extremely cost effective[13].

Magnetic resonance angiography is a useful non-invasive tool in the assessment of foot vessel run-off, especially when there are proximal arterial occlusions limiting the diagnostic value of angiography (Figure 15.8). The use of warm water baths to vasodilate the arterial run off to the feet further enhances the diagnostic quality of the images[14]. However, unlike plain radiographs, MRI gives no clue about arterial calcification, which is important to the surgeon, although less so to the vascular radiologist. In the future it is likely that magnetic resonance proton spectroscopy will provide information about the microvasculature of the diabetic foot.

At the present time, MRI provides accurate cost-effective information about the diabetic foot and should be used in conjunction with plain radiographs, duplex ultrasound and angiography when indicated.

CHRONIC CRITICAL LIMB ISCHAEMIA

The consensus document on critical limb ischaemia[15] contains the following definition:

> Chronic critical leg ischaemia in both diabetic and non-diabetic patients is defined as either of the following two criteria: persistently recurring ischaemic rest pain requiring regular adequate analgesia for more than two weeks, with an ankle systolic pressure ≤50 mmHg and/or a toe pressure of ≤30 mmHg; or ulceration or gangrene of the foot or toes, with an ankle systolic pressure of ≤50 mmHg or a systolic toe pressure of ≤30 mmHg.

It is important not to confuse neuropathic pain with ischaemic rest pain in the diabetic patient. In such patients the toe pressure should always be measured, as the ankle systolic pressure has proved to be unreliable. The arteries are often calcified (Figure 15.1), rigid and incompressible, giving rise to false readings. Critical leg ischaemia should be regarded as a serious complication of diabetes which requires urgent investigation and treatment if amputation is to be avoided. Diabetic patients are at least five times more likely to develop critical limb ischaemia than non-diabetic claudicants, with 10% of elderly diabetic patients developing ischaemic ulcers and gangrene[16].

It is important to differentiate between neuropathic ulceration and neuro-ischaemic ulceration, as the former may be managed conservatively, with a 90% chance of healing. Ischaemic ulcers rarely heal unless an improvement in blood supply is obtained. Neuropathic ulcers are usually found in the presence of normal pulses, they are painless, and they occur most frequently on the plantar aspect of a warm foot. Conversely, ischaemic ulcers are painful, often located on the toes or the borders of the foot and associated with reduced or absent pulses.

Modern treatment of critical limb ischaemia in specialized centres has improved outcomes considerably in recent years. Primary amputation rates are now as low as 20%, and 60% of patients are suitable for some form of revascularization procedure[15].

INVESTIGATION OF VASCULAR DISEASE IN THE DIABETIC PATIENT

Although contrast angiography remains the definitive investigational method in assessment of the peripheral vascular system, the roles of duplex ultrasound and magnetic resonance angiography continue to increase in importance. Within the next few years, the use of diagnostic angiography will decrease and the use of non-invasive techniques, in both diagnosis and intervention, will predominate.

Duplex Ultrasound

Duplex ultrasound combines cross-sectional imaging of arteries and veins with simultaneous colour flow and spectral Doppler information. This allows accurate recording of velocity changes at specific sites within the vessels, and detection of haemodynamically significant stenoses is possible, therefore, without the need for angiography. Such non-invasive assessment of the aorto-iliac and femoropopliteal segments can be performed with a high degree of sensitivity and specificity[17]. Duplex imaging of the tibial vessels demands greater operator skill but, because it can reliably identify significant stenoses and occluded segments, it may be superior to angiography in some cases[18]. The advantage of this non-invasive approach is that only those patients who are likely to benefit from interventional radiological procedures or reconstructive surgery need to go on to have angiography.

Angiography

Angiographic assessment is usually performed by the transfemoral retrograde approach but alternative approaches include transbrachial angiography and intravenous digital subtraction angiography. Under local anaesthesia, the common femoral artery is punctured and a Teflon-coated guidewire with a soft J-tip is advanced into the abdominal aorta. A 4F or 5F gauge catheter with a pigtail shaped end is then advanced over the wire until it lies just below the renal artery origins. With the catheter in place, injections of iodinated contrast are made and images are obtained from the aorta to the ankle, with additional oblique views as required to completely demonstrate the arterial tree and any disease within it. Images are now most commonly obtained using digital subtraction angiography and stored either on X-ray film or digitally on CD-ROM.

Modern angiographic contrast media have a much lower risk of complications and adverse reactions compared with those used a few years ago, although there is still a small risk of anaphylaxis and death. Because of the common association between diabetes and renal impairment, the total volume of contrast injected must always be kept to a minimum. Certain newer agents are claimed to have reduced nephrotoxicity, and although expensive, their use may be justified in such patients. The risk of patients treated by Metformin developing lactic acidosis after contrast examinations has been highlighted by sporadic case reports. Recent studies suggest that this risk is negligible if renal function is normal. Metformin should be withheld for 48 hours prior to the examination if there is evidence of renal impairment then and should be only restarted after repeat serum biochemistry confirms no deterioration[19].

Patterns of Vascular Disease

Typically, vascular disease in the diabetic patient affects the infrapopliteal arteries while sparing the more proximal vessels. Nevertheless, diabetes is only one of a number of factors which predispose to the development of atheroma. The diabetic patient may also be exposed to other risk factors, including smoking, hypertension and familial tendencies, and as a result may develop a pattern of disease affecting the larger, more proximal, vessels and resembling more typical peripheral vascular disease. Therefore, preliminary imaging of the peripheral circulation should be completed, since proximal lesions may have a crucial influence on treatment and outcome. There is little point in dealing with distal crural vessel stenosis if inflow obstruction remains at the femoral or iliac level. In fact, even in the presence of severe distal disease, relief of a significant proximal obstruction may be sufficient to save an ischaemic limb.

INTERVENTIONAL RADIOLOGICAL PROCEDURES

Endovascular procedures are performed routinely in the majority of radiology departments in the UK and increasingly by radiologists who have undergone specialist training in these techniques. Continued improvements in catheter and guidewire technology have contributed significantly to the reduction in morbidity and complication rates associated with radiological treatment of vascular disease. The principal indications for such endovascular intervention in the diabetic patient are severe claudication and critical limb ischaemia, and treatment is most frequently by balloon angioplasty (PTA). A variety of adjunctive treatments may be used in addition to simple balloon PTA, and these are directed towards improving initial success rates and maintaining long-term patency following the initial intervention. Thrombolytic therapy has a particular role in the management of critical ischaemia.

Balloon Angioplasty

Dotter and Judkins first described the technique of balloon angioplasty (PTA) in 1964[20]. A non-deformable balloon mounted on a low-profile angiographic catheter is introduced into the stenosed or occluded portion of the vessel over a previously positioned guidewire. The PTA balloon is then inflated using radio-opaque contrast medium to allow visualization, and pressures of 4–10 atmospheres are then usually sufficient to bring the balloon to its predetermined diameter. Heparin is given at the time of PTA to reduce the risk of acute thrombotic closure of the vessel, and antiplatelet therapy is started before treatment and usually continued indefinitely. The mechanism of balloon PTA is complex and involves disruption and moulding of the atheromatous plaque, longitudinal splitting of the vessel endothelium and disruption of the elastic media. PTA causes mechanical stretching of the vessel, and also results in healing taking place at a cellular level, with the growth of a new intima and remodelling due to macrophage activity at the PTA site. Balloon PTA is a simple procedure that can be performed under local anaesthesia, and as a day case procedure in suitable patients. Morbidity is very low and mortality is virtually zero. Complications are rarely serious or limb-threatening and can often be managed without surgery[21].

The best results are obtained in the iliac arteries, with patency rates approaching 70% at 5 years. The superficial femoral arteries tend to respond less well, especially in the presence of long segment disease with poor distal run-off[22,23]. However, in the setting of critical limb ischaemia, patency can often be restored for long enough to allow distal healing and the development of collateral supply. Furthermore, repeated PTA procedures can be performed, thus continuing to avoid the need for surgery. The use of PTA for tibial vessels in diabetes has increased in the last 5 years, helped by improved technology with very low profile catheter equipment.

Case No. 1

Figure 15.9a shows the angiogram of a 55 year-old diabetic man who was also hypertensive, hypercholesterolaemic and a life-long smoker. He presented with severe claudication. There is a long diffuse stenotic lesion in the distal superficial femoral artery. Angioplasty was performed (Figure 15.9b) and a good post-procedure result was obtained (Figure 15.9c), with marked improvement in the patient's symptoms.

Case No. 2

Figure 15.10a (angiogram) shows the typical appearance of diabetic vascular disease around the knee. The popliteal artery is severely stenosed distally, running into a tibioperoneal trunk which is virtually occluded. Following angioplasty there is in-line flow into the peroneal artery, which

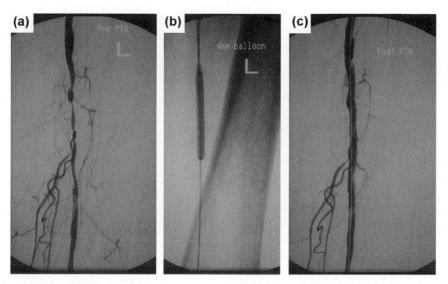

Figure 15.9 (a) Pre-procedure angiogram. (b) Angioplasty balloon inflated. (c) Final result

then runs to the foot (Figure 15.10b). This procedure allowed an ischaemic foot ulcer to heal.

Endovascular Stent Insertion

The major limitation of balloon angioplasty is re-stenosis at the site of the initial lesion, which most often occurs in the first year after treatment. Previously treated occlusions have been shown to have a greater tendency to re-stenosis compared to simple stenotic lesions. A major advance in improving PTA results has resulted from the introduction of vascular stents. Metallic stents are now widely used as an adjunct to balloon PTA. Broadly speaking, they are either self-expanding or balloon-expandable in type. The stent, which is pre-mounted on its delivery system, is introduced over a guidewire to the site of the lesion under fluoroscopic guidance. Usually the diameter of stent chosen is 1 mm greater than the vessel diameter, and its length is chosen to provide complete coverage of the lesion. Deployment of balloon-mounted stents requires inflation of the balloon to a predetermined pressure. Self-expanding stents are deployed by a variety of mechanisms which gradually uncover the stent by retracting a membrane or sheath. Self-expanding stents often require additional balloon expansion to achieve full size. The choice of stent depends on a number of factors, including vessel tortuosity and lesion length.

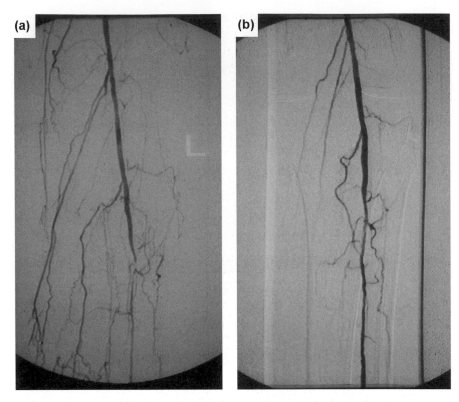

Figure 15.10   (a) Popliteal angiogram showing severe stenosis at the origin of the peroneal artery. (b) Following angioplasty

Stents are used in two main clinical settings. The first of these is in the presence of a suboptimal PTA result or when there is an immediate complication of angioplasty, such as flow-limiting dissection at the PTA site. The second indication for stent use is as a primary treatment in lesions which may respond less well to angioplasty alone. One of the main areas of use of primary stenting has been in the treatment of iliac artery occlusions. The superiority of stenting over balloon angioplasty has been documented in numerous publications[24].

Case No. 3

Figure 15.11a is the angiogram of a 57 year-old smoker who presented with claudication in his right leg after walking approximately 100 yards. The angiogram shows a 5 cm occlusion of the right common iliac artery.

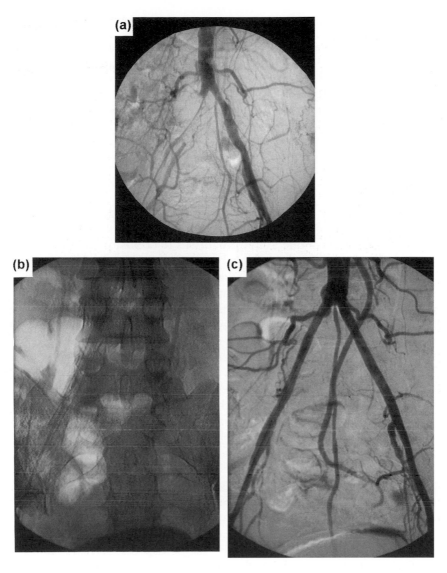

Figure 15.11 (a) Right common iliac occlusion. (b) Long self-expanding stent in place. (c) Post-procedure result showing virtually normal appearance

In Figure 15.11a a wire has been passed through the occlusion. An endovascular stent has been introduced over the wire into the occlusion and the stent has expanded (Figure 15.11b). The angiogram on completion (Figure 15.11c) shows complete restoration of flow and the patient's symptoms were relieved.

Case No. 4

Figure 15.12a shows a short femoral artery occlusion in a 43 year-old poorly controlled diabetic patient. He had already had coronary artery bypass grafting and presented with short-distance claudication, which restricted his ability to work. Balloon angioplasty was performed (Figure 15.12b) but the subsequent result was very poor (Figure 15.12c), with dissection and plaque disruption. Two self-expanding coil stents were therefore implanted to maintain patency (Figure 15.12d) and the patient remains symptom-free.

Thrombolysis

Thrombolysis has an important role in the multidisciplinary approach to the management of critical limb ischaemia. Critical limb ischaemia occurs when a previously stenotic lesion progresses to occlusion, with consequent thrombosis both proximal and distal to the lesion. This may occur both in native vessels, most commonly the superficial femoral artery, and in femoropopliteal grafts. Clinical examination at the time of presentation is important to determine whether the limb is viable prior to starting thrombolysis. Signs of non-viability include progressive sensory loss, muscle paralysis and failure of skin reperfusion after pressure. In the UK, the commonly used thrombolytic agents are streptokinase and recombinant tissue plasminogen activator (rt-PA). Streptokinase is considerably cheaper than rt-PA but is antigenic and is best used only once for each patient. In addition, it has a relatively long half-life of 30 minutes and may be associated with a higher incidence of side effects. rt-PA is approximately four times as expensive as streptokinase but has a shorter half-life of approximately 8 minutes and is non-antigenic.

Following angiography to establish the site of occlusion, a catheter is advanced until its tip is embedded in the thrombus. A guidewire may be used to macerate the clot before infusion of the lytic agent, and sometimes a bolus of rt-PA is given in small aliquots along the length of the thrombus to initiate lysis. A low-dose infusion of thrombolytic agent is then given (typically 0.5–1.0 mg/hour of rt-PA) with concomitant heparinization. Check angiograms are performed at intervals of several hours until clearing of the thrombus load and demonstration of the underlying vessels has been achieved. At this stage, balloon PTA or stent insertion can be performed to correct the underlying lesion, or if this is not possible the patient can go on to surgery. Alternative radiological procedures to catheter-directed thrombolysis include suction embolectomy, in which a large-bore catheter is used to aspirate clots, and mechanical thrombectomy, which uses impeller-driven saline jets to macerate and then aspirate thrombus. These techniques have a limited application but may be useful in cases of severe

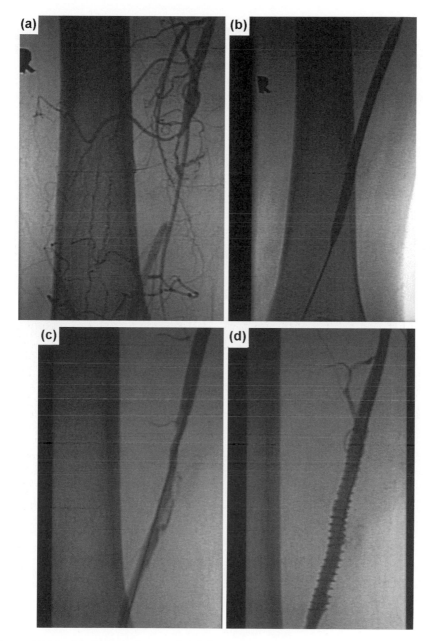

Figure 15.12 (a) Occluded superficial femoral artery. (b) Balloon angioplasty. (c) Result following angioplasty. (d) Result following stenting

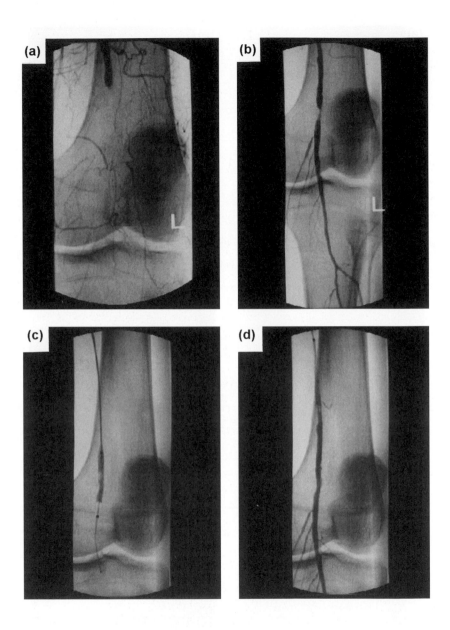

Figure 15.13   (a) Angiogram showing popliteal occlusion. (b) Following overnight thrombolysis. (c) Angioplasty. (d) Final result

ischaemia in which rapid restoration of flow is needed. Thrombolysis is successful in up to 80% of cases in suitable situations, but this is a potentially hazardous therapy with an expected mortality of around 5%. Most complications are haemorrhagic, with a 1–3% risk of haemorrhagic stroke[25,26].

Case No. 5

Figure 15.13a shows the angiogram of a 72 year-old patient who presented with sudden onset of pain and coldness in his right leg. There was complete occlusion of the popliteal artery with no obvious distal vessel filling. Following overnight thrombolysis the artery was patent and a severe stenosis was revealed (Figure 15.13b). Balloon angioplasty was performed (Figure 15.13c) and normal flow was restored (Figure 15.13d).

Other forms of intervention

Many other devices have been described in the treatment of atherosclerotic peripheral vascular disease, including laser angioplasty and atherectomy, but none has been shown to offer any significant advantage over balloon angioplasty. Brachytherapy, the use of irradiation to reduce intimal proliferation, has shown promising early results and is likely to become more widely used in peripheral vessels. The possibility of local administration of endothelial modifying factors to reduce re-stenosis is currently under intensive investigation.

CONCLUSION

Modern imaging techniques play a major part in the assessment of the diabetic patient with foot problems, and the interventional radiologist has a significant role in their management. Close cooperation between the diabetologist, vascular surgeon and interventional radiologist is essential to maximize the chances of a successful outcome for the patient.

REFERENCES

1. Tawn DJ, O'Hare JP, O'Brien IAD, Watt I, Dieppe PA, Corrall RJM. Bone scintigraphy and radiography in the early recognition of diabetic osteopathy. *Br J Radiol* 1988; **61**: 273–9.
2. Yuh WTC, Corson JD, Baraniewski HM et al. Osteomyelitis of the foot in diabetic patients: evaluation with plain film. Tc-MDP bone scintigraphy and MR imaging. *Am J Radiol* 1989; **152**: 795–800.

3. Garcia MJ, Macnamara PM, Gordon T et al. Morbidity and mortality in diabetics in the Framingham population: sixteen year follow-up study. *Diabetes* 1974; **23**: 105–11.

4. Conrad MC. Large and small artery occlusions in diabetics and non-diabetics with severe vascular disease. *Circulation* 1967; **36**: 83–91.

5. Rhodes GR, Rollins D, Sidaway AM et al. Popliteal to tibial *in situ* saphenous vein bypass for limb salvage in diabetic patients. *Am J Surg* 1987; **154**: 245–7.

6. Cofield RH, Morrison MJ, Beabout JW. Diabetic neuropathy in the foot: patient characteristics and patterns of radiographic change. *Foot Ankle* 1983; **4**: 15–22.

7. Kraft E, Spyropoulos E, Finby N. Neurological disorders of the foot in diabetes mellitus. *Am J Radiol* 1975; **124**: 17–24.

8. Mendelson EB, Fisher MR, Deschler TW et al. Osteomyelitis in the diabetic foot: a difficult diagnostic challenge. *Radiographics* 1983; **3**: 248–61.

9. Park HM, Wheat LJ, Siddiqui AR et al. Scintigraphic evaluation of diabetic osteomyelitis: concise communication. *J Nucl Med* 1982; **23**: 569–73.

10. Newman LG, Waller J, Palestro CJ et al. Unsuspected osteomyelitis in diabetic foot ulcers: diagnosis and monitoring by leukocyte scanning with Indium In lll Oxyquinoline. *J Am Med Ass* 1991; **226**: 1246–51.

11. Craig JG, Amin MB, Eyler WR. Osteomyelitis of the diabetic foot: MRI-pathologic correlation. *Radiology* 1997; **203**: 849–55.

12. Croll SD, Nicholas GG, Osbourne MA. Role of magnetic resonance imaging in the diagnosis of osteomyelitis in diabetic foot infections. *J Vasc Surg* 1996; **24**: 266–70.

13. Morrison WB, Schwitzer ME, Wapner KL. Osteomyelitis in feet of diabetics: clinical accuracy, surgical utility and cost-effectiveness of MR imaging. *Radiology* 1995; **196**: 557–64.

14. Blackband SJ, Buckley DL, Knowles AJ. Improved peripheral MR angiography with temperature regulation in healthy patients. *Radiology* 1996; **198**: 899–902.

15. Second European Concensus Document on Chronic Critical Leg Ischaemia. *Circulation* 1991; 84 (suppl IV): 1–26.

16. Krolewski AS, Warren JH. Epidemiology of diabetes mellitus. In Marble A, Kroll LP, Braley RS, Christleib AR, Souldner JS (eds), *Joslin's Diabetes Mellitus*, 12th edn. Philadelphia: Lea and Febiger, 1985; 12–42.

17. Edwards JM, Coldwell DM, Goldman ML, Strandnes DE Jr. The role of duplex scanning in the selection of patients for transluminal angioplasty. *J Vasc Surg* 1991; **13**: 69–74.

18. Larch E, Minar E, Ahmadi R et al. Value of duplex sonography for evaluation of tibio-peroneal arteries in patients with femoro-popliteal obstruction: a prospective comparison with antegrade intra-arterial digital subtraction angiography. *J Vasc Surg* 1997; **25**: 629–36.

19. Nawaz S, Cleveland T, Gaines PA, Chan P. Clinical risk associated with contrast angiography in Metformin-treated patients: a clinical review. *Clin Radiol* 1998; **53**: 342–4.

20. Dotter C, Judkins MP. Transluminal treatment of arteriosclerotic obstruction: description of a new technique and a preliminary report of its application. *Circulation* 1964; **30**: 654–70.

21. Gardiner GA, Meyerovitz MF, Stokes KR, Clouse ME, Harrington DP, Bettmann MA. Complications of transluminal angioplasty. *Radiology* 1986; **159**: 201–8.

22. Johnston W. Iliac arteries: re-analysis of results of balloon angioplasty. *Radiology* 1993; **186**: 207–12.

23. Johnston KW. Femoral and popliteal arteries: re-analysis of results of balloon angioplasty. *Radiology* 1992; **183**: 767–71.

24. Bosch JL, Hunink MGM. Meta-analysis of the results of percutaneous transluminal angioplasty and stent placement for aorto-iliac occlusive disease. *Radiology* 1997; **204**: 87–96.

25. Earnshaw JJ, Westby JC, Gregson RH et al. Local thrombolytic therapy of acute peripheral ischaemic with tissue plasminogen activator: a dose ranging study. *Br J Surg* 1988; **75**: 1196–200.

26. Berridge DC, Makin GS, Hopkinson BR. Local low dose intra-arterial thrombolytic therapy: the risk of stroke or major haemorrhage. *Br J Surg* 1989; **76**: 1230–3.

16

Peripheral Vascular Disease and Vascular Reconstruction

KEVIN G. MERCER and DAVID C. BERRIDGE

St James's University Hospital, Leeds, UK

In diabetic patients the combination of increased risk of peripheral vascular disease (PVD), a propensity for non-occlusive microvascular disease, increased prevalence of concomitant medical disease and the risks of poor wound healing present a complex challenge in vascular surgery. In many ways the general principles of vascular assessment and management still apply. The disease process is, however, substantially altered in diabetes. The high prevalence of concomitant disease and increased risk of postoperative complications (particularly infection) have a significant impact on the surgical decision-making process.

For some patients, therefore, a thorough vascular investigation leading to surgical or radiological intervention will form an important aspect of the management of diabetic foot problems. These patients, however, represent a minority of those attending for continuing foot care with an established medical service (Figure 16.1). Vascular intervention and follow-up represents an adjunct to, not a replacement for, good diabetic foot services.

PERIPHERAL VASCULAR DISEASE IN DIABETES

Diabetes is an important risk factor for the development of peripheral vascular disease. Chronic hyperglycaemia results in atherosclerosis, occurring with a much greater frequency than would be predicted by other risk factors, such as hypercholesterolaemia and smoking.

The Foot in Diabetes, 3rd edn. Edited by A. J. M. Boulton, H. Connor and P. R. Cavanagh.
© 2000 John Wiley & Sons, Ltd.

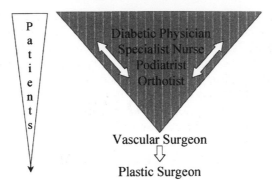

Figure 16.1 Diagrammatic representation of frequency and volume of patient's clinical needs in the management of diabetic foot problems

The atherosclerotic process is pathologically similar to that occurring in non-diabetic individuals; endothelial damage is followed by platelet aggregation, lipid accumulation, smooth muscle proliferation and plaque formation. The precise pathway for accelerated atherosclerosis in diabetes remains unclear and abnormalities of many of the systems involved in atherogenesis have been demonstrated.

Diabetes is associated with a dyslipidaemia involving the development of abnormal, potentially atherogenic, lipid profiles. Hypertriglyceridaemia and abnormalities of low density lipoproteins have both been demonstrated[1,2]. Increased endothelial adhesion molecule expression, in response to hyperglycaemia and oxidative stress, and abnormalities of adhesion of leukocytes and platelets[3] suggest that cell-mediated mechanisms may be involved. However, humoral factors, including pro-inflammatory cytokines and oxygen free radicals, have also been shown to have direct effects on endothelial, basement membrane and vascular smooth muscle cell function[2].

The anatomical distribution of atherosclerosis is altered in diabetes compared with that in the normal population. Iliac disease is more frequent and a particular predilection is seen for occlusion of the superficial femoral artery, profunda femoris and the tibial vessels. Stenoses also occur more frequently as focal and isolated changes in an otherwise relatively healthy arterial tree than in the non-diabetic population. The atherosclerotic process usually spares the arteries in the foot, and microvascular atherosclerosis is not present as frequently as has been suggested[4]. At the level of the microvasculature there are some functional abnormalities, with thickening of the capillary basement membrane producing abnormalities of nutrient exchange. These abnormalities are, however, very rarely so severe that significant benefit would not be gained from improved arterial flow[5].

Atherosclerosis in diabetes is characterized by early calcification of the media, resulting in hardening of the arterial walls. This is not to be confused with Mönckeberg's sclerosis, which is not necessarily associated with atherosclerosis. The relative incompressibility of arteries in diabetes can result in misleading clinical findings. When measuring the ankle brachial pressure index (ABPI), flow may be detectable below a cuff exerting pressures above systolic pressure, even when the true ankle arterial pressure is substantially reduced due to incompressible calcified arteries.

Another major abnormality of PVD in diabetes is the impairment of the development of collateral circulation, which results in an increased susceptibility to the effects of lesions in the principal vessels. It is this, rather than microvascular disease, which is now thought to result in the disproportionate effects of arterial lesions on distal nutrition. It has been suggested that "no occlusive microvascular disease of the diabetic foot exists that precludes revascularization." [5].

Detailed vascular investigation is therefore not only indicated in cases of a diabetic foot with signs of vascular insufficiency, but also in cases of delayed healing where initial examination appears to have excluded significant PVD. Relative sparing of foot arteries from atherosclerosis, peripheral pulse preservation with ischaemia, and the relative importance of focal lesions in diabetes all contribute to the high risk of clinically significant PVD in the absence of conventional clinical signs.

THE MULTIDISCIPLINARY TEAM

The management of peripheral vascular disease in diabetes is best achieved using a multidisciplinary team (Figure 16.2). The investigation of the vascular system to detect ischaemia and to identify significant vascular lesions will involve the vascular surgeon, the vascular laboratory and the vascular radiologist. Revascularization of the ischaemic limb may best be

Vascular Service

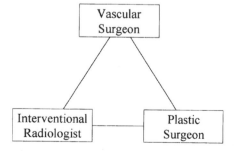

Figure 16.2 Trimodal vascular service

achieved by radiological intervention, local surgical procedures, bypass or combined procedures. The team approach allows the identification of the most appropriate treatment from an early stage.

In some cases assessment and treatment may also involve plastic surgery. The resolution of large ulcers or rapid, uncomplicated healing after a foot sparing amputation may be enhanced by tissue transfer techniques. These range from local tissue rotation techniques and the use of split skin grafts to the use of free myocutaneous flaps, which bring healthy tissue from the forearm or shoulder regions. These methods can, in appropriate cases, provide immediate coverage of a defect with healthy, well-perfused tissue[6].

For the patient undergoing these interventions, the question of multi-disciplinary nursing care is an important one. Patients will, at different phases of revascularization, require varying amounts of attention from the diabetologist, vascular surgeon, radiologist and plastic surgeon, podiatrist and chiropodist and nursing staff, which will at different phases favour one unit or another. The changes in the patient's medical status and requirements may be reflected in movement to the unit which addresses their most acute needs.

CLINICAL PRESENTATION

Diabetic patients may present to the vascular surgeon with symptoms of claudication and rest pain in the same way as non-diabetic individuals. PVD is graded on the basis of symptomatic criteria (Table 16.1), ranging from Grade 0, with minimal symptoms on maximal exercise testing, to Grade 3, with critical ischaemia leading to tissue loss[7].

Acute Presentation

Diabetic patients presenting with foot ulceration and infection comprise a more difficult diagnostic problem. In the non-diabetic population with PVD

Table 16.1   Presentation of lower limb ischaemia in diabetics

Chronic limb ischaemia
  Grade 0   Mild claudication
  Grade 1   Moderate to severe
                  claudication without
                  tissue loss or ischaemic
                  rest pain
Chronic critical ischaemia*
  Grade 2   Ischaemic rest pain
  Grade 3   Tissue loss due to ischaemic
                  ulceration or gangrene
	The acutely presenting diabetic foot may be associated with any degree of chronic limb ischaemia. Ischaemia may be critical or insignificant in the aetiology of ulceration infection and tissue necrosis

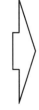

*Classification of chronic critical ischaemia based on reference 7.

the majority of ulceration represents Grade 3 disease. The investigation of ulcers requires assessment of the relative aetiological contributions of peripheral neuropathy, peripheral vascular disease and infection. Ulceration will occur as a result of Grade 3 disease but may also be present in the absence of arterial insufficiency or with Grade 0, 1 or 2 PVD. In these patients rapid assessment is indicated in order to establish the degree of ischaemia and the scope for vascular intervention. In suitable patients the relief of foot ischaemia improves wound healing and contributes to prevention of uncontrolled infections which would, if allowed to develop, lead inevitably to amputation.

SELECTING PATIENTS FOR VASCULAR RECONSTRUCTION

Ulceration in the diabetic foot is multifactorial, with a principal contribution from peripheral neuropathy and variable elements of ischaemia and infection. Selection of patients for vascular intervention to facilitate ulcer healing depends on the identification of patients in whom ischaemia is a significant contributor to ulcer formation and failure to heal. In the non-diabetic population, the diagnosis of significant lower limb ischaemia is made based on elements of the history, physical examination and non-invasive investigation.

In some diabetic patients a history of intermittent claudication, rest pain and eventual tissue loss accompanied by loss of pulses in a pale cool limb may suggest ischaemia, and non-invasive assessment may reveal a reduced ABPI and reduced transcutaneous oxygen tension. In these patients ischaemia is a likely contributor to an ulcer and investigations to identify remediable lesions are indicated.

Significant neuropathy, infection and the presence of ulceration may, however, mask the symptoms and signs of peripheral vascular disease or make interpretation difficult. Claudication and rest pain may not be present and tissue loss may not be ischaemic in origin. Skin changes can result from neuropathy, pulses may be impossible to assess under inflamed, ulcerated, oedematous skin, and cold and pallor may be masked by infection. Segmental pressure measurement is also potentially unreliable. In many cases, therefore, the clinical picture may not clearly identify the ischaemic limb.

The most reliable non-invasive investigations to detect ischaemia are the ABPI of the peroneal artery, which is relatively spared from calcification of the media; toe pressures; and analysis of the Doppler waveform. Reduced toe pressure and damping of the Doppler waveform may both indicate significant ischaemia in the difficult clinical picture. Colour duplex

sonography is gaining increasing reliability in the non-invasive investigation of PVD, and magnetic resonance angiography (MRA) shows great
promise as a modality of the future.

NON-INVASIVE INVESTIGATION

Doppler Pressures

The systolic arterial blood pressure at the ankle is measured using
sphygmomanometer, with an appropriately sized cuff, and a hand-held
Doppler probe. The cuff is applied to the lower calf and the Doppler probe
positioned to detect pulsatile flow in each artery at the ankle in turn. The
cuff is inflated and deflated to detect the pressure at which blood flow
ceases. The highest of the three systolic pressures is expressed as a ratio to
the Doppler systolic pressure measured in the brachial artery to give the
ABPI for each lower limb. A reduction in ABPI reflects a reduction in
perfusion pressure in the foot and the degree of ischaemia in peripheral
vascular disease.

Doppler pressures can also be measured segmentally using cuffs applied
to the thigh, upper calf and lower calf to infer the level of occlusion as
femoropopliteal, proximal or distal tibial vessel. Interpretation of Doppler
pressures in diabetes is, however, complicated by the problem of tibial
arteries becoming incompressible because of calcification of the intima,
which occurs independently of occlusive arterial disease. In this situation
flow can be maintained distal to compression by a cuff exerting a pressure
well above systolic. In diabetes, therefore, Doppler pressures correlate
poorly with symptoms and angiographic findings. The ankle pressure
measured in the peroneal artery may be more sensitive in detecting PVD
because it is relatively spared from intimal calcification.

The peripheral systolic pressure may also be measured in the toes using
digit cuffs and photoplethysmography. A combination of ankle and toe
pressures has been shown to predict primary wound healing[8]. Toe
pressures, however, can false-positively suggest peripheral vascular
disease, as reduced pressures have been demonstrated in limbs affected
by peripheral neuropathy in the absence of significant PVD or ischaemia.

Transcutaneous Oxygen Tension (TcP$_{O_2}$)

The partial pressure of oxygen (P_{O_2}) in tissues reflects the balance between
oxygen supply from the circulation and utilization. Tissue oxygen tension is
reduced in ischaemia due to peripheral vascular disease and can be
measured non-invasively in the vascular laboratory. The partial pressure of
oxygen equilibrates transcutaneously with an electrolyte solution in a

chamber held in contact with the skin. The TcP_{O_2} is measured using a probe to measure the P_{O_2} in the solution. A low TcP_{O_2} reflects the degree of tissue ischaemia and increases with successful intervention. In diabetes, TcP_{O_2} is lower than in the matched arteriopathic patients, a TcP_{O_2} of less than 40 mmHg is associated with failure of wound healing, and increased TcP_{O_2} after intervention predicts success of angioplasty and wound healing more accurately than changes in ABPI[9].

Doppler Waveform Analysis

In peripheral vascular disease, the normal, triphasic, waveform detectable using Doppler waveform analysis is damped distal to haemodynamically significant lesions. In diabetes, damping of the waveform may indicate PVD; however, diabetic neuropathy has been shown to be related to abnormalities of Doppler waveform in the dorsalis pedis artery in the absence of PVD[10].

Colour Duplex Sonography (CDS)

Ultrasound of the peripheral vascular system has been greatly enhanced by duplex-Doppler imaging. Ultrasound imaging, enhanced by colour flow representation and Doppler waveform analysis, can be used to detect and characterize haemodynamically significant lesions in larger vessels with 90% accuracy and predicts final surgical intervention as accurately as does angiography. It has therefore been suggested that CDS may replace contrast angiography in the investigation of PVD[11]. Ultrasound resolution at present limits its use in assessing distal vessels for limb salvage procedures; however, no single modality can accurately identify foot vessels as suitable for a distal anastomosis.

Contrast Angiography

Non-invasive investigation, using a combination of modalities, can in most cases detect clinically significant ischaemia and will identify most lesions of the larger vessels that are amenable to intervention. At present, however, despite full non-invasive investigation it is impossible to exclude surgically correctable lesions because of the problems of imaging disease in, and determining patency of, distal vessels.

Angiography offers a further imaging modality which may help with the assessment of the distal vasculature but also provides a "road map" for planning surgical intervention. It is therefore indicated in cases of delayed ulcer healing as well as those in which preliminary vascular assessment has identified significant ischaemia. Best quality images are obtained with intra-arterial digital subtraction angiograms, with antegrade studies if necessary.

Magnetic Resonance Angiography (MRA)

The developing technology of magnetic resonance imaging is now beginning to offer accurate vascular imaging as an alternative to contrast angiography. The development of gadolinium enhancement and protocols for time-of-flight analysis has resulted in high-resolution MRA which may, in the future, replace angiography[12]. MRA can now accurately detect haemodynamically significant stenoses and occlusions and can resolve images of digital vessels and run-off vessels 1 mm in diameter. Availability of MRA currently prevents its routine use; in selected cases, however, it may offer an important imaging modality and increasing use seems likely.

PRE-OPERATIVE ASSESSMENT

One of the aims of the St Vincent Declaration on diabetes care made by the World Health Organization and International Diabetic Federation in 1991 was a reduction in rates of major lower limb amputation for diabetic gangrene[13]. Achieving this goal requires a rigorous approach to limb salvage based on medical, paramedical and surgical intervention and care. The elderly diabetic population in whom diabetic foot diseases occur are affected by many other medical problems. Assessment and control of these factors is important for successful limb salvage and patient survival after vascular reconstruction.

Ischaemic Heart Disease

Pre-operative assessment of patients for peripheral vascular reconstruction should routinely include assessment of cardiac status, including history of hypertension, angina and myocardial infarction (MI) and ECG. In diabetic patients, previous symptomatic ischaemic heart disease (IHD) carries a four-fold risk of cardiac complication. However, previously asymptomatic individuals contribute significantly to the 5% overall risk of MI or cardiac death[14]. Previous "silent" MI may produce an unsuspectedly poor cardiac reserve, and slow post-operative recovery may reflect a peri-operative ischaemic event.

Cerebrovascular Disease

Previous severe disabling stroke would be a relative contra-indication to major vascular reconstruction for limb salvage for patients who would return rapidly to their usual state of wheelchair mobility by considering primary amputation.

Renal Impairment

Impaired renal function as a result of renal artery or small vessel disease is an important factor in vascular assessment. Contrast arteriography carries with it significant risks of renal failure or increased renal impairment, particularly in patients with existing impaired renal function and diabetes. For these patients it is particularly important to maintain good urine output, using intravenous fluids to maintain hydration. Diuretics are used in some regimens for renal protection; however, loop diuretics have been linked to adverse effects on renal function in some studies. MRA and CO_2 arteriography[15] may, in the future, be important modes of investigation in patients at particular risk of renal complications. Close operative monitoring of renal function is also essential in this group of patients.

Proliferative Retinopathy

Diabetic retinopathy may influence decisions regarding the use of thrombolysis to salvage occluded grafts. Thrombolysis carries a risk of sight-threatening occular haemorrhage.

Diabetic Control

In the presence of significant sepsis, diabetic control is frequently lost and some patients are at potential risk of developing diabetic keto-acidosis. The acute presentation of the diabetic foot may also be heralded by development of uncontrolled diabetes. Methods of diabetes control in the peri-operative period vary and several methods can be utilized. In the setting of poor glycaemic control due to sepsis, a regimen of intravenous dextrose and potassium with an intravenous sliding scale of insulin based on blood glucose measurements is frequently employed.

Risk of Infection

Some of the factors that contribute to the development of foot ulcers also result in increased risks of complications following surgical intervention. Long-standing diabetes is associated with poor wound healing, which may be related to poor nutrient transfer due to small vessel disease. Additionally, diabetes, particularly when poorly controlled, is associated with increased susceptibility to wound infection. The combination of poor wound healing and susceptibility to wound infection may require an alternative antibiotic policy and extra vigilance for wound-related complications. The risks of wound-related complications are also important with respect to the use of prosthetic graft materials for reconstruction.

VASCULAR SURGERY FOR THE DIABETIC FOOT

General Considerations

Major vascular reconstruction requires prolonged anaesthesia and represents a significant risk of major postoperative morbidity and mortality, particularly in patients with other long-term complications. Surgical planning should therefore include consideration of the minimal intervention that will achieve successful healing and control of symptoms and, if vascular reconstruction is indicated, whether the probability of success and risk of complications are acceptable. Planning surgery should attend particularly to the arterial inflow to the limb, the availability of a suitable distal outflow vessel for anastomosis, and the surgery required to remove devitalized or infected tissue from the distal extremity to allow healing.

Consideration should also be given to the alternatives to general anaesthesia that are available in high-risk patients. Techniques of regional anaesthesia, including spinal and epidural methods, may be suitable for selected patients and selected operations, although not when cephalic and basilic veins are to be obtained and used as a graft conduit.

An important aspect of planning surgical intervention is the immediacy of the clinical situation. The presentation ranges from chronic ulceration to fulminant limb-threatening infection. In chronic cases, vascular reconstruction may only be a consideration if more conservative methods fail to achieve ulcer healing. More acute presentations will require a rapid assessment of the prospect for limb salvage, the role of tissue debridement and vascular intervention.

The Emergency Diabetic Foot

For patients presenting with rapidly progressive tissue loss due to infection and/or ischaemia, the disease process represents a significant risk of limb loss and mortality. A rapid assessment is required of whether the degree of necrosis and infection can be controlled by local debridement or minor amputation and, second whether ischaemia is an aetiological factor. In the acute situation, the diagnosis of ischaemia may not be possible before intervention to control localized infection and, if major amputation is not required due to extensive necrosis of the weightbearing areas, drainage and debridement can be undertaken as a primary procedure.

After local control of infection, and because of the difficulties of diagnosing ischaemia non-invasively, an intensive vascular assessment will frequently be indicated. Colour duplex ultrasound may satisfactorily identify lesions suitable for angioplasty in many situations; however, angiography will be more readily available and will, in any case, be required to perform angioplasty and assess the arterial system for reconstructive surgery. Depending upon the patient's premorbid condition, the extent of the necrosis and infection, and the pattern of any arterial disease, a decision can be made as to the best combination of angioplasty, stent insertion, debridement, endovascular and vascular surgical reconstruction.

Planning Vascular Surgery (Table 16.2)

Inflow

Planning vascular surgery in suitable patients follows the basic principle of correction of haemodynamically significant proximal lesions before more distal disease. The success of any reconstruction below the inguinal ligament is largely dependent on satisfactory inflow and in some cases, even with significant distal arterial disease, improved inflow to a limb may be sufficient to allow healing. Radiological intervention, such as percutaneous transluminal angioplasty (PTA) and stenting of iliac lesions, is dealt with in Chapter 15.

Surgical approaches to inflow disease are divided into those designed to improve flow through native vessels and operations that bypass diseased or

Table 16.2 Cascade of surgical and radiological intervention for PVD (proximal before distal)

Focal lesions stenosis/short segment occlusion	Optimization of inflow and limb perfusion by radiological intervention
Iliac disease without iliac inflow	Aorto-(bi-)iliac
	Aorto-(bi-)femoral
	Axillo-(bi-)femoral
Iliac disease with ipsilateral inflow	Ipsilateral iliofemoral
Iliac disease with contralateral inflow	Contralateral iliofemoral
	Femoro-femoral cross-over
Femoral artery bifurcation disease	Profundaplasty
	Endarterectomy
Femoropopliteal disease	Femoropopliteal (AK)
	Femoropopliteal (BK)
Popliteal trifurcation disease	SFA/popliteal–crural
	Femorocrural
Crural disease	SFA/popliteal pedal
	Femoropedal

SFA=superficial femoral artery.

occluded vessels. Focal stenosis due to atheroma can reduce flow through native vessels and may not always be suitable for radiological intervention. This commonly occurs at the bifurcation of the common femoral artery into profunda femoris and the superficial femoral artery. In this position PTA risks occluding the branch arteries, which can worsen the situation. The stenosis can be corrected by a surgical angioplasty. The exposed and clamped artery is opened longitudinally over the stenotic segment, atheroma is removed from the three vessels by careful endarterectomy, and the arteriotomy closed using a patch of native vein or synthetic material such as dacron. The arteriotomy and patch closure can be extended onto the profunda femoris to perform a profundaplasty.

Operations to improve inflow by bypassing iliac occlusive disease include iliofemoral bypass, contralateral or unilateral as appropriate, and femoro-femoral cross-over. Similarly, for bilateral disease, transabdominal aorto-(bi-)iliac or (bi-)femoral bypass represent major surgical interventions, whereas axillo-(bi-)femoral bypass offers a less invasive, but haemodynamically inferior, procedure. Improved proximal inflow may be sufficient to promote healing and relieve symptoms. Once satisfactory inflow has been achieved, infra-inguinal reconstruction may be appropriate to improve more distal circulation.

Infra-inguinal Reconstruction

Bypass of arterial occlusions distal to the inguinal ligament requires a suitable inflow vessel, without any more proximal obstruction to flow, and a suitable distal vessel for the outflow anastomosis. In diabetes, arterial disease may be isolated to the popliteal trifurcation or proximal tibial vessels and inflow may, therefore, more frequently be taken from the distal superficial femoral or proximal popliteal arteries than in the general vascular population[16–19].

The longevity of the graft is partially dependent upon the level and quality of the outflow vessel (Figures 16.3, 16.4). The distal vessel may be identified by dependent Doppler ultrasound, pulse-generated run-off or on arteriographic images and these all give information about the quality of the distal vessel and the run-off from it.

The decision as to the level of the distal anastomosis depends upon the level and quality of the available distal vessels. Patency is better for grafts to more proximal vessels. This observation, however, may reflect the more limited disease pattern seen in patients with suitable vessels at this level. Anastomosis to a diseased vessel is technically demanding and risks early graft occlusion because of disease close to the anastomosis and, therefore, anastomosis to a healthy, more distal vessel is essential if one is available (Figures 16.3, 16.4). For distal vascular reconstructions, an important

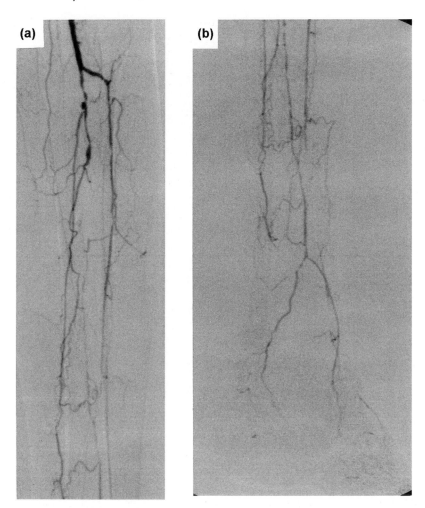

Figure 16.3 Selection of outflow vessel for infra-inguinal reconstruction. The digital subtraction angiogram shows a patent below knee popliteal artery but with severely diseased run-off in all three tibial vessels (a) which occlude in the calf. Collateral vessels reconstitute just above the ankle in a peroneal artery with patent, but diseased, anterior and posterior branches. In this case a graft to the below knee popliteal is at high risk of occlusion due to poor run-off (b); however, the less than perfect ankle vessel makes a decision regarding distal anastomosis a difficult one

component of arterial run-off is the dorsal pedal arch. An angiographically intact arch is an important determinant of the success and survival of a graft to the distal vessels[20].

In diabetic patients, the prevalence of disease in the tibial vessels dictates a femorodistal approach more frequently than in the general population.

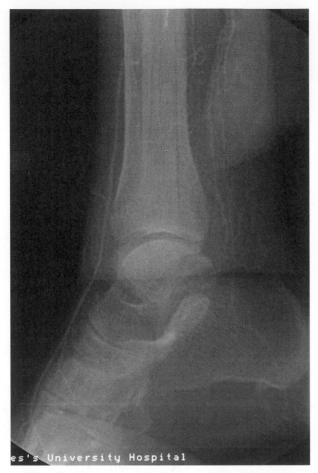

Figure 16.4 Healthy distal vessel for outflow anastomosis. In a limb displaying otherwise severe atheromatous disease, a patent and angiographically healthy anterior tibial/dorsalis pedis artery running into a patent pedal arch is available for distal anastomosis

The relative sparing of foot vessels from the atherosclerotic process in diabetes makes femoropedal surgery a relatively frequent option in reconstruction.

Choice of Conduit—Autogenous Vein Should be Used Whenever Possible

Infra-inguinal bypass is technically feasible using either autogenous vein or synthetic materials, such as expanded polytetrafluoroethylene (PTFE), as a conduit. General vascular surgical practice favours the use of autogenous vein whenever possible because long-term patency is significantly better for vein grafts. In diabetic patients, the preferential use of autogenous vein is particularly important because of an increased risk of occlusion[21]. Such patients are also at increased risk of prosthetic graft infection, which carries a significant risk of amputation and death.

The ipsilateral long saphenous vein (LSV) offers the first source of autogenous vein; a satisfactory vessel may be used, employing *in situ*, reversed or non-reversed techniques, depending upon the quality and dimensions of the vessel and the anatomical bypass type. In the absence of a suitable vessel, however, the contralateral LSV, the short saphenous, basilic and cephalic veins or grafts spliced using vein from different sources are all available as sources of autogenous material before a synthetic graft must be contemplated.

The result of these deliberations should be a planned procedure that will provide durable revascularization to the extremity and improve the rate and probability of healing of that extremity. The patient should understand the principles of the procedure, the potential benefits and also the risks associated with the surgery.

Surveillance

Occlusion of infra-inguinal bypass grafts leading to recurrent foot ischaemia requires major intervention. Thrombolytic therapy may achieve graft patency but there is a significant risk of haemorrhagic complications locally and systemically, including fatal or disabling intracerebral bleeding. Patients in whom thrombolysis cannot be used or in whom it fails will require further bypass surgery or risk amputation[22].

In order to reduce graft failure rates, graft surveillance is undertaken to detect haemodynamically significant lesions in inflow or outflow vessels or the graft itself. In the outpatient situation, repeated measures of the ABPI may detect a falling foot perfusion and indicate the need for further investigation. The gold standard for non-invasive graft surveillance, however, is duplex scanning[23,24]. A postoperative duplex scan performed in the first week after operation followed by further scans at intervals of 4 weeks, 3, 6, 9 and 12 months, and 6 monthly thereafter, can be used to detect lesions requiring correction to prevent graft failure. Detected lesions are further investigated, frequently with angiography, and amenable lesions corrected by radiological or surgical means. Successful correction is followed by continued graft surveillance (Figure 16.5).

Results of Infra-inguinal Reconstruction in Diabetics

With close attention to pre-operative assessment, surgical planning, surgical technique and interventional graft surveillance, excellent rates of secondary

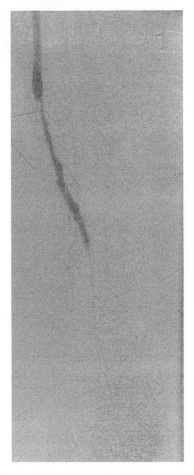

Figure 16.5 High grade stenosis in femoro-distal bypass graft. Three years after a femoro-dorsalis pedis graft using a composite vein graft a high grade stenosis, which required surgical intervention, was detected, on duplex surveillance, at the junction between the two segments of vein used

graft patency (82–98%) and limb salvage (76–89%) can be achieved (Table 16.3). Graft patency and limb salvage rates are similar to those for non-diabetic patients[31–33].

ADJUNCTIVE PLASTIC SURGERY

For the majority of patients undergoing peripheral vascular reconstruction, improved tissue perfusion and good nursing care will allow healing of an ulcer or minor amputation wound. Even in cases where a minor amputation

Table 16.3 Results of infra-inguinal bypass in diabetic patients

Reference	n	DM (%)	Details	Follow-up (months)	Primary patency (%)	Secondary patency (%)	Limb salvage (%)	Survival (%)
25	54	100	65%, distal	24	66	75	83	84
26	56	100	Pedal with infection	36	92	–	98	84
27	33	100	Pedal	12	76	89	89	82
18	124	100	Popliteal-distal	36	85	89	–	–
16	32	100	Popliteal-distal	36	75 (24 months)	89	82	–
17	75	100	Below knee inflow	60	72	76	–	–
28	384	95	Pedal		–	82	87	57
19	156	95	Pedal		–	87	92	–
29	96	94	Pedal	18	–	82	87	80
30	46	80	Pedal	24	72	–	89	–

wound has been left open because of local residual infection, delayed closure or healing by secondary intention will frequently eventually achieve a satisfactory result.

In some cases, however, healing may be achieved more rapidly using adjunctive plastic surgical techniques. Early resolution of the pain from ulcers or amputation sites is an aid to early mobilization and, therefore, rehabilitation. An intact epithelial surface is also an important barrier to further infection, which may delay wound or ulcer healing.

Split Skin Grafting

Split skin grafting may be useful in order to expedite healing of ulcers and areas of wound breakdown where healthy granulation tissue is present. The graft, which consists of the epidermis and superficial capillary dermis, is cut from the donor area using a dermatome and transferred to the recipient site. The donor site heals by regrowth of the skin from epidermal appendages not removed by the dermatome, such as hair follicles. Perforation of the graft and an appropriate dressing prevent separation of the graft from the healthy vascular bed and ensure maximum "take".

Free Tissue Transfer[6]

In cases where deep ulceration or infection require extensive debridement or minor amputation, surgery may leave bone exposed and remaining healthy tissue may not be sufficient to achieve primary or secondary closure. In these cases, secondary healing will also be delayed and there is a particular risk of limb-threatening infection where bone is exposed; such wounds are unsuitable for split skin grafting because of the lack of a highly vascular recipient site. In some of these cases early primary or secondary closure can be achieved by free tissue transfer.

Free tissue transfer involves the isolation of a pedicle of tissue consisting of blood supply, overlying skin and the underlying vascular bed, frequently a muscle. The vessels of the myocutaneous flap are anastomosed to suitable inflow and drainage vessels. These may be native vessels or, in the case of vascular surgical cases, inflow may be from a graft. The flap can then be used to close the skin defect on the limb.

Donor sites for free flaps include the radial aspect of the forearm, the parascapular region, latissimus dorsi, temporalis and rectus abdominis. In each of these sites tissue can be obtained with a reliable anatomic blood supply. Removal of the tissue and supplying vessels does not compromise local blood supply or significantly affect the function of the remaining muscle groups. Choice of donor site depends upon the area and volume of skin coverage required and factors related to patient and surgeon preferences.

Myocutaneous free flaps achieve rapid coverage of the tissue defect and provide a mass of healthy tissue with a good blood supply in the area of ischaemic damage. The operative procedure, however, is associated with marked haemodynamic and surgical stresses and frequently requires a second prolonged anaesthetic. The procedure is frequently best delayed until the bypass graft has demonstrated early patency and satisfactory radiological imaging. This also allows control of local infection by the initial debridement and revascularization and further debridement of non-viable tissue at the time of second operation, and reduces the risk of loss of the flap due to early failure of graft.

SYMPATHECTOMY

In some cases, arterial disease is so extensive as to preclude any sort of arterial reconstruction and for some of these patients, who have extensive infection or necrosis, major amputation is required. For others, however, although circulation is tenuous, the ulcers are painful and healing is extremely slow, although limb loss is not inevitable. In these patients interruption of the sympathetic nerve supply to the vessels of the lower limb, producing vasodilatation, can be used to increase limb blood flow. Open lumbar sympathectomy using an extraperitoneal operative approach has largely been superseded by sympathetic ablation, by injection of phenol under fluoroscopic control. The procedure produces rapid increases in blood flow and limb temperature and is associated with pain relief and ulcer healing in 58% of patients[34]. Benefit may still be obtained in the diabetic patient who appears to have already lost sympathetic tone.

REFERENCES

1. O'Neal DN, Lewicki J, Ansari MZ, Matthews PG, Best JD. Lipid levels and peripheral vascular disease in diabetic and non-diabetic subjects. *Atherosclerosis* 1998; **136**: 1–8.
2. Kamal K, Powell RJ, Sumpio BE. The pathobiology of diabetes mellitus: implications for surgeons. *J Am Coll Surg* 1996; **183**: 271–89.
3. Brown AS, Hong Y, de Belder A et al. Megakaryocyte ploidy and platelet changes in human diabetes and atherosclerosis. *Arterioscler Thromb Vasc Biol* 1997; **17**: 802–7.
4. LoGerfo FW, Gibbons GW. Vascular disease of the lower extremities in diabetes mellitus. *Endocrinol Metabol Clin N Am* 1996; **25**: 439–45.
5. Gibbons GW. Vascular evaluation and long-term results of distal bypass surgery in patients with diabetes. *Clin Podiat Med Surg* 1995; **12**: 129–40.
6. Karp NS, Kasabian AK, Siebert JW, Eidelman Y, Colen S. Microvascular free-flap salvage of the diabetic foot: a 5-year experience. *Plastic Recon Surg* 1994; **94**: 834–40.
7. Rutherford RB, Baker JD, Ernst C et al. Recommended standards for reports dealing with lower extremity ischemia: revised version. *J Vasc Surg* 1997; **26**: 517–38.
8. Apelqvist J, Castenfors J, Larsson J, Stenstrom A, Agardh C-D. Prognostic value of systolic ankle and toe blood pressure levels in outcome of diabetic foot ulcer. *Diabet Care* 1989; **12**: 373–8.
9. Hanna GP, Fujise K, Kjellgren O et al. Infrapopliteal transcatheter interventions for limb salvage in diabetic patients: importance of aggressive interventional approach and role of transcutaneous oximetry. *J Am Coll Cardiol* 1997; **30**: 664–9.
10. Chew JT, Tan SB, Sivathasan C, Pavanni R, Tan SK. Vascular assessment in the neuropathic diabetic foot. *Clin Orthopaed Rel Res* 1995; **3/2**: 95–100.
11. Aly S, Sommerville K, Adiseshiah M, Raphael M, Coleridge SP, Bishop CC. Comparison of duplex imaging and arteriography in the evaluation of lower limb arteries. *Br J Surg* 1998; **85**: 1099–102.
12. Velazquez OC, Baum RA, Carpenter JP. Magnetic resonance angiography of lower-extremity arterial disease. *Surg Clin N Am* 1998; **78**: 519–37.
13. Krans HMJ, Porta M, Keen H and Staehr Johansen K. *Diabetes Care and Research in Europe: the St Vincent Declaration Action Programme Implementation Document*, 2nd edn. Copenhagen: World Health Organization.
14. Hood DB, Weaver FA, Papanicolaou G, Wadhwani A, Yellin AE. Cardiac evaluation of the diabetic patient prior to peripheral vascular surgery. *Ann Vasc Surg* 1996; **10**: 330–5.
15. Seeger JM, Self S, Harward TR, Flynn TC, Hawkins IF Jr. Carbon dioxide gas as an arterial contrast agent. *Ann Surg* 1993; **217**: 688–97.
16. Mohan CR, Hoballah JJ, Martinasevic M et al. Revascularization of the ischemic diabetic foot using popliteal artery inflow. *Int Angiol* 1996; **15**: 138–43.
17. Woelfle KD, Lange G, Mayer H, Bruijnen H, Loeprecht H. Distal vein graft reconstruction for isolated tibioperoneal vessel occlusive disease in diabetics with critical foot ischaemia—does it work? *Eur J Vasc Surg* 1993; **7**: 409–13.

18. Stonebridge PA, Tsoukas AI, Pomposelli FB Jr et al. Popliteal-to-distal bypass grafts for limb salvage in diabetics. *Eur J Vasc Surg* 1991; **5**: 265–9.
19. Pomposelli FB Jr, Jepsen SJ, Gibbons GW et al. A flexible approach to infrapopliteal vein grafts in patients with diabetes mellitus. *Arch Surg* 1991; **126**: 724–9.
20. O'Mara CS, Flinn WR, Neiman HL, Bergan JJ, Yao JS. Correlation of foot arterial anatomy with early tibial bypass patency. *Surg* 1981; **89**: 743–52.
21. Williams MR, Mikulin T, Lemberger J, Hopkinson BR, Makin GS. Five year experience using PTFE vascular grafts for lower limb ischaemia. *Ann R Coll Surg Engl* 1985; **67**: 152–5.
22. Berridge DC, al-Kutoubi A, Mansfield AO, Nicolaides AN, Wolfe JH. Thrombolysis in arterial graft thrombosis. *Eur J Vasc Endovasc Surg* 1995; **9**: 129–32.
23. Moody P, Gould DA, Harris PL. Vein graft surveillance improves patency in femoro-popliteal bypass. *Eur J Vasc Surg* 1990; **4**: 117–21.
24. Bergamini TM, George SMJ, Massey HT et al. Intensive surveillance of femoropopliteal–tibial autogenous vein bypasses improves long-term graft patency and limb salvage. *Ann Surg* 1995; **221**: 507–15.
25. Kwolek CJ, Pomposelli FB, Tannenbaum GA et al. Peripheral vascular bypass in juvenile-onset diabetes mellitus: are aggressive revascularization attempts justified? *J Vasc Surg* 1992; **15**: 394–400: discussion, 400 *et seq*.
26. Tannenbaum GA, Pomposelli FB Jr, Marcaccio EJ et al. Safety of vein bypass grafting to the dorsal pedal artery in diabetic patients with foot infections. *J Vasc Surg* 1992; **15**: 982–90.
27. Isaksson L, Lundgren F. Vein bypass surgery to the foot in patients with diabetes and critical ischaemia. *Br J Surg* 1994; **81**: 517–20.
28. Pomposelli FB Jr, Marcaccio EJ, Gibbons GW et al. Dorsalis pedis arterial bypass: durable limb salvage for foot ischemia in patients with diabetes mellitus. *J Vasc Surg* 1995; **21**: 375–84.
29. Pomposelli FB Jr, Jepsen SJ, Gibbons GW et al. Efficacy of the dorsal pedal bypass for limb salvage in diabetic patients: short-term observations. *J Vasc Surg* 1990; **11**: 745–51: discussion, 751–2.
30. Quinones-Baldrich WJ, Colburn MD, Ahn SS, Gelabert HA, Moore WS. Very distal bypass for salvage of the severely ischemic extremity. *Am J Surg* 1993; **166**: 117–23: discussion, 123.
31. Rosenblatt MS, Quist WC, Sidawy AN, Paniszyn CC, LoGerfo FW. Results of vein graft reconstruction of the lower extremity in diabetic and nondiabetic patients. *Surg Gynecol Obstet* 1990; **171**: 331–5.
32. Karacagil S, Almgren B, Bowald S, Bergqvist D. Comparative analysis of patency, limb salvage and survival in diabetic and non-diabetic patients undergoing infrainguinal bypass surgery. *Diabet Med* 1995; **12**: 537–41.
33. Panayiotopoulos YP, Tyrrell MR, Arnold FJ, Korzon-Burakowska A, Amiel SA, Taylor PR. Results and cost analysis of distal (crural/pedal) arterial revascularization for limb salvage in diabetic and non-diabetic patients. *Diabet Med* 1997; **14**: 214–20.
34. Mashiah A, Soroker D, Pasik S, Mashiah T. Phenol lumbar sympathetic block in diabetic lower limb ischemia. *J Cardiovasc Risk* 1995; **2**: 467–9.

17

Charcot Foot: an Update on Pathogenesis and Management

ROBERT G. FRYKBERG

Des Moines University, Des Moines IA, USA

Neuro-arthropathy was first described in 1868 by J.-M. Charcot[1] and is sometimes called a Charcot joint or Charcot foot. Our current understanding of the pathogenesis and management of this condition has been enhanced by several key papers and thorough reviews of the subject over the previous three decades[2–7]. Although there has been an ultimate consolidation of purported aetiologic theories of neuro-arthropathic joints, a review of past and present literature reveals that there have been no novel changes in our approach to this disorder since the early classic works. However, the past 20 years have brought widespread attention to the diabetic neuro-arthropathic foot, and the reported increase in frequency of this condition may be due primarily to increased detection. Neuro-arthropathy is now recognized as an important complication of long-standing diabetes and peripheral neuropathy and is generally acknowledged as a predisposing risk factor for foot ulceration and subsequent amputation[7,8]. Many of these consequences can be averted through early detection of the acute neuro-arthropathic foot, a thorough understanding of its pathophysiology and a rational approach to management.

NATURAL HISTORY AND PATHOGENESIS

Much of the current understanding of the aetiopathogenesis of the neuro-arthropathic foot is based on clinical observation and case studies. There are

The Foot in Diabetes, 3rd edn. Edited by A. J. M. Boulton, H. Connor and P. R. Cavanagh.
© 2000 John Wiley & Sons, Ltd.

still few, if any, prospective observational studies that have systematically examined the variety of putative casual factors. Thus, much of the following discussion is based on authoritative opinion.

Neuro-arthropathy can be defined as a *relatively* painless, progressive and destructive arthropathy in single or multiple joints due to underlying neurologic deficits. Peripheral joints are most often affected, although involvement of the spine can occur. The location of the affected joint is dependent upon the nature of the disease causing the underlying neuropathy[7]. Many diseases can cause neuro-arthropathy, including tertiary syphilis (as Charcot originally described), diabetes mellitus, syringomyelia and leprosy (Hansen's disease) (Table 17.1). With this century's decline in frequency of patients with tabes dorsalis and the concomitant rise in numbers of persons with diabetes, the latter has become the most frequent cause of neuro-arthropathy. Certain diseases also have a predilection for specific sites of involvement. Tabes dorsalis, for instance, usually presents as a monoarticular involvement of large joints of the lower extremities such as the hip or knee. Conversely, syringomyelia involves the joints of the upper extremities, i.e. the shoulder, elbow and cervical vertebrae. In diabetes mellitus, the joints of the foot and ankle are characteristically involved.

Although some have postulated an intrinsic osseous defect in the neuropathic extremity, there have been no conclusive studies indicating a primary defect other than a relative osteopenia due to autonomic neuropathy[9–12]. It is likely that the pathogenesis of the neuro-arthropathic foot may be directly attributed to neuropathy and trauma. The neuropathic component consists of the classic sensorimotor polyneuropathy of diabetes involving both sensory and motor nerves[3,7,8]. There is some loss of peripheral sensation, which results in absent or diminished pain, vibratory sensation, proprioception and temperature perception. Additionally, the autonomic peripheral nerves are impaired, resulting in a "sympathetic failure" and attendant bone arteriovenous shunting, hypervascularity and demineralization[10,12]. The insensitivity of the distal extremity and the putative weakening of bone due to the neurally initiated "vascular reflex" place the foot at risk for injury and subsequent development of neuro-arthropathy.

Table 17.1 Diseases with potential for causing neuro-arthropathic joints

Diabetes mellitus	Congenital insensitivity to pain
Tertiary syphilis	Hysterical insensitivity to pain
Leprosy (Hansen's disease)	Paraplegia
Syringomyelia	Familial dysautonomia
Myelodysplasia	Peripheral nerve lesions
Pernicious anaemia	Spinal cord injuries
Multiple sclerosis	

When extrinsic trauma occurs, such as a trivial twisting or blunt injury, the osteopenic bone is ostensibly more likely to fracture (although this has not been studied prospectively). Absence of the protective sense of pain allows continued weightbearing on the injured foot, with consequent hyperaemic and inflammatory response to injury, resulting in increased blood flow and massive oedema. The insensitive joints are subjected to their extreme ranges of motion as capsular and ligamentous stretching or tearing result from the primary insult and subsequent joint effusions. Instability increases as weightbearing continues, with progressive joint laxity and eventual subluxation, even in the absence of a primary fracture. Dislocated articular surfaces grind on adjacent bone, causing osteochondral fragmentation and severe degeneration of joint architecture. The hypervascular response to injury promotes even more softening and resorption of bone. Further trauma (weightbearing) to these osteoporotic areas produces further destruction of the compromised joint, and a vicious cycle ensues. (Figure 17.1)

Often, an intra-articular or extra-articular fracture initiates the destructive process. Additionally, amputation of the great toe, often a consequence of osteomyelitis or gangrene, may lead to neuropathic joint changes in the adjacent lesser metatarsal–phalangeal joints (Figure 17.2). Presumably, this is a stress-related factor secondary to an acquired biomechanical deficiency[13]. Since intra-articular infections can also be implicated in the pathogenesis of neuro-arthropathy, it becomes apparent that any type of injury or inflammatory process introduced to a neuropathic joint has the potential for producing a neuro-arthropathic joint[3].

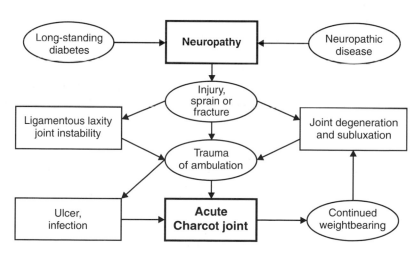

Figure 17.1 Pathogenesis of the neuro-arthropathic (Charcot) foot

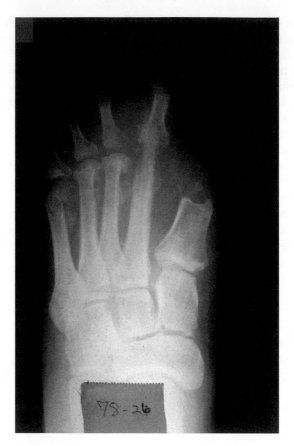

Figure 17.2   Osteolysis following great toe amputation

Eichenholtz[14] has divided the disease process into three stages based on pathologic findings. The *stage of development* is characterized by the acute destruction of the joint, with debris formation, osteochondral fragmentation, capsular distention, ligamentous laxity and subluxation. The *stage of coalescence* is marked by absorption of much of the debris and fusion of fragments to adjacent bone. Finally, *the stage of reconstruction* involves the remodelling of bone ends and fragments. This results in a lessening of the sclerosis and an attempt to restore joint architecture. Clinically, it is easier to separate the natural history of neuro-arthropathy into only two stages: *acute* or *chronic*. These distinctions will also facilitate and direct treatment[7,15]. The *acute* stage represents the active or destructive phase of the disease process, during which the joint is being actively destroyed. This would be consistent with Eichenholtz's "stage of development". The *chronic* (quiescent) stage represents the onset of the coalescence and reconstruction stages during which the body attempts to heal and restore stability to the involved joint(s)[6].

The fate of any neuro-arthropathic joint is greatly dependent upon the amount of destruction that has taken place during the acute process. This is directly a function of the amount of trauma or weightbearing sustained by the joint while in the stage of development. If such stress is continually introduced to the compromised neuropathic joint, the destructive cycle will be perpetuated, healing will be greatly prolonged, and the foot will maintain a poor prognosis. In these situations, the result is often significant deformity or pseudo-arthrosis, with attendant instability, abnormal weightbearing surfaces, ulceration and infection. If, however, the disease is diagnosed early and strict non-weightbearing is instituted, there will be an arrest in the joint destruction and an early conversion to the quiescent stage, with the benefit that there will be less morbidity and a greater likelihood of stable fusion or reconstruction taking place.

CLINICAL FEATURES

Various studies of diabetic neuro-arthropathic feet indicate a high incidence in patients with a duration of diabetes of 12 years or more, regardless of age[7,15–18]. Although most are in their sixth or seventh decade, these patients can range in age from their early 20s to late 70s, depending again on diabetes duration. There is no apparent predilection for either sex. In the majority of patients only one foot is affected, although bilateral involvement can be expected in 9–25% of cases[7,15,17,19,20]. Usually the diabetes has been poorly controlled, regardless of treatment or type of diabetes. Since neuropathic individuals might initially present with active neuro-arthropathic feet of several months' duration, they should be questioned carefully for even a remote history of injury. Almost invariably, there will be a history of previous trauma, which might include ligamentous sprains or fractures and surgery. One recent series reported that 73% of subjects could not remember a specific foot injury prior to onset of symptoms[15].

Neuropathy is always present to some degree, whether of recent onset or of long-standing duration. In Cofield's[17] large study of patients with peripheral neuropathy, 29% had bone and joint changes consistent with neuro-arthropathy. Neuropathic manifestations include loss or diminution of sensation to vibration, light touch, pin-prick and proprioception. Biothesiometer examination should reveal vibration thresholds of >25 volts and aesthesiometry deficits usually include loss of cutaneous perception of the 10 g Semmes–Weinstein monofilament. Deep tendon reflexes are often absent and the patients might have neuropathic symptoms, such as lancinating pains or muscle cramping. Peripheral and

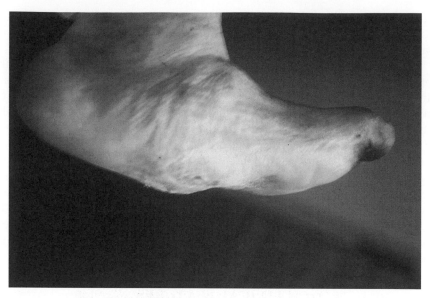

Figure 17.3   Rocker bottom deformity

central autonomic dysfunction might be evident through the appearance of excessively dry skin due to anhidrosis, orthostatic hypotension, abnormal cardiovascular autonomic function, gastroparesis or nocturnal diarrhoea[10,19].

The patient will often present with a markedly swollen foot which makes it difficult to wear ordinary footwear. A history of recent injury will often have preceded the onset of the swelling. Characteristically, neuro-arthropathic feet have been described as painless. However, pain or discomfort often accompanies the foot deformity, but to a degree much less than might be expected for such extensive pathology[21]. On examination, the foot might appear to be grossly deformed, with the classic "rocker bottom" subluxation of the midfoot (Figure 17.3). In early acute cases, however, minimal deformity will usually be present and might consist only of a prominence on the medial border of the foot. Ankle neuro-arthropathy, especially in later presentations, will be evidenced by medial or lateral deviation, with its associated instability (Figure 17.4). Regardless of specific site of involvement, the foot will reveal an element of hypermobility and crepitus due to the joint effusions, subluxations and destructive process taking place within it. The entire foot will often be erythematous, warm to the touch, and demonstrate signs of anhidrosis. A temperature gradient of 2–5°C from the affected to the contralateral foot has been a consistent finding with the acute neuro-arthropathic foot[7,8,12,15]. Almost invariably, the pulses will be bounding, a finding that, in association with the other clinical characteristics listed, makes the diagnosis probable, even prior to

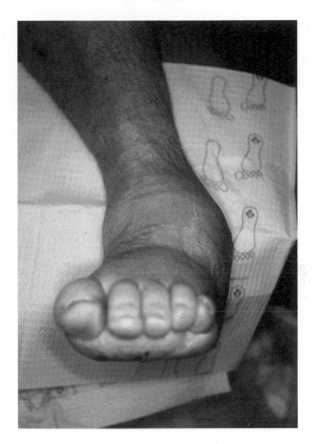

Figure 17.4 Neuro-arthropathic ankle with angular deviation

radiographic examination. A neurological examination should reveal the impaired sensory status of the extremity, as previously described. Infection can also play a role in the pathogenesis of neuro-arthropathy, and the examiner may find an infected neuropathic ulcer adjacent to the affected joint. Clinical history should reveal whether the ulcer developed as a consequence of the deformity or if, in fact, the neuro-arthropathic joint resulted from a pre-existing infected ulceration. The clinical findings attendant on acute neuro-arthropathy are summarized in Table 17.2.

RADIOGRAPHIC FINDINGS

On radiographic examination, neuro-arthropathic joints take on the appearance of severely destructive forms of degenerative or atrophic arthritidies. Generally, radiographic changes can be categorized broadly as

Table 17.2   Clinical findings in acute neuro-arthropathic feet

Neuropathic	Vascular	Cutaneous	Structural
Absent or diminished Pain	Bounding pulses	Ulceration Infection	Rocker bottom deformity
Vibration Proprioception	Oedema		Medial tarsal prominences
Light touch Reflexes	Erythema Warmth	Hyperkeratoses	Ankle deformity Hypermobility Crepitus
Anhidrosis	Autonomic Microcirculatory disturbances	Dry skin	Digital subluxation

*Certain findings will be related specifically to site of involvement or degree of deformity and might not always be present.

Table 17.3   Radiographic findings in diabetic neuro-arthropathy

Stage	Atrophic	Hypertrophic	Miscellaneous
	Phalangeal "hour-glassing"	Osteochondrial fragmentation	Soft tissue oedema
Acute	Metatarsal head osteolysis "sucked candy, pencil-pointing"	Intra-articular debris	Joint effusions
	Mortar and pestle deformities		Fractures
	Aggressive osteolysis in rearfoot		Subluxations
	Osteopenia		Medial calcification
Quiescent	Bone loss	Marginal osteophytes	Deformity
	Osteopenia	Periosteal new bone	Reduced swelling
		Absorption of debris	Subchondral
		Ankylosis/fusion	sclerosis
		Healed fractures with abundant bone callus	

Modified from Table 2 in Frykberg RG, Kozak GP: Neuropathic Arthopathy in the diabetic foot. *Am Fam Physician* 1978; **17**: 105–113.

either hypertrophic or atrophic responses to injury, both of which can be detected on serial radiographs of neuro-arthropathic feet[4,7] (Table 17.3). The tubular bones of the forefoot frequently react with atrophy or osteolysis of bone, often described as a "sucked candy" or "mortar and pestle" appearance of the metatarsophalageal (MTP) joint or interphalangeal joints[3,22] (Figure 17.5). Nonetheless, late changes might indeed include evidence of periosteal proliferation or periarticular spurring. This anatomic distinction is not absolute, however, since acute neuro-arthropathy of the rearfoot (i.e. subtalar and ankle joints) is often marked by aggressive demineralization and osteolysis of articular and periarticular bone

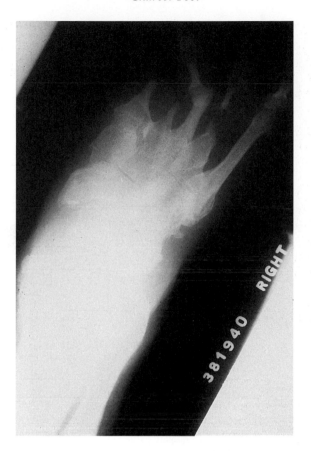

Figure 17.5 Osteolysis of forefoot indicating atrophic changes after undergoing ray amputations. These findings are typical of the forefoot pattern

(Figure 17.6). These changes are consistent with the underlying pathogenesis and vascular reflex theory of the disease, in which the precipitating insult to the joint results in a compensatory hyperaemia, resorption and softening of bone[7,8]. These early responses to trauma, typically seen in neuro-arthropathic joints, corroborate the need for a good vascular supply and have refuted the errant notion that this is an ischaemic process[2,3]. Joint effusions, subluxations, osteopenia, periarticular fractures and soft tissue oedema will also accompany atrophic joint changes, and are all characteristic of active neuro-arthropathy.

Hypertrophic changes, which seem to predominate in the chronic or quiescent stages, are most evident in the solid bones of the midfoot and rearfoot (Figure 17.7). These findings have the appearance of an exaggeration of those found in advanced osteoarthritis, i.e. cartilage

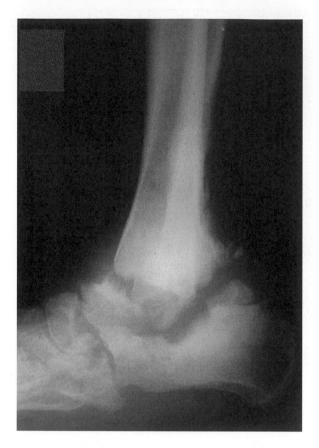

Figure 17.6 Atrophic changes found in acute neuro-arthropathy of the ankle and subtalar joints

fibrillation, loose body formation, subchondral sclerosis and marginal osteophytic proliferation[3]. Proliferation of new bone, healing of neuropathic fractures, ankylosis of involved joints and a partial restoration of stability will characterize findings in the late or reparative stages of neuro-arthropathy. If the constant trauma of continued weightbearing is not eliminated from the cycle, these latter events may not occur, and although some hypertrophic changes will be visible on radiographs, the foot might easily become a "chronically active" neuro-arthropathic foot.

Newman has described six non-infective changes of bones and joints that he found in neuropathic diabetic patients and for which he used the all-inclusive term "osteopathy"[22]. In addition to classic neuro-arthropathy, the main conditions Newman found included osteoporosis, new bone

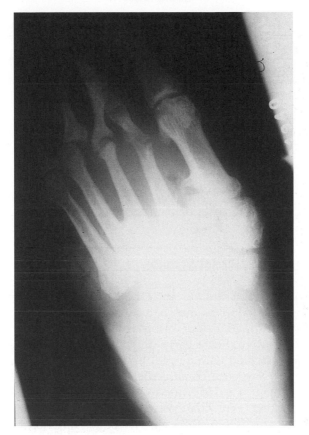

Figure 17.7 Hypertrophic changes typically found in the midfoot. Atrophic changes are also seen in the forefoot

formation, bone loss (atrophy), pathological fracture and spontaneous dislocation. From the preceding discussion, it should be evident that each of these isolated findings is often part of the pathology found in neuro-arthropathy. Similar findings were also reported by Cavanagh et al[23], who determined that diabetic patients with neuropathy were significantly more likely to develop bony abnormalities than non-neuropathic diabetics and age-matched non-diabetic control subjects. Since neuropathy seems to be the common thread amongst the radiographic changes in these two separate studies, the role of this complication in the aetiology of neuro-arthropathy and other bone conditions in diabetes is now well established. Table 17.4 further summarizes the categories of bone and joint changes typical in patients with diabetic neuropathy.

Table 17.4 Types of diabetic neuropathic bone and joint changes

	Features
I	Osteolysis
	Hyperaemic, infective, post-injury
II	Neuropathic fractures
	Pathological fractures
	Stress fractures
	Calcaneal insufficiency avulsion fractures
III	Neuro-arthropathy
	Neuro-arthropathy
	Atrophic-acute, hyperaemic, destructive
	Hypertrophic-chronic, sclerotic, reparative
	Spontaneous dislocations
	Talonavicular, subtalar, metatarsophalangeal, tarsometatarsal

OTHER DIAGNOSTIC STUDIES

Although usually unnecessary in establishing the diagnosis, other diagnostic imaging modalities may be useful in early clinical situations in which a neuro-arthropathic foot disorder is suspected but plain radiographs remain negative. Since early diagnosis requires a high degree of clinical suspicion coupled with a careful patient history, ostensibly normal radiographs in the presence of an acutely swollen neuropathic foot may warrant further imaging in addition to serial radiographs[21]. While highly sensitive in detecting joint changes, technetium bone scans alone have proved quite unreliable in this regard, since autonomic neuropathy promotes a general increase in radio-isotope uptake in the feet of neuropathic patients[24]. With a high percentage of false-positive readings in this patient population, bone scans have a complementary low specificity for both neuro-arthropathy and osteomyelitis[25,26]. Since joint hyperactivity is frequently mistaken for osteomyelitis, especially in the presence of an overlying ulceration, bone scans must be interpreted with caution in the neuropathic patient. In this clinical situation, combinations of indium labelled leukocyte scans, bone and gallium scans might be used to delineate non-infected neuro-arthropathy from osteomyelitis[18,25–27]. Whereas indium scans might have a higher specificity for bone infection, gallium can localize in neurotrophic joints much the same as does technetium, thereby reducing its utility. Johnson, however, reports a 91% accuracy in detecting osteomyelitis, even in the presence of neuro-arthropathy, by combining technetium bone scans with indium-labelled leukocyte scans[25]. Magnetic resonance imaging (MRI) and CT scanning might also be of use in detecting early bone and joint changes, but the role of MRI in reliably distinguishing neuro-arthropathy from osteomyelitis is disputed[18,27,28] (Figure 17.8).

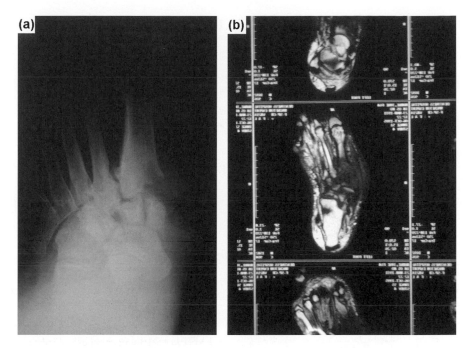

Figure 17.8 (a) Neuro-arthropathy with associated osteomyelitis in the presence of a long standing neuropathic ulcer which probes to bone. (b) MRI of same patient showing diffuse inflammation of medial midfoot on T-1 weighted image. Osteomyelitis was confirmed histopathologically

PATTERNS OF NEUROARTHROPATHY

Patterns of destruction within the tarsus of neuropathic feet of leprosy patients were eloquently reported by Harris and Brand[4]. They identified five different patterns of "tarsal disintegration" corresponding to sites of infection or pathomechanical stresses placed upon the anaesthetic feet: (a) posterior pillar, involving a collapse of the calcaneus; (b) central disintegration of the talus; (c) anterior pillar–medial arch, the classic neuro-arthropathic midfoot involving fracture of the head of the talus, navicular, or medial cuneiform; (d) anterior pillar–lateral arch with cuboid–lateral ray subluxation or deterioration; (e) cuneiform–metatarsal base (Lisfranc's joint) fracture or subluxation. Forefoot involvement, however, was not categorized in this scheme, which dealt exclusively with Hansen's disease patients[4].

Although several other authors have subsequently presented slightly different classification patterns for diabetic neuro-arthropathic feet, Sanders and Frykberg have suggested a categorization of diabetic neuro-arthropathy based on the anatomical site of involvement[7,8]. Pattern I (forefoot)

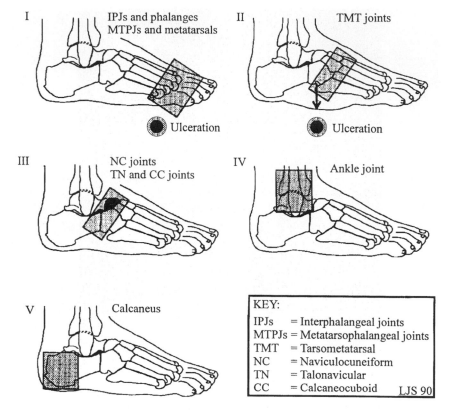

Figure 17.9 Five anatomic patterns of diabetic neuropathic neuro-arthropathy. See text for detailed description. Reproduced from reference 7 by permission of W.B. Saunders Company

includes osteolytic changes within the phalanges, metatarsophalangeal joints and distal metatarsals. Typical of this pattern are the atrophic findings of "pencil pointing" of metatarsal heads or hourglass resorption of phalangeal diaphyses (Figure 17.9). Pattern II (tarsometatarsal joints) is perhaps the most common presentation in diabetes and directly corresponds to pattern 5 of Harris and Brand[4]. This site of involvement (Lisfranc's joint) typically results from mechanical trauma which fractures and/or subluxes the base of the metatarsal(s) (Figure 17.5). Early changes might often be quite subtle, consisting of only a 1 or 2 mm lateral deviation of the second metatarsal base (Figure 17.10). Failure to diagnose this harbinger of neuro-arthropathy and failure to restrict weightbearing will frequently lead to midfoot collapse. Pattern III includes Chopart's joint (talonavicular and/or calcaneocuboid) or the naviculocuneiform joints, frequently involving two or three of these articulations upon initial

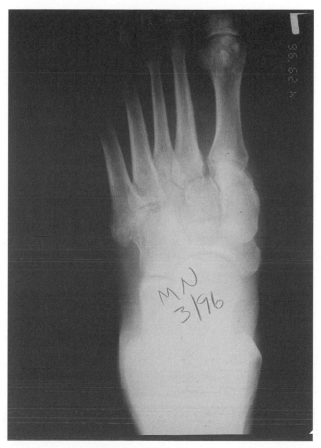

Figure 17.10 Pattern II neuro-arthropathy is often initiated by this very subtle dislocation of the 2nd metatarsal-cuneiform joint

presentation (Figure 17.11). As Newman[5] and Lesko and Maurer[29] have reported, isolated dislocation of the talonavicular joint, with or without associated fracture, is also an important variant of this pattern, resulting in marked instability. Perhaps due to predisposing ligamentous laxity and subsequent rupture, such isolated soft-tissue changes without attendant bone destruction might indeed be considered as related but separate entities from true neuro-arthropathy. Pattern IV is usually marked by aggressive osteolysis with instability of the ankle and/or subtalar joints (Figure 17.6). Typically, ankle joint involvement might develop following a malleolar or talar fracture. In Figure 17.12, the patient initially developed subtalar instability and dislocation subsequent to a peroneal tendon rupture. After unsuccessful subtalar arthrodesis, he went on to develop a typical pattern

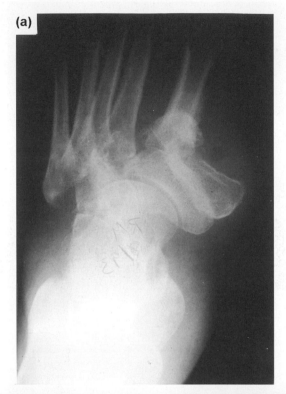

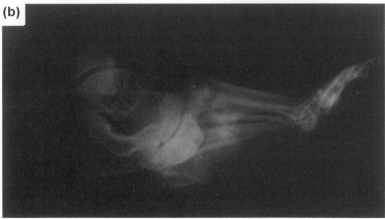

Figure 17.11 (a) Pattern III neuro-arthropathy involving subtle changes in the talonavicular, calcaneocuboid, and navicular-cuneiform joints in association with Pattern II changes (this is the same foot as illustrated in Figure 17.3). (b) Lateral view showing rocker-bottom subluxation

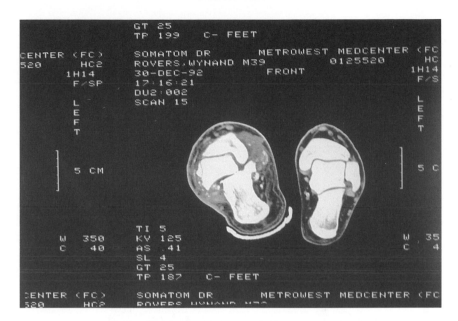

Figure 17.12 This CT scan shows a subtalar dislocation in this neuropathic patient who ruptured his peroneal tendons several weeks previously

IV neuro-arthropathy despite prolonged bracing (Figure 17.13). Pattern V is consistent with Harris and Brand's[4] "posterior pillar" presentation and includes neuropathic fractures of the body or posterior process of the calcaneus (Figure 17.14). Kathol et al[30] have used the term "calcaneal insufficiency avulsion" (CIA) fracture to describe this pattern. Since these neuropathic fractures do not usually involve any joints, the more appropriate term *"osteopathy"* is used rather than "arthropathy" when referring to this pattern.

Multiple sites and patterns of involvement are frequently manifest with initial presentation of neuro-arthropathic patients, which precludes classification by a single pattern. Frequencies of patterns of involvement have recently been reported as 3% in the forefoot (Pattern I), 48% at the tarsometatarsal joints (Pattern II), 34% at Chopart's joint (Pattern III), 13% at the ankle joint (Pattern IV) and 2% with calcaneal insufficiency avulsion fractures (Pattern V)[15]. These percentage frequencies are in general agreement with other reported studies[17,20]. Although not yet studied prospectively, classification by type might be helpful in determining management and predicting outcome. Whereas Pattern I presents with little instability or deformity, outcomes with healing usually result in little morbidity. Pattern V is not complicated with joint involvement, and

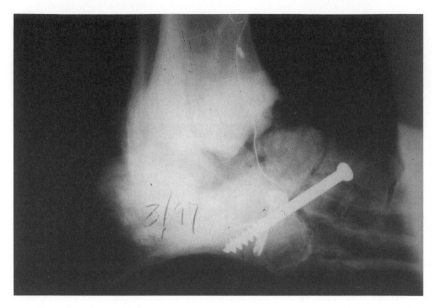

Figure 17.13 Pattern IV neuro-arthropathy developed in same patient as in Figure 17.12 after failing an initial subtalar arthrodesis

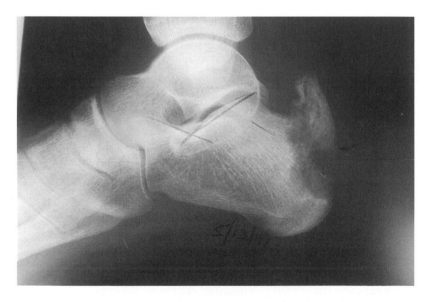

Figure 17.14 Pattern V osteopathy demonstrating the classical calcaneal insufficiency avulsion fracture of the posterior process

although sometimes requiring internal fixation, healing usually results in a stable foot with little deformity. Conversely, acute presentations of Patterns III or IV can have marked instability and aggressive destruction of bone. Even with prolonged non-weightbearing and immobilization, major surgical intervention is usually necessary, followed by another extended period of immobilization[15,29].

MANAGEMENT

Early diagnosis of this disorder is critical, since neuro-arthropathic joints that are detected and treated at an early stage in their development will result in less bony destruction. Hence, the recommended approach to management of acute neuro-arthropathy is based upon the need to prevent further trauma and to promote eventual healing with stability and a minimum of deformity[3,7,8]. Although our diagnostic acumen and our understanding of the underlying pathophysiology have improved in recent years, the basic tenets of managing neuro-arthropathic joints have not significantly changed in the past 60 years. The general goals and objectives for the treatment of the neuro-arthropathic foot are outlined in Table 17.5.

Acute Stage

Prevention of further trauma is the primary goal in treating the acute neuro-arthropathic foot. Once the destructive forces have been eliminated from the pathogenic cycle, the acute process can subside and allow conversion to the reparative, quiescent stage. This imperative requires an initial period of non-weightbearing to eliminate all stress from the injured foot. Although total bed rest may not be a viable option at this time, elevation with complete off-loading using crutches or a wheelchair will result in a fairly

Table 17.5 General goals and objectives for managing the diabetic neuro-arthropathic foot

Convert from active to quiescent stage
  Non weightbearing is essential to prevent further trauma
    Bedrest, crutches, wheelchair
Prevent further deformity
  Immobilization
    Elastic or compressive soft bandage
    Cast, cast brace, posterior splint
Provide protected ambulation
  Special footwear
    Healing sandal, moulded insoles, patellar tendon-bearing brace
    Extra-depth shoes, custom-made shoes

rapid reduction in oedema. Weekly foot assessments with dermal thermometry should note the gradual normalization of temperatures on the affected side and will indicate efficacy of management[2,3,7,8,15]. Serial radiographs might also be taken to assess the reduction of soft tissue oedema, absorption of debris, fracture healing and a general arrest of the destruction of joint architecture and periarticular bone[3,21].

Immobilization and protection are also critical components of care in the acute stage, often consisting of total contact casts, prefabricated braces, posterior splints, or soft casts. These modalities will prevent motion, prevent further deformity, and lead to a rapid reduction in oedema, especially when applied during the period of non-weightbearing. Prophylactic immobilization of the contralateral extremity has also been advocated to prevent subsequent development of neuro-arthropathy on that side caused by the increased stress of unilateral weightbearing[16]. Once adequate resolution of acute changes (oedema, aching and temperature elevation) occurs, gradual protected partial weightbearing with one of the aforementioned modalities can commence. Gradual weaning from non-weightbearing to protected partial weightbearing to full protected weightbearing over the course of 3 months or so is recommended, as indicated by the patient's progress[3]. Prospective, randomized studies of contrasting treatments have not yet been performed to elucidate which treatments, at which times, will be most beneficial in this stage. Several centres report success with the application of total contact walking casts without an initial period of strict non-weightbearing[15,19,21]. Due to a rapid reduction of oedema, these casts must be changed weekly or bi-weekly to ensure proper fit, avoid ulceration and to carefully evaluate the progress of treatment. Immobilization must be continued until the quiescent stage has been achieved and healing has taken place. This might require a period of 3–6 months, depending upon the pattern and severity of pre-existing destruction[3,15,19,23]. Serial radiographs will provide evidence of healed fractures without progression of deformity, while the clinical examination should reveal lessening of the temperature gradient between the two feet and a significant reduction in oedema.

In recent years there has been interest in the study of altered bone mineral density (BMD) in patients with diabetes, especially in those persons with peripheral neuropathy. Autonomic neuropathy presumably results in excess bone blood flow, leading to an osteoclast-mediated decrease in peripheral bone mass[11,24]. In diabetic patients with neuro-arthropathy, the local reductions in BMD have been attributed to increased osteoclastic activity, which outpaces osteoblastic bone formation to an even greater degree than found in neuropathic subjects without neuro-arthropathic changes[12,31]. Due to methodological deficiencies in these studies (markers were measured only after the onset of neuro-arthropathy), cause and effect cannot be proved. However, these findings have led to investigation into the use of bisphosphonates as a treatment for acute diabetic neuro-arthropathy[32]. These pyrophosphate analogues are potent inhibitors of osteoclastic bone resorption and are widely used in the treatment of osteoporosis and Paget's disease. In their uncontrolled study of six patients with active neuro-arthropathic arthropathy treated with infusions of pamidronate, Selby et al[32] found significant reductions in foot temperature and alkaline phosphatase levels compared to baseline. Aside from its small size and lack of a control group, this study did not measure serum markers of osteoclastic activity or attempt to control for concurrent treatment effects from simple off-loading. Until definitive controlled studies are performed which address these deficiencies, bisphosphonate use can only be considered as an unproved ancillary treatment for active neuro-arthropathy.

Quiescent Stage

Once the active neuro-arthropathic foot has converted to the chronic or quiescent stage and radiographic evidence of bone healing is present, full weightbearing can commence without the need for rigid immobilization. Frequently, however, removable prefabricated walking braces, custom ankle–foot orthoses, or patellar tendon-bearing braces might be used as an interim step in graduating from non-weightbearing or casting to full weightbearing in shoes or healing sandals[3,7,8,15,21,33] (Figure 17.15). Crutch walking with partial weightbearing might also be beneficial during this transition period. Care must be exercised to prevent neuropathic fracture of the osteopenic bone, especially if a prolonged period of non-weightbearing has taken place. Although unusual, reactivation of the acute process in the same or adjacent joints might ensue from such trauma precipitated by premature unrestricted ambulation. One report suggests that transient skin temperature elevations at this stage might be treated with a return to casting until temperatures normalize[15].

Footwear requirements are usually determined by the amount of deformity present in these high-risk feet. Regardless, all neuro-arthropathic feet will require constant attention to appropriate footwear and lifelong surveillance against foot ulceration. In feet with minimal deformity, comfort, extra-depth or athletic shoes (trainers) might suffice, while those patients with grossly deformed or rocker bottom feet will require custom-moulded shoes[3,21]. In all cases, however, custom insoles should be fabricated to cushion the foot, providing a commensurate reduction in plantar pressures and protection from ulceration.

Reconstructive surgery has gained popularity in recent years as an alternative to amputation to provide stability and improved alignment, or to remove bony prominences causing recurrent ulcerations[7,8,15,19,21,34,35]. As

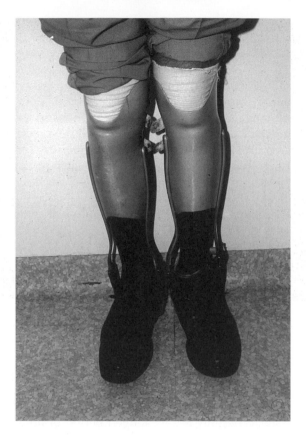

Figure 17.15 Patellar tendon-bearing braces used to partially off-weight the ankle used during the early quiescent phase

previously indicated, however, *appropriate* surgical stabilization for selected patients with neuro-arthropathy has been practised for many years. However, such surgery is recommended only in cases where conservative measures have failed to provide stable ambulation or when recurrent ulceration makes footwear accommodation for pedal deformity unlikely. Furthermore, surgical treatment should be considered only during the chronic or subacute stages, since such intervention during the acute process adds additional trauma to the joint, which can result in even more bone resorption. One exception to this rule seems to be early fusions for isolated joint subluxations without accompanying bone destruction[5,29]. Most authors agree with the need for a period of rest and/or immobilization prior to surgical intervention to allow oedema and local temperatures to subside.

Once the quiescent stage has been reached and non-surgical measures have not resulted in satisfactory outcomes, surgical operations can be

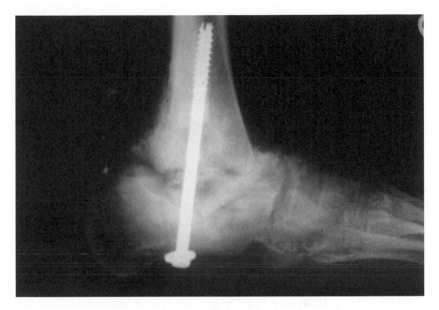

Figure 17.16 Calcaneo-tibial fusion with autogenous bone graft was performed in this patient with severe Pattern IV neuro-arthropathy. One month after operation

performed which directly address the problems encountered. When instability of the ankle, rearfoot or midfoot predominate, arthrodesis utilizing rigid internal fixation should be performed to provide the necessary alignment and stability required for safe ambulation[4,34,35] (Figure 17.16). When recurrent plantar or midfoot ulcerations are the primary complications of management, simple exostectomies with debridement or excision of the ulcer can often suffice[7,34]. Osteomyelitis underlying ulcerations should preferably be managed by debridement, exostectomy and antimicrobial therapy, rather than primary arthrodesis. Frequently, coexistent contractures of the Achilles tendon, causing an accentuation of deformity and plantar pressure, require lengthening concurrently with the osseous procedures[7,34]. Postoperatively, most patients are initially kept non-weightbearing and then casted for an additional period of 1–6 months, depending upon the procedure performed[15,35]. When healing is complete, there can be a gradual return to protective footwear, as previously discussed. Generally, the operated foot should be treated much the same as an acute neuro-arthropathic foot, utilizing the aforementioned management protocols. Surgery on these feet is not without associated risks, attesting to the complexities of the patients themselves. Hardware failure, pseudoarthrosis, infection, subsequent amputation and even death can occur in the peri-operative period[7,8,15,34,35]. Careful patient selection, combined with expertise and close postoperative monitoring, are essential for obtaining optimal surgical outcomes while minimizing complications.

CONCLUSION

Although not all neuro-arthropathic feet can be prevented, the progression and subsequent destruction of the foot can be attenuated through early detection and appropriate management. This requires a thorough under-standing of the underlying pathophysiology, natural history and accepted standards of management. The ultimate goal of treatment is to maintain a useful extremity, free from ulceration, which will allow the patient to function as normally as possible throughout his/her lifetime. While longitudinal studies have not been forthcoming regarding the survival of these patients, they are certainly at risk for numerous other complications of diabetes. Prevention of ulceration and subsequent amputation is therefore a key objective in managing persons with this disorder. Constant vigilance on the part of both patient and health care providers is necessary to ensure that, once healed, the neuro-arthropathic foot is protected from further injury through appropriate footwear and careful attention to preventive foot care.

REFERENCES

1. Charcot J-M. Sur quelques arthropathies qui paraissent dependre d'une lesion du cerveau ou de la moelle epiniere. *Arch Physiol Norm Pathol* 1868; **1**: 161–78.
2. Edelman SV, Kosofsky EM, Paul RA, Kozak GP. Neuro-neuroarthropathy (Charcot's joints) in diabetes mellitus following revascularization surgery: three case reports and a review of the literature. *Arch Intern Med* 1987; **147**: 1504–8.
3. Frykberg RG, Kozak GP. The diabetic Charcot foot. In Kozak GP, Campbell DR, Frykberg RG, Habershaw GM (eds), *Management of Diabetic Foot Problems*, 2nd edn. Philadelphia: WB Saunders, 1995; 88–97.
4. Harris JR, Brand PW. Patterns of disintegration of the tarsus in the anaesthetic foot. *J Bone Joint Surg* 1966; **48B**: 4–16.
5. Newman JH. Spontaneous dislocation in diabetic neuropathy. *J Bone Joint Surg* 1979; **61B**: 484–8.
6. Sanders LJ, Frykberg RG. Charcot foot. In Levin ME, O'Neal LW, Bowker JH (eds), *The Diabetic Foot*, 5th edn. St Louis, MI: Mosby Yearbook, 1993; 149–80.
7. Sanders LJ, Frykberg RG. Diabetic neuropathic neuroarthropathy: the Charcot foot. In Frykberg RG (ed.), *The High Risk Foot in Diabetes Mellitus*. New York: Churchill Livingstone, 1991; 297–338.
8. Sanders LJ, Mrdjenovich D. Anatomical patterns of bone and joint destruction in neuropathic diabetics. *Diabetes* 1991; **40**(suppl 1): 529A.
9. Childs M, Armstrong DG, Edelson G. Is Charcot arthropathy a late sequela of osteoporosis in patients with diabetes mellitus? *J Foot Ankle Surg* 1998; **37**: 437–9.

10. Cundy TF, Edmonds ME, Watkins PJ. Osteopenia and metatarsal fractures in diabetic neuropathy. *Diabet Med* 1985; **2**: 461–4.

11. Forst T, Pflitzner A, Kann P, Schehler B, Lobmarm R, Schafer H, Andreas J, Bockisch A, Beyer J. Peripheral osteopenia in adult patients with insulin-dependent diabetes mellitus. *Diabet Med* 1995; **12**: 874–9.

12. Young MJ, Marshall A, Adams JE, Selby PL, Boulton AJM. Osteopenia, neurological dysfunction, and the development of Charcot neuroarthropathy. *Diabet Care* 1995; **18**: 34–8.

13. Frykberg RG. Biomechanical considerations of the diabetic foot. *Lower Extremity* 1995; **2**: 207–14.

14. Eichenholtz SN. *Charcot Joints*. Springfield, IL: Charles C Thomas, 1966.

15. Armstrong DG, Todd WF, Lavery LA, Harkless LB, Bushman TR. The natural history of acute Charcot's arthropathy in a diabetic foot specialty clinic. *Diabet Med* 1997; **14**: 357–63.

16. Clohisy DR, Thompson RC. Fractures associated with neuropathic arthropathy in adults who have juvenile-onset diabetes. *J Bone Joint Surg* 1988; **70A**: 1192–200.

17. Cofield RH, Morison MJ, Beabout JW. Diabetic neuroarthropathy in the foot: patient characteristics and patterns of radiographic change. *Foot Ankle* 1983; **4**: 15–22.

18. Seabold JE, Flickinger FW, Kao S, Gleason TJ, Kahn D, Nepola J, Marsh JL. Indium-111 leukocyte/technetium-99m-MDP bone and magnetic resonance imaging: difficulty of diagnosing osteomyelitis in patients with neuropathic neuroarthropathy. *J Nucl Med* 1990; **31**: 549–56.

19. Klenerman L. The Charcot joint in diabetes. *Diabet Med* 1996; **13**: S52–4.

20. Sinha S, Munichoodappa C, Kozak GP. Neuro-arthropathy (Charcot joints) in diabetes mellitus: clinical study of 101 cases. *Medicine* 1972; **52**: 191–210.

21. Caputo GM, Ulbrecht J, Cavanagh PR, Juliano P. The Charcot foot in diabetes: six key points. *Am Fam Phys* 1998; **57**: 2705–10.

22. Newman JH. Non-infective disease of the diabetic foot. *J Bone Joint Surg* 1981; **63B**: 593–6.

23. Cavanagh PR, Young MJ, Adams JE, Vickers KL, Boulton AJM. Radiographic abnormalities in the feet of patients with diabetic neuropathy. *Diabet Care* 1994; **17**: 201–9.

24. Edmonds ME, Clarke MB, Newton S, Barrett J, Watkins PJ. Increased uptake of bone radiopharmaceutical in diabetic neuropathy. *Q J Med (New Ser)* 1985; **57**: 843–55.

25. Johnson JE, Kennedy EJ, Shereff MJ, Patel NC, Collier BD. Prospective study of bone, indium-111-labeled white blood cell, and gallium-67 scanning for the evaluation of osteomyelitis in the diabetic foot. *Foot Ankle Int* 1996; **7**: 10–16.

26. Schauwecker DS, Park HM, Burt RW, Mock BH, Wellman HN. Combined bone scintigraphy and indium-111 leukocyte scans in neuropathic foot disease. *J Nucl Med* 1988; **29**: 1651–5.

27. Longmaid HE, Kruskal JB. Imaging infections in diabetic patients. *Infect Dis Clin N Am* 1995; **9**: 163–182.

28. Beltran J, Campanini S, Knight C, McCalla M. The diabetic foot: magnetic resonance imaging evaluation. *Skel Radiol* 1990; **19**: 37–41.

29. Lesko P, Maurer RC. Talonavicular dislocations and midfoot arthropathy in neuropathic diabetic feet: natural course and principles of treatment. *Clin Orthop Rel Res* 1989; **240**: 226–31.

30. Kathol MH, El-Koury GY, Moore TE. Calcaneal insufficiency avulsion fractures in patients with diabetes mellitus. *Radiology* 1991; **180**: 725–9.
31. Gough A, Abraha H, Li F, Purewal TS, Foster AVM, Watkins PJ, Moniz C, Edmonds ME. Measurement of markers of osteoclast and osteoblast activity in patients with acute and chronic diabetic Charcot neuroarthropathy. *Diabet Med* 1997; **14**: 527–31.
32. Selby PL, Young MJ, Boulton AJM. Bisphosphonates: a new treatment for diabetic Charcot neuroarthropathy? *Diabet Med* 1994; **11**: 28–31.
33. Mehta JA, Brown C, Sargeant N. Charcot restraint orthotic walker. *Foot Ankle Int* 1998; **19**: 619–23.
34. Myerson MS, Henderson MR, Saxby T, Short KW. Management of midfoot diabetic neuroarthropathy. *Foot Ankle Int* 1994; **15**: 233–41.
35. Sammarco GJ, Conti SF. Surgical treatment of neuroarthropathic foot deformity. *Foot Ankle Int* 1998; **19**: 102–9.

18

Prophylactic Orthopaedic Surgery—Is There A Role?

PATRICK LAING

Wrexham Maelor Hospital, Wrexham, UK

Prophylactic surgery in the diabetic foot is normally categorized as non-emergency surgery. The complications of diabetic foot ulceration can be so devastating that the concept of such surgery to prevent ulceration, or re-ulceration, is inviting. All too frequently we see feet which are suffering from repeated breakdown and creeping amputation. Surgery, though, is most often used in the acute situation as a reaction to infection or gangrene and less rarely in an elective attempt to prevent future problems. Although classified as non-emergency surgery, early aggressive surgery in the acute situation, which limits the extent of amputation and avoids more proximal limb loss, is regarded by some as equally prophylactic[1].

Neuropathy and ischaemia are the two main risk factors for development of diabetic foot ulceration. However, the initiating factor in ulceration is usually pressure of some description. In a foot with a poor blood supply, ischaemic ulcers may develop due to quite low pressures. Conversely, higher pressures are required in a neuropathic foot that has a good blood supply but lacks protective sensation. The neuropathic foot is frequently cavus in shape with clawed toes and callosities under the heel and metatarsal heads in which high pressures develop. The clawing of the toes leads to dorsal friction and increased pressures as the protruding interphalangeal joints rub against the toe box of the shoe. In a normal foot the toes take 30% and sometimes up to 50% of the load transmitted through the foot, but with severe clawing the toes become non-weightbearing, increasing the load under the metatarsal heads. In

The Foot in Diabetes, 3rd edn. Edited by A. J. M. Boulton, H. Connor and P. R. Cavanagh.
© 2000 John Wiley & Sons, Ltd.

Ellenberg's[2] series 90% of diabetic ulcers occurred under pressure-bearing areas of the foot. Studies such as that by Veves et al[3] have shown that high plantar pressures are predictive of plantar ulceration. In their group of 86 diabetic patients, plantar ulceration occurred in 35% of those with high foot pressures but in none of those with normal pressures. Yet, despite such studies, it is not possible to predict with absolute accuracy which patients will develop ulceration. Two-thirds of Veves' group of patients with high pressures did not develop ulceration. In a large-scale screening of over 1000 patients in a diabetic clinic in Liverpool, about 25% of patients were deemed "at risk" of ulceration but only 2.8% had a history of previous ulceration[4]. Our screening methods are, therefore, generally highly sensitive but low in specificity. Even if we could identify with accuracy those patients with high pressures under the foot who were certain to ulcerate, the initial treatment or protection should always be conservative, i.e. non-operative. It must also be remembered that pressure is defined as force divided by area. Insoles and shoes can redistribute pressure over the whole foot and reduce peak pressures at critical points. Surgery is normally ablative to some degree and will reduce the total area of the foot, thus increasing the overall pressure. Transfer lesions may then occur, leading to further surgery and a spiral of events.

However, shoes and insoles have a significant failure rate in preventing primary ulceration or re-ulceration. Edmonds[5] found a 25% recurrence rate in both neuropathic and ischaemic ulcers, even with patients who accepted and wore special shoes and insoles. For those who wore their own shoes, over half the neuropathic group and 83% of the ischaemic group re-ulcerated. This is not surprising because, as already noted, ulceration in the diabetic foot largely occurs because of pressure on the at-risk foot and, unless those pressures are adequately modified, then re-ulceration will occur. The risks of recurrent ulceration are ascending infection, osteomyelitis, wet and dry gangrene and amputation. Helm[6] noted that nearly half the ulcer recurrences in his series were secondary to an underlying biomechanical problem or bony prominence. Myerson[7] found 19 of 22 ulcer recurrences had an underlying fixed deformity or osseous prominence.

Before considering surgery it is important to assess the patient as a whole and also to consider the underlying aetiology of the recurrent ulceration. In assessing any ulceration we use the Liverpool classification (Table 18.1) as this is a practical way of approaching the problem. Primarily we must consider whether the underlying aetiology is neuropathic, ischaemic or neuro-ischaemic, i.e. a combination of both and accurate assessment of vascular status, as described in Chapter 16, is essential. It is vitally important not to proceed with any surgery unless there is a good expectation that any wound will heal. The foot shown in Figure 18.1 was referred from another hospital, having already undergone three operations,

Table 18.1 Liverpool classification of diabetic foot ulcers

Primary
 Neuropathic
 Ischaemic
 Combination of both, i.e. neuro-ischaemic
Secondary
 Uncomplicated
 Complicated, i.e. presence of cellulitis, abscess or osteomyelitis

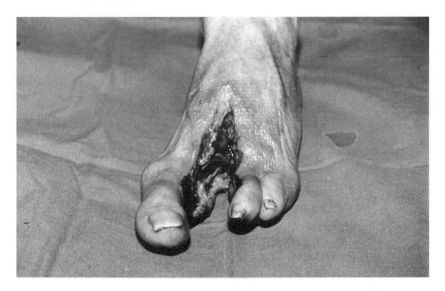

Figure 18.1 "Lobster foot" following multiple surgery

starting with the amputation of an infected toe. The failure of each wound to heal was followed by more radical surgery, producing the "lobster foot" illustrated, which was still not healing because the underlying problem was peripheral vascular disease. The amount of blood supply required to heal a surgical wound is several times that required to keep the skin intact in the first place. Figure 18.2 shows a foot with hallux valgus in which an ulcer was present over the medial aspect of the first metatarsophalangeal joint in a middle-aged diabetic patient with neuropathy. This, however, is a classic site for ischaemic ulceration and the ulcer was caused by pressure from the shoe on his hallux valgus deformity. Pressure from a shoe upper is highest at the points where the radius of curvature is lowest, i.e. over the first and fifth metatarsal heads. The ulcer had a necrotic appearance to it and his ankle brachial pressure index was significantly low. An arteriogram

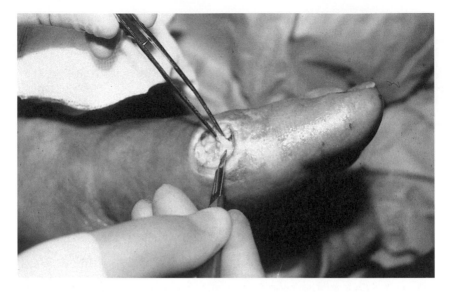

Figure 18.2 Necrotic ischaemic ulcer over first metatarsophalangeal joint being debrided

showed a stenosis amenable to angioplasty, following which his pressure index improved to 1.07. We were then able to debride the ulcer down to good bleeding bone and heal it (Figure 18.3). Improving the blood supply prior to surgery can be vitally important in avoiding, or limiting the extent of, any subsequent amputation and ensuring that wounds such as this one will heal and not simply end up as a larger non-healing wound. In this case the necrotic ulcer was stable, with no cellulitis or spreading infection. If acute infection is present, then urgent surgery is required to control infection and prevent it spreading. If that can be achieved it may then be possible to improve the circulation prior to performing any definitive closure or distal amputation.

Second, if ulceration is present, we must assess whether the ulcer is uncomplicated or complicated, i.e. whether cellulitis or deep infection, such as an abscess or osteomyelitis, is present. It should be noted that a positive wound swab from an ulcer does not necessarily imply infection because all ulcers become colonized with bacteria, both aerobic and anaerobic. Clearly, deep infection requires immediate treatment but identification of under-lying osteomyelitis is important, as this will influence the amount of any bony resection. Although it has been suggested that osteomyelitis can be successfully treated with antibiotics alone[8], it has been our experience that it is difficult to eradicate true osteomyelitis without resecting the infected bone. This has been the experience of others[9] and studies comparing

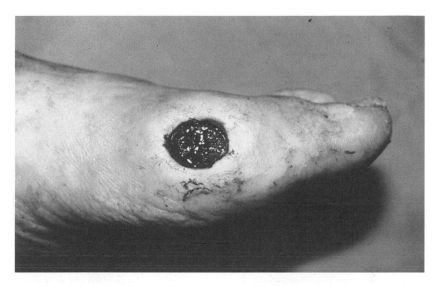

Figure 18.3 Ulcer in Figure 18.2 following debridement and now with good bleeding base

conservative surgery and medical treatment alone have shown benefit from surgery[10]. The controversy arises from the difficulties in diagnosing osteomyelitis with any certainty from plain radiographs. The changes of diabetic osteopathy, which include periosteal reactions, osteoporosis, juxta-articular cortical defects and osteolysis, can mimic the changes of osteomyelitis (see Chapter 15).

Which patients then may benefit from surgery? Our main indication for elective prophylactic surgery in the diabetic foot is recurrent ulceration in the presence of a fixed deformity. The fixed deformity may be clawed toes with recurrent ulceration or it may be intractable ulceration under the metatarsal heads due to gross forefoot deformity (Figure 18.4). In neuro-arthropathic feet it may be recurrent plantar midfoot ulceration due to a rocker bottom deformity. Often the most difficult patient to treat successfully with shoes and insoles is the middle-aged patient who is overweight and still very active, trying to hold down a manual job. Such a patient has frequently had previous ulceration and surgery and may already have lost some toes. What is often noticeable about these feet is how the plantar skin under the metatarsal heads has lost the elasticity seen in a normal foot and how the fat pads under the metatarsal heads have been drawn forward and atrophied. The loss of elasticity is due partly to the glycosylation of collagen in the skin and partly to scar tissue from previous ulceration. Scar tissue lacks the elasticity of normal skin and is more prone to break down with shearing forces.

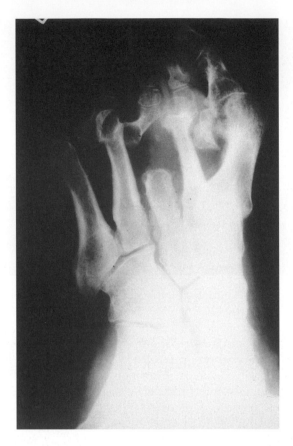

Figure 18.4 X-ray showing deformed forefoot with dislocated toes and previous partial ray amputation

For the patient with intractable plantar ulceration under the metatarsal heads, we may do a forefoot arthroplasty with resection of the metatarsal heads. The foot is approached through 2–3 dorsal incisions between the metatarsal heads and the metatarsal heads resected. The undersurface of the metatarsal neck is chamfered to provide a smooth surface when weightbearing and pushing off. Figure 18.5 shows this being done in a patient who required a forefoot arthroplasty with amputation of his remaining toes. The site of chronic ulceration can be left open to drain and heal and Figure 18.6 shows the end result. When fashioning skin flaps, it is important to leave sufficient plantar skin to cover the end of the foot, as the plantar skin is best adapted for withstanding the stresses of weightbearing. In resecting the metatarsal heads one aims for a gentle crescent along the resected heads (Figure 18.7). If the majority of toes are still present, then

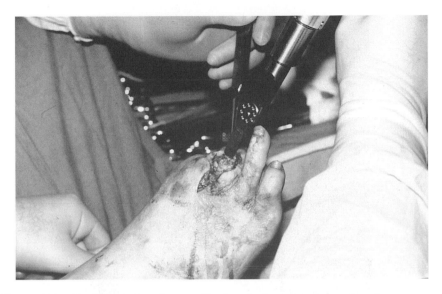

Figure 18.5 Forefoot arthroplasty with chamfering of metatarsal necks

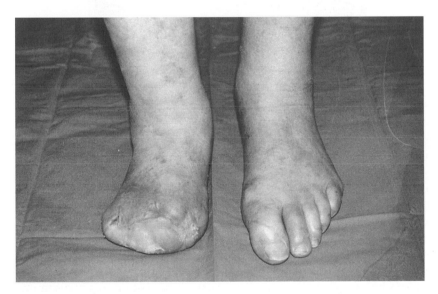

Figure 18.6 End result forefoot arthroplasty with resection of remaining toes

these can usually be preserved. If there is gross deformity or only a couple of defunctioned toes are left, then it is better to amputate these at the same time, because otherwise they will inevitably protrude and be liable to further injury. When assessing patients with intractable forefoot ulceration

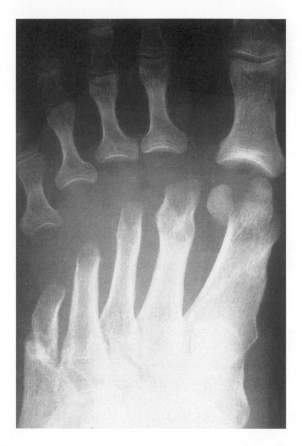

Figure 18.7 X-ray of forefoot arthroplasty showing gentle crescent of resected metatarsal heads (note previous surgery to metatarsals)

it is important to look at the tendo achilles, as equinus deformity or tightness of this tendon restricts ankle joint dorsiflexion and leads to greater pressure under the metatarsal heads during the toe-off phase of walking. Lengthening a tight tendo achilles can facilitate ulcer healing and result in a lower rate of recurrence[11].

Individual toe problems may be addressed in different ways, depending on the pathology. Clawing usually affects all the lesser toes but sometimes an individual toe will be clawed or hammered, causing chronic ulceration. Our first line of treatment will be to try to improve the diabetic footwear and provide sufficient space in the toe-box of the shoe. If surgery is required, then the toe can be straightened by an interphalangeal fusion, or simply by resection of the head of the proximal phalanx, along with a tenotomy of the extensor tendon and a dorsal capsulotomy of the metatarsophalangeal joint. If the toe is markedly subluxed or dislocated at the metatarsophalangeal joint, then it will be more appropriate to do a Stainsby-type procedure with a proximal hemiphalangectomy of the proximal phalanx of the toe. If there is a fixed mallet deformity of the toe, then a terminal Syme procedure with resection of the distal phalanx is sometimes indicated. It is not unusual for a patient to present with digital gangrene which is sometimes associated with ulceration and soft tissue gas on the X-ray, indicating spreading infection. Soft tissue gas does not necessarily mean clostridial infection, as many organisms, both aerobic and anaerobic, produce soft tissue gas in diabetic patients[12]. In neuropathic feet the overall circulation may be good but septic thrombi in digital vessels can cause gangrene. Dry gangrene of the toe can be left to demarcate and proceed to autoamputation, but wet gangrene, as in this case, requires prompt amputation to stop infection spreading. Infection in the foot can spread along the tissue planes of tendons and in diabetic patients infection can often spread with great rapidity, particularly if the patient continues walking. The effectiveness of the inflammatory response may be reduced in diabetic patients. Microvascular studies have shown an impaired response to minor thermal injury, and leukocyte action may also be impaired[13,14].

We usually use a racquet incision to disarticulate the toe (Figure 18.8) and then leave the wound open to heal by secondary intention. Primary closure of an infected diabetic wound generally leads to chronic infection. If the associated metatarsal is involved with osteomyelitis, then it may be

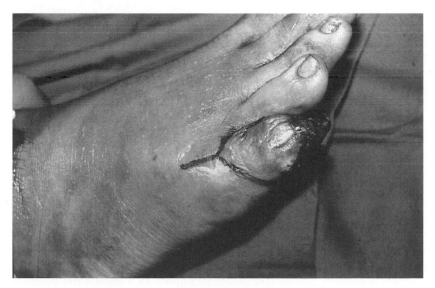

Figure 18.8 Disarticulation of gangrenous toe using racquet incision

necessary to do a partial ray amputation. Ray amputations are discussed in Chapter 19.

In the past the literature has suggested that prophylactic surgery in diabetic patients carries a high rate of complications. Gudas[15] did a 5 year retrospective study of 32 procedures considered to be prophylactic surgery in diabetic patients. His complication rate was over 30% and occurred largely in areas where ulceration had previously been present for one year under a metatarsal head. Petrov et al[16] looked at the results of removal of all the metatarsal heads in 12 diabetic patients and 15 rheumatoid patients. There was an ulcer recurrence rate of 25% in the diabetic patients, marginally less than in the rheumatoid patients. In the diabetic patients, recurrence was most frequent under the third and fourth metatarsal heads and occurred between 1 and 2 years following surgery. This is a significant complication rate, as any revision surgery will shorten the foot further and produce more complications. Quebedeaux et al[17] looked at unilateral first ray amputations in 25 diabetic patients at a mean of approximately 3 years following surgery. Prior to amputation the lesser toes on the operated side had been normal. At follow-up there were significantly more deformities of the lesser toes of the ipsilateral foot and more new ulcerations than in the contralateral foot with an intact first ray. Murdoch et al[18] reviewed the subsequent course after 90 great toe and first ray amputations in diabetic patients; 60% of all patients had a second amputation at a mean of 10 months after the first and 17% subsequently had a below-knee and 11% a transmetatarsal amputation. These figures partly reflect the progress of the disease, but on the contralateral side only 5% had a below-knee or transmetatarsal amputation. As you reduce the weightbearing area of the foot you shift the pressure elsewhere. Armstrong et al[19], however, carried out a retrospective review of resectional arthroplasty on single lesser toes and compared the results in 31 diabetic patients with 33 non-diabetic patients. At a mean of 3 years postoperatively, only one of the diabetic patients had re-ulcerated. However, diabetic patients with a previous history of ulceration were more likely to have a postoperative infection than non-diabetic patients or those with no history of ulceration.

Before considering surgery, it is also important to consider why non-operative treatment has failed. Although we work closely with our orthotist, pressure-relieving windows in insoles may not be in the correct place. The normal foot changes considerably in shape between a non-weightbearing and a weightbearing position. As the plantar arch flattens on weightbearing, the metatarsal heads move forward and the lesser metatarsal heads also move laterally. These changes are probably less pronounced in the severe diabetic foot because of generalized stiffness, but some flattening will occur. The insole in Figure 18.9 shows the position of the weight-relieving window and the actual position of the metatarsal head.

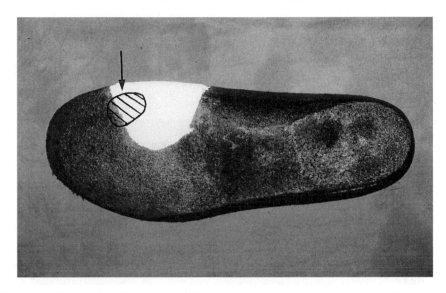

Figure 18.9 Insole with weight relieving window placed too proximally—actual site of ulcer is cross-hatched and indicated with arrow

It can be seen that the window is not under the ulcer and the edge effect from the window can create ulceration in itself.

Recurrent ulceration and osteomyelitis of the calcaneum pose a particular problem. The heel is not so easy to unload, with either a plaster cast or footwear and insoles, as the forefoot. It is difficult keeping the pressure off the heel, even in a resting position, and patients with neuropathy are not always very compliant because of a lack of sensory feedback. Ulceration is therefore difficult to heal, becomes chronic and often leads to underlying osteomyelitis. Because of these problems, many patients have ended up with a below-knee amputation. A surgical alternative, however, can be a partial or even total calcanectomy through a midline plantar incision, known as Gaenslen's incision (Figure 18.10). It is necessary to remove sufficient calcaneum to either clear existing osteomyelitis or provide enough slack to allow approximation of the skin following ulcer excision. Extensive excision of the calcaneum will also remove the distal attachment of the tendo achilles which, in any case, may be necrotic if involved in the ulcerated area. The tendon is debrided and allowed to retract proximally. Postoperatively, patients will usually require a moulded ankle–foot orthosis but generally are able to mobilize well, with much lower energy requirements than if a below-knee amputation had been performed. Although originally described by Gaenslen in 1931, there have been few series reporting results of these procedures in diabetic patients. The

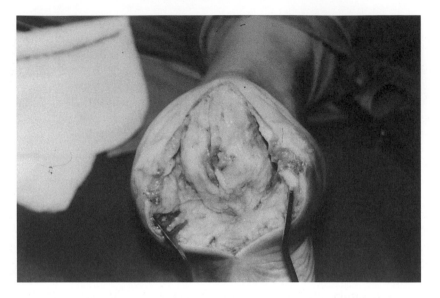

Figure 18.10   Gaenslen's incision for partial calcanectomy showing the exposed calcaneum

operation failed in eight of the 18 diabetic patients reported by Crandall and Wagner[20]. More recently Smith et al[21] reported that six of their seven diabetic patients went on to complete wound healing with no loss of their pre-operative ability to walk. Baumhauer et al[22] reported a series of eight patients undergoing total calcanectomy for calcaneal osteomyelitis, of whom six were diabetic. Five of the diabetic patients healed and one required a below-knee amputation. The minimum acceptable pre-operative ankle brachial pressure index in both Smith's and Baumhauer's series was greater than 0.45.

The neuro-arthropathic foot is a special challenge. It develops in less than 1% of diabetic patients, and is a chronic, relatively painless, degenerative process affecting the weightbearing joints of the foot. The patient will often present with a hot, swollen, erythematous foot. Such a foot is not entirely painless, but the pain experienced is not in proportion to the degree of swelling or bony changes apparent on X-ray. The main danger is that it will be mistaken for infection and osteomyelitis, and operated on inappropriately. Radiological investigations can be misleading, as the appearances on plain radiographs and magnetic resonance imaging scans of the neuro-arthropathic foot can be mistaken for infection. It is possible to have an infected neuro-arthropathic foot, but this is very rare in the acute presentation. The neuro-arthropathic foot goes through three stages, described by Eichenholtz[23]. In Stage I there is acute inflammation associated with hyperaemia and erythema, the bone dissolves and fragments and fractures and dislocations are common. In Stage II there is bony coalescence, decreasing swelling, and radiographic evidence of periosteal new bone formation is present. In Stage III, bony consolidation and healing occurs. This whole process is variable, but may take 2–3 years to run its full course. The joints most commonly affected are the midtarsal joints (60% of patients), the metatarsophalangeal (30%) and the ankle joint (10%). In the acute neuro-arthropathic foot, i.e. Eichenholtz Stage I, surgery is almost always contra-indicated. The bone is osteopenic and the literature abounds with cases of internal fixation which have failed in the acute neuro-arthropathic foot. The one exception to this may be the acute midfoot dislocation, which is severe and unstable. Myerson[24] has reported that this can be reduced and fixed, provided no bony fragmentation is present. Prophylactic surgery is therefore almost exclusively confined to the late stages of the disease, to treat recurrent ulceration due to bony prominences or to stabilize a foot which is unbraceable. The neuro-arthropathic foot frequently ends up with a rocker bottom deformity with a bony prominence prone to ulceration (Figure 18.11). A deformity such as this can be treated with excision of the bony exostosis through a lateral or medial incision away from the weightbearing plantar surface. Late deformity, such as that in Figure 18.12 in the hindfoot, may warrant surgery to stabilize the foot in a plantigrade

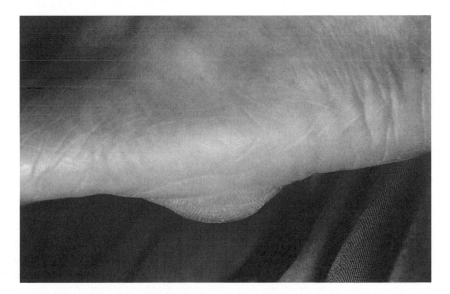

Figure 18.11 Neuro-arthropathic foot with midfoot plantar bony prominence

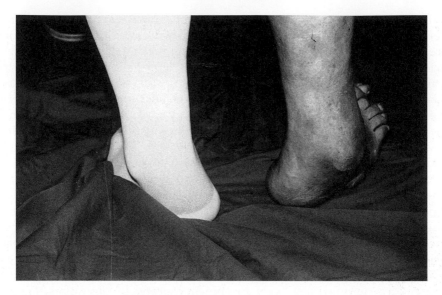

Figure 18.12 Neuro-arthropathic ankle with hindfoot varus and recurrent ulceration on the lateral border

position. This patient had recurrent ulceration along the lateral border of his foot which was impossible to keep healed in footwear. Prior to surgery his ulceration was healed in a plaster cast, as there is a higher rate of infection when operating with open ulceration. He then had an open fusion of his ankle joint, correcting the marked varus deformity and allowing the whole foot to be swung round into a plantigrade position (Figure 18.13). Although a good blood supply is a prerequisite for the initial development of a neuro-arthropathic foot, it is still important to assess the vascular state before surgery, as ischaemia may have supervened by the time such a foot has reached the chronic stage.

Surgery on neuro-arthropathic feet is not without complications. In the past there have been few series of diabetic patients with significant numbers but many complications and pseudarthroses have been reported. Stuart and Morrey[25] reported a series of hindfoot and midfoot fusions in 13 diabetic patients, nine of whom had neuro-arthropathy. Of these nine, two had non-unions, two had below-knee amputations and there were three deep infections. Papa[26] reported on 29 diabetic patients with neuro-arthropathy who all underwent fusion of the ankle, subtalar or transverse tarsal joints. Although salvage was successful in 93% of their patients (in that they did not undergo amputation), there were 20 complications in 19 of the patients and 10 pseudarthroses. However, the majority of these pseudarthroses were

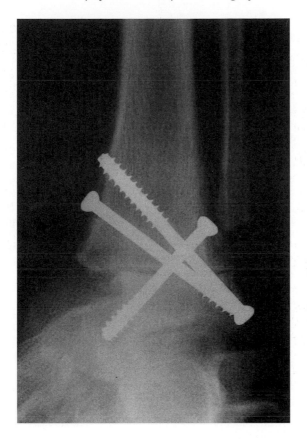

Figure 18.13 Post-operative X-ray of Figure 18.12 showing ankle fusion held with three large cancellous screws

stable and presumably not painful because of the underlying neuroarthropathy. Most recently, Sammarco[27] has reported results in 26 patients (21 diabetic) with neuro-arthropathic fracture leading to significant deformity and requiring reconstruction. All feet were improved and no patient subsequently required amputation. However, there were six non-unions plus other complications. Surgery of the neuro-arthropathic foot is thus not for the occasional foot surgeon, but nowadays can be a viable alternative to amputation for failed non-operative care.

In conclusion, prophylactic surgery in the diabetic foot has a valuable place but should always follow adequate non-operative treatment. It should be apparent that our general philosophy with diabetic foot surgery is to preserve as much of the foot as possible in order to maximize the weightbearing area. The ultimate prophylaxis is not surgery but refined identification of the at-risk patient, education, protection and prevention of primary ulceration.

REFERENCES

1. Tan JS, Friedman NM, Hazelton-Miller C, Flanagan JP, File TM. Can aggressive treatment of diabetic foot infections reduce the need for above-ankle amputation? *Clin Infect Dis* 1996; **23**: 286–91.
2. Ellenberg M. Diabetic neuropathic ulcer. *J Mt Sinai Hosp* 1968; **35**: 585–94.
3. Veves A, Murray MJ, Young MJ, Boulton AJM. The risk of foot ulceration in diabetic patients with high foot pressure: a prospective study. *Diabetologia* 1992; **35**: 660–3.
4. Klenerman L, McCabe C, Cogley D, Crerand S, Laing P, White M. Screening for patients at risk of diabetic foot ulceration in a general diabetic outpatient clinic. *Diabet Med* 1996; **13**: 561–3.
5. Edmonds M. Experience in a multidisciplinary diabetic foot clinic. In Connor H, Boulton AJM, Ward JD (eds), *The Foot in Diabetes*, 1st edn. Chichester: Wiley, 1987; 121–33.
6. Helm PA, Pullium G. Recurrence of neuropathic ulceration following healing in a total contact cast. *Arch Phys Med Rehabil* 1991; **72**: 967–70.
7. Myerson M, Papa J, Eaton K, Wilson K. The total-contact cast for management of neuropathic plantar ulceration of the foot. *J Bone and Joint Surg* 1992; **74**A: 261–9.
8. Venkatesan P, Lawn S, Macfarlane RM, Fletcher EM, Finch RG, Jeffcoate WJ. Conservative management of osteomyelitis in the feet of diabetic patients. *Diabet Med* 1997; **14**: 487–90.
9. Le Quesne LP. Surgical aspects of the diabetic foot. In Connor H, Boulton AJM, Ward JD (eds) *The Foot in Diabetes*, 1st edn. Chichester: Wiley, 1987: 69–79.
10. Ha Van G, Siney H, Danan J-P, Sachon C, Grimaldi A. Treatment of osteomyelitis in the diabetic foot. Contribution of conservative surgery. *Diabet Care* 1996; **19**: 1257–60.
11. Lin SS, Lee TH, Wapners KL. Plantar forefoot ulceration with equinus deformity of the ankle in diabetic patients: the effect of tendo-achilles lengthening and total contact casting. *Orthopaedics* 1996; **19**: 465–75.
12. McIntyre KE. Control of infection in the diabetic foot: the role of microbiology, immunopathology, antibiotics and guillotine amputation. *J Vasc Surg* 1987; **5**: 787–90.
13. Rayman G, Williams SA, Spencer PD, Smaje LH, Wise PH, Tooke JE. Impaired microvascular hyperaemic response to minor skin trauma in type 1 diabetes. *Br Med J* 1986; **292**: 1295–8.
14. Pecoraro RE, Chen MS. Ascorbic acid in diabetes mellitus. *Ann N Y Acad Sci* 1987; **498**: 248–58.
15. Gudas CJ. Prophylactic surgery in the diabetic foot. *Clin Pod Med Surg* 1987; **4**: 445–58.
16. Petrov O, Pfeifer M, Flood M. Recurrent plantar ulceration following pan metatarsal head resection. *J Foot Ankle Surg* 1996; **35**: 573–7.
17. Quebedeaux TL, Lavery DC, Lavery LA. The development of foot deformities and ulcers after great toe amputation in diabetes. *Diabet Care* 1996; **19**: 165–7.
18. Murdoch DP, Armstrong DG, Dacus JB, Laughlin TJ, Morgan CB, Lavery LA. The natural history of great toe amputations. *J Foot Ankle Surg* 1997; **36**: 204–8.

19. Armstrong DG, Stern S, Lavery LA, Harkless LB.   Is prophylactic diabetic foot surgery dangerous? *J Foot Ankle Surg* 1996; **35**: 585–9.
20. Crandall RC, Wagner FW.   Partial and total calcanectomy. A review of thirty-one consecutive cases over a ten-year period. *J Bone Joint Surg* 1981; **63**A: 152–5.
21. Smith DG, Stuck RM, Ketner L, Sage RM, Pinzur S.   Partial calcanectomy for the treatment of large ulcerations of the heel and calcaneal osteomyelitis. An amputation of the back of the foot. *J Bone and Joint Surg* 1992; **74-A**: 571–76.
22. Baumhauer JF, Fraga CJ, Gould JS, Johnson JE.   Total calcanectomy for the treatment of chronic calcaneal osteomyelitis. *Foot Ankle Int* 1998; **19**: 849–55.
23. Eichenholtz SN.   *Charcot Joints*. Springfield, IL: Charles C. Thomas, 1966.
24. Myerson M.   Salvage of diabetic neuropathic arthropathy with arthrodesis. In Helal B, Rowley DI, Cracchiolo A, Myerson M (eds), *Surgery of Disorders of the Foot and Ankle*. London: Martin Dunitz, 1996, 513–22.
25. Stuart MJ, Morrey BF.   Arthrodesis of the diabetic neuropathic ankle joint. *Clin Orthop* 1990; **253**: 209–11.
26. Papa J, Myerson M, Girard P.   Salvage, with arthrodesis, in intractable diabetic neuropathic arthropathy of the foot and ankle. *J Bone Joint Surg* 1993; **75**A: 1056–66.
27. Sammarco GJ, Conti SF. Surgical treatment of neuroarthropathic foot deformity. *Foot Ankle Int* 1998; **19**: 102–9.

19

Amputations in Diabetes Mellitus: Toes to Above Knee

JOHN H. BOWKER and THOMAS P. SAN GIOVANNI*

Jackson Memorial Medical Center, Miami, FL
and *Boston Children's Hospital, Boston, MA, USA

The surgeon who deals even occasionally with disorders of the foot and ankle in diabetic patients will inevitably face the need for amputation of part or all of the foot. Most often this need arises as an emergency as a result of infection, with or without concomitant ischaemia. Much less often, amputation may be required following failure of conservative or operative treatment of Charcot neuro-arthropathy. This chapter will serve as an introduction to this much-neglected area of care, which has happily been dynamized over the past few years by significant advances in materials science, resulting in continual improvement in partial foot prostheses, foot orthoses and footwear. Descriptions of the most commonly utilized procedures will be given, followed by a discussion of their expected functional outcomes.

Until the latter part of the twentieth century, partial foot amputations and disarticulations were done almost exclusively for trauma. When dry gangrene due to ischaemia or wet gangrene related to infection occurred, the usual treatment was a major lower limb amputation. More often than not, the transfemoral level was chosen, since the rationale was to amputate at a level where primary healing could safely be anticipated. Failure of primary healing due to wound ischaemia or infection posed a very real danger of death in the pre-antibiotic era, when the emphasis was on survival, not functional rehabilitation. The most common cause for partial foot ablations today is infection (wet gangrene) in persons with diabetes mellitus. The initiating aetiology is most often a normal bony prominence

The Foot in Diabetes, 3rd edn. Edited by A. J. M. Boulton, H. Connor and P. R. Cavanagh.
© 2000 John Wiley & Sons, Ltd.

combined with sensory neuropathy and inappropriate footwear, producing ulcerations which penetrate the full thickness of the skin into the bones and joints of the foot. Thermal injuries from hot foot soaks or baths, automobile floor boards or transmission tunnels, solar radiation, fireplaces or floor-furnace grids are also common. Dry gangrene, in contrast, is frequently seen as a result of dysvascularity with attendant sensory neuropathy, with smoking often an aggravating factor in all of these situations.

With advances in fields such as nutrition, wound healing and tissue oxygenation, as well as vascular and amputation surgery techniques, the surgeon now has the opportunity to consider the foot rather than the tibia or femur as the level of choice for amputation in selected cases of diabetic infection, with or without peripheral vascular disease[1]. A question that remains is how to best take advantage of these advances in order to conserve tissue commensurate with optimum future function. Unfortunately, many surgeons still consider a transverse ablation, such as a transmetatarsal amputation, to be the ideal solution for forefoot infection, even if only a ray (toe and metatarsal) is involved, analogous to the automatic selection of a transfemoral over a transtibial amputation in the past.

A major challenge today is to the attitude of the surgeon toward amputation as a treatment modality. It is now to be considered as a reconstructive procedure, not a failure of medical science or personal skills to be treated off-handedly by assigning it to the most junior surgical trainee to do without close intra-operative supervision. Indeed, the procedure should be regarded as the first step in returning the patient to his/her former functional status. As such, there is no longer any excuse for a poorly-fashioned residuum. Instead, modern amputation surgery results in the creation of a modified locomotor end-organ that will interface comfortably with a prosthesis, orthosis or modified shoe and provide the most efficient, energy-conserving gait possible. To this end, a well-planned amputation or disarticulation conserves all tissue commensurate with good function and the diagnosis; obviously, amputation must be done proximal to gangrenous tissue or an otherwise irreparably damaged body part. The next consideration is the creation of a soft-tissue envelope for the residual skeleton, which will be just mobile enough to absorb shear and direct (normal) forces during prosthetic usage. In foot ablations, the soft tissue envelope is ideally formed of plantar skin, subcutaneous tissue and investing fascia. Muscle tissue, although an integral part of the soft-tissue envelope in more proximal amputations, is not available at these levels.

Proper contouring of bone ends, by removal of sharp edges and corners, will prevent damage to the soft tissue envelope from within as it is compressed between the bony structure and the prosthesis, orthosis or shoe. Above all else, adherence of skin directly to bone must be minimized to prevent ulceration from shear forces during walking. In foot amputations and disarticulations, this is best accomplished by avoiding, insofar as possible, coverage with split skin grafts on the distal, lateral and plantar surfaces of the residuum, because split grafts in these areas often ulcerate. In contrast, split grafts placed dorsally, even directly on bony surfaces covered with granulation tissue, can last indefinitely with reasonable care. Because the skin often has compromised vascularity, it should never be handled with forceps during surgery. Attention must also be directed to prevention of equinus contracture of the ankle joint in all transverse ablations proximal to the metatarsophalangeal joints.

DETERMINING THE LEVEL OF AMPUTATION

There are a number of factors that influence the level of amputation or disarticulation. Some are not controllable and/or reversible by the efforts of the surgeon and some are. In regard to the former, amputation must be done proximal to the level of gangrenous tissue or an irreparably damaged body part; thus, the location of the lesion is critical. For example, it is extremely difficult to recommend a level distal to the tibia in cases of gangrenous changes of the heel pad. Conversely, while tissue oxygen perfusion is often a major determinant of level, it can sometimes be improved by the vascular surgeon. Before attempting the distal procedures described in this chapter, therefore, thorough evaluation of arterial blood flow is essential. In the case of foot abscesses, prompt incision and drainage in the emergency department will, by controlling proximal spread of pus under pressure, tend to preserve the greatest length at the time of definitive debridement. There are other factors that are at least partially controllable and/or reversible, some with strong behavioural overtones, such as tobacco usage or poor serum glucose control. Although these should not dictate amputation level selection, they do deserve adequate pre-operative evaluation and assiduous correction. In patients with uncontrollable psychosis or a history of major non-compliance with foot care programmes, the surgeon may be deterred from performing a Syme ankle disarticulation, a procedure which requires a high degree of patient compliance, both in the immediate postoperative period and long-term, for success to be assured. Lack of protective sensation alone should not be a factor resulting in a higher amputation level, since it can be compensated for by the appropriate use of protective interfaces in prostheses, orthoses and shoes.

FACTORS AFFECTING WOUND HEALING

Tissue oxygen perfusion may be profoundly decreased by the chronic use of vasoconstrictors. The use of caffeine and especially tobacco products should, therefore, be actively discouraged. A study by Lind et al[2] showed a marked increase in complications after primary amputations of the lower limb in patients who continued to smoke cigarettes postoperatively. This group's rate of infection and re-amputation was 2.5 times higher than in cigar smokers and non-smokers. The authors also concluded that smoking should cease at least 1 week before surgery to allow platelet function and fibrinogen levels to normalize[2]. Another potentially controllable factor influencing wound healing is nutritional status, as reflected by the level of serum albumin. Levels below 30 mmol/l can be indicative of starvation, severe renal disease with loss of protein in the urine, acute stress or a combination of these factors. Wound-healing potential is also diminished in patients who are immunosuppressed, as indicated by the total lymphocyte count, which should be at least 1500/mm[3]. Of these measures, serum albumin appears to be the more significant.

FUNCTION AND COSMESIS

Because the heel lever is intact, the partial foot or Syme amputee can continue to bear weight directly on the residual foot in a manner which approximates the normal in regard to proprioceptive feedback, in contrast to the transtibial amputee, who must interpret an entirely new feedback pattern. The ease with which normal walking function may be prosthetically restored is relative to the loss of forefoot lever length and associated muscles. This ranges from full-length, as in the case of single ray (toe and metatarsal) amputation, to virtually none in the case of midtarsal (Chopart) disarticulation. In addition to preserving weightbearing and proprioceptive functions, partial foot amputations result in the least disruption of body image and may only require shoe modifications or a limited prosthesis or orthosis.

POSTOPERATIVE MANAGEMENT

The most important part of postoperative management is compliance with the programme on the part of the patient. This includes avoiding weightbearing on the affected foot until the wound is sound enough for suture removal (usually 3–4 weeks). Since this is virtually impossible for the average diabetic patient to achieve by hopping, another strategy is required. By allowing touch-down weightbearing on the affected foot using a walking frame, only the weight of the limb is transferred through the foot. This compensates for the patient's poor balance due to loss of lower limb proprioception and truncal obesity. The foot should be kept elevated whenever the patient is not engaged in essential walking to reduce the negative effect of wound oedema on healing. During the first few weeks, the wound should be evaluated weekly. In the case of closed wounds, the protective rigid cast can be finally removed at 3 weeks with resumption of ankle and subtalar motion. In the case of open wounds, it is often possible to allow protected weightbearing, using heel-bearing weight-relief shoes. Once sound healing has been achieved, the emphasis must shift to prevention of recurrence. In recent years, great advances in the long-term protection of feet following toe, ray and transmetatarsal amputations have been made through organized pedorthic care[3]. At more proximal levels in the foot (tarsometatarsal and midtarsal), the residuum becomes progressively more difficult to capture for successful late stance phase gait activity. Here, successful fitting may require the skills of an orthotist, prosthetist and pedorthist.

MANAGEMENT OF LIMB-THREATENING EMERGENCIES

Ischaemia (Dry Gangrene)

Ischaemia of the foot often results from peripheral vascular disease with diabetes mellitus. When this presents as dry gangrene, it is extremely important to avoid the use of wet dressings, soaks and debriding agents. These measures often result in conversion of a localized, relatively benign condition to limb-threatening wet gangrene. While the necrotic areas remain dry, there is ample time to allow the completion of tissue demarcation and initial evaluation of vascular perfusion. If arterial circulation proximal to the necrosis is found to be significantly impaired, evaluation by a vascular surgeon is advised regarding the possibility of arterial bypass or recanalization with concomitant distal amputation. If blood flow cannot be improved, amputation at the appropriate level should be done promptly to optimize prosthetic rehabilitation by minimizing deconditioning due to immobility. In selected cases, maximum tissue preservation can be achieved by allowing auto-amputation of the necrotic portions. This is especially true if gangrene is limited to the digits. The entire process may take many months (Figure 19.1A,B).

Infection (Wet Gangrene)

All further weightbearing should be prohibited as soon as the patient is seen to avoid the spread of pus proximally along tissue planes. The wound is then probed with a sterile cotton-tipped applicator. If bone is contacted, a presumptive diagnosis of osteomyelitis can be made[4]. This is easily confirmed by coned-down radiographs. Bone scans are expensive and rarely required, in the authors' experience. Initial aerobic and anaerobic cultures should be taken at this time, allowing presumptive selection of antibiotics, pending the result of cultures and antibiotic sensitivities.

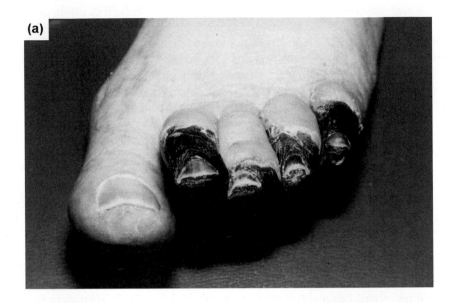

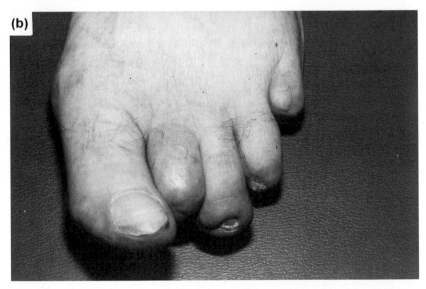

Figure 19.1 (a) Left foot of a 77 year-old diabetic male with a 30 year history of smoking. Note dry gangrene of four lateral toes. Vascular reconstruction was not feasible due to cardiac status. (b) The final result at 6 months, showing considerable salvage of toe tissue by allowing completion of auto-amputation without surgical interference. Reproduced from reference 22 by permission of Butterworth-Heineman

Broad-spectrum antibiotics should be given intravenously, due to the polymicrobial nature of most diabetic foot infections (Chapter 12).

The initial abscess drainage should be done promptly in the emergency department with ankle block anaesthesia, or without it if sensory loss from diabetic neuropathy is profound. The decompressive incision(s) must respect normal weightbearing surfaces, such as the heel pad, lateral sole and skin directly plantar to the metatarsal heads. The incision should be longitudinally orientated to avoid as many neural and vascular structures as possible. By unnecessarily extending a midsole incision into the heel pad or proximal to the ankle joint, a later procedure, such as a Syme ankle disarticulation, may be severely compromised. Control of serum glucose should be promptly initiated, although this may be difficult to accomplish in the presence of infection. Treatment of the infection with antibiotics alone, on the other hand, will be only partially effective because of the inhibitory effect of hyperglycaemia on leukocyte functions and the thrombosis of blood vessels in an abscessed area. This interdependence of serum glucose level and infection control reinforces the need for prompt surgical debridement of all necrotic and infected tissue, including bone.

Prior to definitive debridement in the operating room under ankle block anaesthesia, it is important to get a non-invasive evaluation of the arterial circulation. This and plain radiographs will quickly determine the options available for foot salvage. Nonetheless, the surgeon cannot be certain of the full proximal extent of an infective process or the viability of remaining tissues at the beginning of debridement. The patient and family must understand that the procedure is, therefore, somewhat exploratory in nature and, based upon further information obtained during the exploration, the surgeon will be as conservative as possible in removal of tissue.

Both dorsal and plantar incisions may be required to gain fully open drainage of all abscess pockets. All of the central plantar spaces can be opened by a single extensile plantar incision, which begins posterior to the medial malleolus and ends distally between the first and second metatarsal heads. Distal infections may track across the entire distal foot pad, requiring a transverse incision at the base of the toes. Following removal of patently necrotic tissue, the dorsal and plantar surfaces of the foot should be firmly stroked toward the wound, from proximal to distal along tissue planes, to empty and thus discover pockets of pus. These recesses are then probed to their proximal end, widely opened and thoroughly debrided. If the infection involves the midfoot extensively, but spares the heel pad, an open Syme ankle disarticulation may be done. Spread of infection along tendon sheaths proximal to the ankle joint or into the heel pad or ankle joint generally precludes anything but an open ankle disarticulation as a prelude to transtibial amputation.

In addition to obviously infected and necrotic tissue, all poorly vascularized tissues, such as tendons, joint capsules, volar plates and articular cartilage, should be treated as foreign bodies and removed as part of a thorough debridement. Otherwise, the wound may remain open, often for months, until these sequestrate. All visually uninvolved, well-vascularized tissue should be saved for secondary reconstruction regardless of its configuration. The "guillotine" approach to amputation, in contrast, will preclude creative use of otherwise salvageable tissues in preserving forefoot length. All wounds should be *lightly* packed with saline-moistened gauze to allow free wicking of the infective fluids to the surface. Thrice daily wet saline gauze dressings start the next day.

In cases where the infective process is purulent, the surgeon must be willing to redebride the foot. This may become necessary for several reasons. First, it is sometimes difficult to be certain that all involved tissue has been removed. Second, some areas of skin, optimistically left, may now be frankly necrotic. Third, the infection may have persisted; therefore, every 24–48 hours, the surgeon should manually strip the infected areas from proximal to distal to locate pockets of infection which may have escaped initial detection and require redebridement. Secondary debridements can be done either at the bedside or more formally in the operating room.

POSTOPERATIVE MANAGEMENT OF OPEN AMPUTATIONS

Damp saline gauze dressings, gently packed into all recesses of the wound, are excellent for most open amputations. This method possesses the advantages of low cost and ease of execution. Requiring only "clean" technique, it is easily taught to patient and family prior to discharge. The basic method consists of a dressing change every 8 hours. This allows the gauze to dry enough to adhere to the wound surface and debride detritus with each change. If the wound is producing an excess of fluid, the gauze may be used dry until this ceases. Conversely, if the wound is too dry, or if a vital tendon or joint capsule is exposed, a wet-to-wet method is useful. Four hours after each dressing change, the dressing is rewetted exteriorly with saline to prevent critical tissues from ever drying. Repeated exposure of the wound surface to povidone–iodine or hydrogen peroxide can be cytotoxic to granulation tissue. If *Pseudomonas* colonization occurs, as evidenced by a greenish tinge to the dressings, a 0.25% acetic acid solution can be used to suppress it for a few days *only*, because its fibroblast toxicity exceeds its bactericidal activity.

Conversely, if the wound has little or no initial purulence and is visually clean following debridement with no compromised tissue, a primary loose closure can generally be done. If the wound has sufficient volume (e.g. great toe, ray or transmetatarsal ablations), it can be closed over a Kritter flow-through irrigation system as follows: a 14-gauge polyethylene venous catheter is passed into the depths of the wound from an adjacent site by means of its integral needle. The catheter is sutured to the skin and connected to a bag of normal saline solution. The fluid exits the wound between widely-spaced simple skin sutures and is collected in an absorbent dressing. The irrigation continues for 3 days at the rate of 1 litre/24 hours. The outer layers only of the dressing are changed every 4–5 hours[5]. On the third day, the surgeon should gently compress the edges of the wound. If there is any sign of purulence, the sutures can be easily removed and the wound packed, but this should be an uncommon occurrence if patients have been carefully selected. The advantages of this method are that it allows primary healing, usually within 3 weeks, and avoids the need for secondary closure or the several months required for healing by secondary intention. In addition, skin grafting is avoided, resulting in better cosmesis.

Before discharging the patient to outpatient status, the surgeon should await initial formation of granulation tissue throughout the depths of the wound. The diabetologist will have been consulted at the time of admission to assist in preoperative control of serum blood glucose levels and to get the patient on a management programme that will continue to assist wound healing after discharge by decreasing tissue glycation. The infectious disease specialist will have been consulted in cases of unusual infection. All possible factors that will likely delay healing should be corrected, such as malnutrition and the use of vasoconstrictors, like nicotine and caffeine. Weightbearing should be limited to the absolute minimum, and then only with a weight-relief shoe. The patient is taught to reduce wound-site oedema by avoiding dependency on the foot. Adequate postoperative nutritional support must include sufficient caloric intake to compensate for poor initial serum albumin level, as well as the catabolic effects of infection and bed rest. Supplements such as iron, zinc and vitamin C provide essential elements for collagen formation in wound healing[6]. Oral hyperalimentation will require appropriate adjustment in hypoglycaemic medication to prevent iatrogenic hyperglycaemia.

PARTIAL FOOT AMPUTATIONS AND DISARTICULATIONS

If the criteria for level selection are met and the standards for wound healing are correctly factored in, no amputation level in the foot need be excluded on the basis of associated diabetes mellitus. Longitudinal, rather than transverse, amputation should be the goal whenever achievable. By only narrowing the foot, rather than shortening it, postoperative fitting of shoes is greatly simplified. Conversely, the surgeon should also consider the distinct possibility that a failed forefoot amputation done for infection may forfeit the chance for a Syme ankle disarticulation, so he/she must be reasonably sure that a partial foot amputation is the logical initial procedure. Specific amputations and disarticulations, starting with the toes, will now be considered, followed by discussion of the expected functional outcome at each level.

Toe Disarticulations

Method

In cases of osteomyelitis of the distal phalanx of the great toe, sufficient skin can often be salvaged to permit an interphalangeal disarticulation. To achieve closure of the wound without tension, it may be necessary to trim the condyles of the proximal phalanx as well as to shorten it slightly. The proximal phalanx will aid with balance through preservation of the flexor hallucis brevis–sesamoid complex (windlass mechanism). The metatarso-phalangeal joint is the next site of election when more than the distal portion of the proximal phalanx is infected. To avoid future plantar ulceration, the sesamoids, with their fibrocartilaginous plate, should be excised. The articular cartilage should also be removed and the head carefully rounded with a file.

Osteomyelitis of the distal phalanx of a lesser toe often follows ulceration of a fixed mallet toe deformity in association with loss of protective sensation. It is most commonly noted in the second toe in persons with a long second metatarsal bone, especially following disarticulation of the great toe. Removal of the infected distal phalanx shortens the toe, which then no longer projects beyond the adjacent toes, reducing the risk of future ulceration.

Disarticulation of the second toe at the metatarsophalangeal joint may create a special problem by removing the lateral support it provides to the great toe. A hallux valgus (bunion) deformity is likely to follow (Figure 19.2A,B). To avoid this iatrogenic bony prominence in an insensate foot, it is usually better to remove the second metatarsal through its proximal metaphysis along with the toe (ray amputation). The forefoot can then narrow as the first and third metatarsals approximate each other, resulting in a good cosmetic and functional result (Figure 19.3). If toes three or four alone are disarticulated, the adjacent ones will tend to close the intervening space, thus restoring a smooth contour to the distal forefoot. Leaving a lesser toe isolated by removing the toes on either side should be avoided

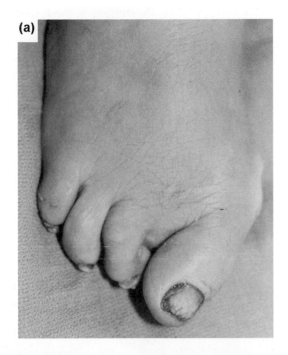

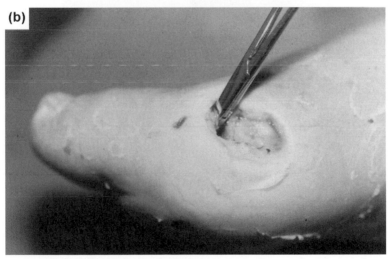

Figure 19.2 Result following disarticulation of right second toe in an 87 year-old diabetic male. (a) Note hallux valgus deformity secondary to loss of lateral support of second toe. (b) Note ulcer penetrating first metatarsophalangeal joint. The great toe was salvaged by excision of the joint (see also Figures 19.8, 19.9)

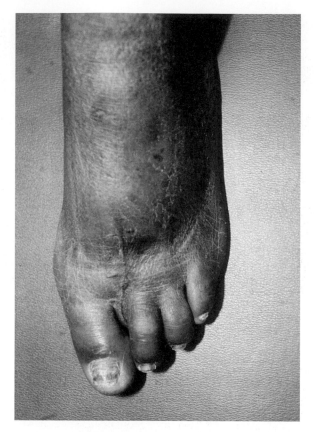

Figure 19.3 Left foot of diabetic female with second ray resection for osteomyelitis shows no significant hallux valgus because of lateral support provided by third toe after postoperative forefoot narrowing. Reproduced from reference 5 by permission of W. B. Saunders Company

because of the increased susceptibility to injury of the isolated and functionless toe (Figure 19.4).

Expected Functional Outcome

Following toe disarticulations, ambulatory function should approach normal, provided that a shoe with a firm sole and moulded soft insert incorporating any required filler has been fitted.

Function will be most affected by disarticulation of the great toe at the metatarsophalangeal joint, because the specialized function of the first ray in the final transfer of weight during late stance phase is lost. Mann et al[7] found that, following removal of the great toe, the end-point of progression

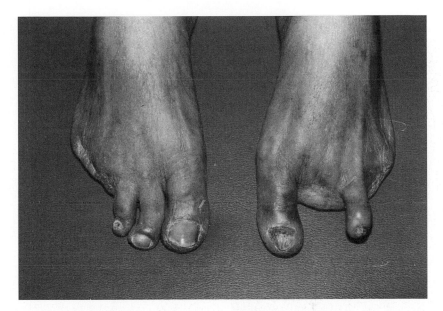

Figure 19.4 Note striking difference in distal forefoot contours of right and left feet. On the right, the remaining lesser toes are protected by the great toe. On the left, the fourth toe is constantly exposed to minor trauma and does not contribute to propulsion or foot length like the great toe. It should have been removed with the other lesser toes. Reproduced from reference 19 by permission of W. B. Saunders Company

of the moving centre of plantar pressure during stance had shifted from the second metatarsal head to the third, despite a dropping of the first metatarsal head, due to loss of the great toe's stabilizing windlass mechanism associated with the flexor hallucis brevis complex. Loss of lesser toes, in contrast, appears to cause little clinical difficulty.

Ray Amputations

Method

A ray amputation is a longitudinal excision of a toe and its metatarsal. In regard to the first (medial) ray, shortening should be as limited as possible, leaving the maximum metatarsal shaft length to allow effective orthotic restoration of the medial arch (Figure 19.5A,B). Preservation of first metatarsal length is generally relatively easy, because the usual cause of septic arthritis of the metatarsophalangeal joint is a penetrating ulcer plantar to the first metatarsal head/sesamoids. Only a portion of the head may need to be removed to eradicate the infection, preserving all uninvolved portions of the shaft. The extent of osteomyelitis in a metatarsal

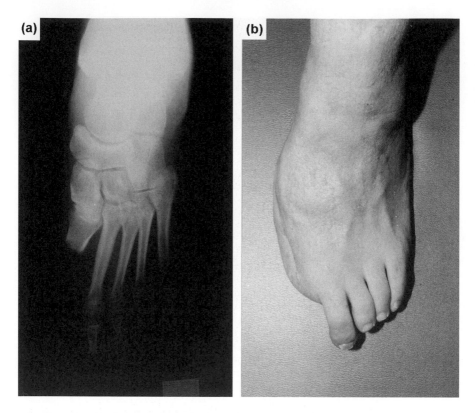

Figure 19.5 (a) Radiograph of left foot after radical first ray amputation for diabetic infection. There is insufficient metatarsal shaft remaining to allow effective medial orthotic support. (b) Note planovalgus position of foot secondary to loss of medial column support. Reproduced from reference 20 by permission of W. B. Saunders Company

can generally be determined visually. The bone should be bevelled on the plantar aspect to avoid a high-pressure area during roll-over at the end of the stance phase of gait.

Single lesser ray amputations will affect only the width of the forefoot. Resection may be carried out through the proximal metaphysis, where the involved ray intersects with the adjacent metatarsals. The fifth metatarsal should be transected obliquely with an inferolateral-facing facet. The uninvolved portion of the shaft is left to retain the insertion of the peroneus brevis muscle. At times, multiple lateral ray resections are required in cases of massive forefoot infection. In this situation, the lateral metatarsals can be divided in an oblique fashion, with each affected metatarsal being cut somewhat longer as one progresses toward the first ray (Figure 19.6). If all

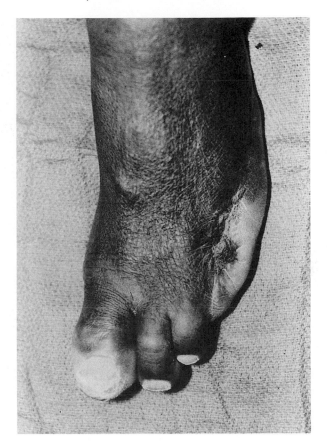

Figure 19.6 Left foot of diabetic male with fourth and fifth ray amputations. He functions well in a depth shoe with custom-moulded inlay with lateral filler. Reproduced from reference 21 by permission of W. B. Saunders Company

rays but the first are involved, it can be left as the only complete ray (Figure 19.7). With proper pedorthic fitting, this is preferable to a transmetatarsal amputation.

Expected Functional Outcome

First ray amputation, involving major removal of the first metatarsal, is devastating to barefoot stance and gait because an intact medial column is essential to proper foot balance during stance and forward progression. The greater the length of first metatarsal shaft preserved, the more effective the orthotic restoration of the medial arch can be. This is

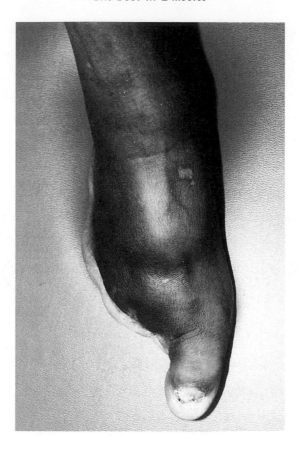

Figure 19.7 Right foot of a diabetic male with the lateral four rays excised in an oblique fashion for a severe diabetic foot abscess. The first ray was left intact. Good function was present with customized footwear

accomplished by means of a custom-moulded non-rigid foot orthosis, fitted into a shoe with a rigid rocker bottom. Single lesser ray amputation will provide an excellent result from both the functional and cosmetic points of view. In these cases, only the width of the forefoot is affected, while roll-over function and overall foot balance during terminal stance appear to remain essentially normal. Removal of several lateral rays, if done as conservatively as possible, can be adequately compensated for with proper pedorthic fitting. Preservation of even the first ray alone will retain roll-over function at the end of stance as well as full foot length in the shoe. Barefoot walking appears to be severely impaired in all but the single lesser ray amputations.

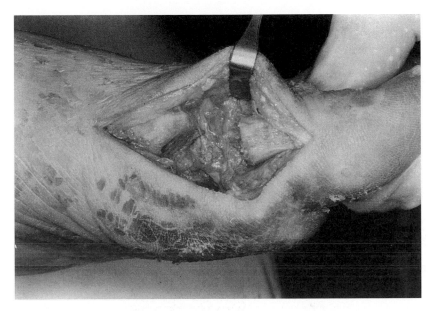

Figure 19.8 Intra-operative medial view of the left forefoot showing excision of chronically infected first metatarsophalangeal joint. Note plantar bevel of the metatarsal metaphysis. Joint infection had followed penetration from plantar ulcer. Reproduced from reference 1 by permission of W. B. Saunders Company

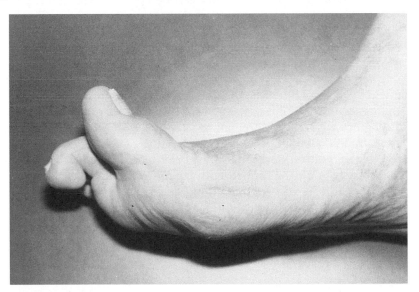

Figure 19.9 Right foot of diabetic male 14 months following excision of first metatarsophalangeal joint for septic arthritis. Adequate active dorsiflexion is demonstrated due to preservation of the extensor hallucis longus tendon

Excision of First Metatarsophalangeal Joint

There are instances in which a penetrating ulcer has destroyed the first metatarsophalangeal joint, leaving the great toe viable. In this instance, in lieu of a first ray amputation, the joint alone can be removed through a medial longitudinal incision. Of course, all relatively avascular tissues, including the sesamoid complex, remaining articular cartilage, joint capsule and flexor tendons, as well as infected cancellous bone, should be removed (Figure 19.8). If the wound is sufficiently clean at the conclusion of the procedure, it can be closed loosely over the Kritter flow-through irrigation system, as described above. The cosmetic result is much better than following great toe amputation, although the stabilizing windlass mechanism is lost with the excision of the flexor hallucis brevis complex. Active dorsiflexion of the great toe is retained by preservation of the extensor hallucis longus tendon (Figure 19.9).

Transmetatarsal Amputation

Method

This should be considered whenever most or all of the first metatarsal bone must be removed, or two or more medial rays, or more than one central ray, must be excised to control infection. For maximum function, it is important to save all metatarsal shaft length that can be covered with good plantar skin distally (Figure 19.10A,B). Residual dorsal defects can be easily closed with split skin grafts. With avoidance of shear forces and with properly fitted footwear, these dorsal grafts rarely ulcerate. To assist in preserving forefoot length and in assuring distal coverage of the metatarsal shafts with a durable soft tissue envelope, the transverse plantar and dorsal incisions are made at the base of the toes. The metatarsal shafts should be bevelled on the plantar surface to reduce distal plantar peak pressures during roll-over. In addition, if passive ankle dorsiflexion is absent with the knee extended, a concomitant percutaneous fractional lengthening of the Achilles tendon is indicated to also reduce these pressures. Prior to discharge, a well-padded total contact cast should be applied with the foot in a plantigrade or slightly dorsiflexed position to protect the wound and prevent equinus deformity. The cast is changed weekly until the wound is sound, usually at 6 weeks, when a shoe with filler and stiff rocker sole can be fitted. In case of an associated "drop foot", common in diabetic patients, a well-padded ankle–foot orthosis will be necessary.

Expected Functional Outcome

Durham and associates reported that 53% of 43 open transmetatarsal amputations healed by wound contraction or split skin grafting at a mean

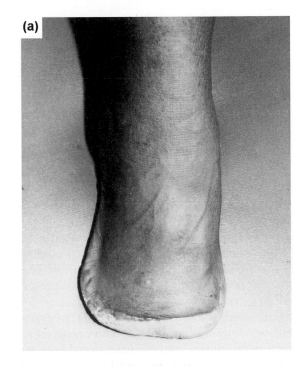

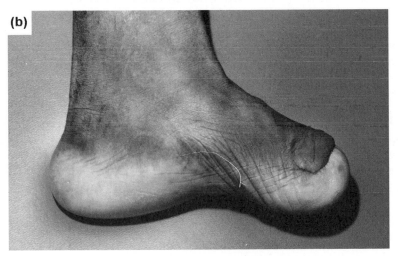

Figure 19.10 Ideal transmetatarsal amputation. (a) Dorsal view. (b) Medial view. Note placement of distal plantar flap, overall length of residual forefoot, maintenance of medial arch and absence of equinus deformity. Reproduced from reference 19 by permission of W. B. Saunders Company

time of 7.1 ± 5.6 months. Ninety-one per cent (21 of 23 patients) became independent walkers, but they provided no long-term data regarding durability of the scarred or grafted wounds[8]. Following transmetatarsal amputation, the shoe sole will require a steel shank or carbon fibre stiffener with rocker to avoid distal stump ulcers from the shoe wrapping around the end of the residual foot. A distal filler will also be needed to maintain the integrity of the toebox. Some patients who are not too concerned about cosmesis will elect for a custom-made short shoe, but this will cause an unequal "drop-off" gait due to the shortened forefoot lever arm.

Tarsometatarsal (Lisfranc) Disarticulation

Method

This disarticulation, described by Lisfranc in 1815, can be used in cases of diabetes mellitus if one is very selective, since infection uncontrolled at this level will risk the failure of a Syme ankle disarticulation. To help maintain a muscle-balanced residual foot, it is important to preserve the tendon insertions of the peroneus brevis, peroneus longus and tibialis anterior muscles. They will help to counterbalance the massive triceps surae complex, preventing equinus deformity. This contracture can also be avoided by doing a primary percutaneous fractional heel cord lengthening, followed by application of a cast with the foot in a plantigrade or slightly dorsiflexed position. Another method that the author now uses successfully in lieu of heel cord lengthening is cast immobilization of the residual foot in dorsiflexion for 3–4 weeks, to weaken the triceps surae relative to the ankle dorsiflexors (Figure 19.11).

Expected Functional Outcome

This level represents a major loss of forefoot length, with a corresponding decrease in barefoot walking function. To restore fairly normal late stance phase walking function, an intimately-fitting fixed-ankle prosthesis or orthosis, combined with a rigid rocker bottom shoe, is required.

MIDTARSAL (CHOPART) DISARTICULATION

Method

This disarticulation is through the talonavicular and calcaneocuboid joints. It can only occasionally be used in diabetic foot infections because of its proximity to the heel pad, as discussed under tarsometatarsal disarticulation. All active dorsiflexion function is lost at the time of disarticulation, but can be restored to this extremely short residual foot by attachment of the

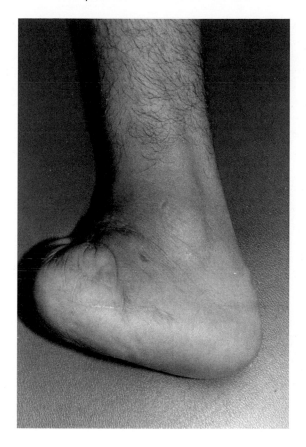

Figure 19.11 Lateral views of right foot of male with Lisfranc disarticulation, demonstrating range of ankle dorsiflexion available with preservation of midfoot insertions of extrinsic muscles

tibialis anterior tendon to the anterolateral talus[9]. To maintain balance between dorsiflexors and plantar flexors, excision of 2–3 cm of the Achilles tendon is effective in preventing equinus deformity. A well-padded total contact cast should be applied with the hindfoot in slight dorsiflexion, with appropriate changes for about 6 weeks to prevent equinous deformity of the hindfoot and allow secure healing of the tendon to the talus. The authors have treated several cases of equinus deformity following Chopart disarticulation in which the tibialis anterior tendon was not surgically attached to the talus. Active dorsiflexion with restoration of heel pad weightbearing was obtained by partial Achilles tendon excision and cast immobilization, as described above, with resulting comfortable plantigrade

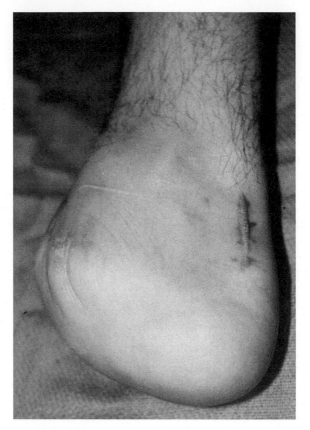

Figure 19.12 Medial view of right foot of 17 year-old male with Chopart disarticulation. He presented with distal stump pain while walking in prosthesis secondary to severe equinus deformity. Photograph taken 3 weeks after excision of 2 cm of the Achilles tendon to restore the heel pad to a plantigrade position. Maximum active dorsiflexion is demonstrated

gait. This simple salvage procedure avoids revision to a Syme or higher level (Figure 19.12).

Expected Functional Outcome

This disarticulation also allows direct end-bearing without a prosthesis, but has no inherent roll-over function. This is in contrast to the Syme level, where the prosthesis is essential to heel-pad stability and leg-length equality. As in Lisfranc disarticulation, an intimately-fitted rigid ankle prosthesis or orthosis fitted into a shoe with a rigid rocker sole is required to permit adequate late stance phase gait.

Syme Ankle Disarticulation

Method

This procedure, described by Syme in 1843, permits distal end-weightbearing on the preserved heel pad and thus may be considered a type of partial foot ablation. The chief indication is inability to salvage a more distal level in an infected foot with an adequate posterior tibial artery, the main source of flow to the heel pad. It is also indicated if an infection is too close to the heel pad to risk failure of a Lisfranc or Chopart disarticulation. Syme ankle disarticulation can also be a reasonable choice in certain cases of severe neuroarthropathic (Charcot) destruction of the ankle joint. It offers the patient a much more rapid return to weightbearing status than ankle arthrodesis, because it requires no fusion or fibrous ankylosis of bones (Figure 19.13A,B,C). Contraindications include inadequate blood flow to the heel pad, infection involving the heel pad compartments, or ascending lymphangitis uncontrolled by systemic antibiotics. A low serum albumin due to malnutrition or diabetic nephropathy, as well as decreased immunocompetence, can also seriously impede healing[10,11]. Uncompensated congestive heart failure will prevent healing by keeping the wound tissues oedematous[10]. A past history of reckless non-compliance or overt psychosis should alert the surgeon to the likelihood of failure of this procedure.

This operation, although not difficult, must be meticulously done, with careful attention to preservation of the posterior tibial neurovascular structures and the integrity of the vertically orientated fat-filled fibrous chambers of the heel pad, which provide shock absorption on heel strike. If infection is close to the heel pad, the wound can be left open for 7–10 days before closure to determine whether drainage and antibiotics have been effective. If infection has not been controlled, a long transtibial amputation is done without further delay. Closure must be snug, but not tight, with the heel pad perfectly centred under the leg. The heel pad flap can be accurately secured under the tibia by suturing the plantar fascia to the anterior tibial cortex through drill holes. Closed wound irrigation, using a modified Foley catheter inserted through a lateral stab wound, is continued for 3 days. A carefully moulded non-weightbearing cast, holding the heel pad centred and slightly forward, is applied immediately after removal of the catheter. The cast is changed weekly for 4–5 weeks, at which time a temporary prosthesis, consisting of a cast with walking heel, is applied. This is changed whenever loose, but at least every 2 weeks, until limb volume has stabilized. A definitive prosthesis is then applied. At no time is the patient allowed to bear weight without a prosthesis.

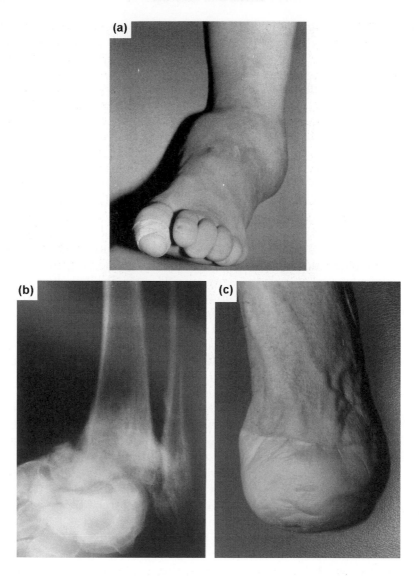

Figure 19.13 Feet of 32 year-old female with type 1 diabetes one year after undisplaced bimalleolar fracture of left ankle treated in cast for 6 weeks. She was insensate to just below the knees. (a) Anterior view showing severe medial displacement of left foot. Pressure ulcer was present over lateral malleolus from misguided use of ankle–foot orthosis to control this irreducible, increasing deformity. (b) Anteroposterior radiograph showing foot displacement with ankle joint and hindfoot dissolution. (c) Stump appearance 8 years after surgery. She actively wears her prosthesis 14–16 hours daily. Reproduced from reference 19 by permission of W. B. Saunders Company

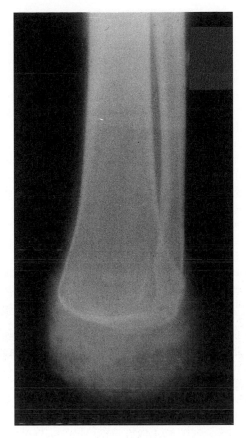

Figure 19.14 Syme procedure: radiograph of Syme stump. Note the thickness of the heel pad, which provides excellent end-weightbearing within the prosthetic socket

Expected Functional Outcome

In that the Syme ankle disarticulation preserves heel-pad bearing along normal proprioceptive pathways, minimal prosthetic gait training is required. The stump is also remarkably activity-tolerant, even if insensate, provided that the socket holds the heel pad directly under the tibia (Figure 19.14). This position must then be maintained by careful prosthetic follow-up as the inevitable calf atrophy occurs. The Syme level is more energy-efficient than the transtibial level[12]. Although the prosthesis is more difficult to contour anatomically in its distal half, in relation to its transtibial counterpart, the patient's ability to engage comfortably in a wide variety of activities should lead to much wider use of this procedure than at present.

Transtibial Amputation

Method

Despite the manifest functional advantages of partial foot ablations and the desire of the surgeon to conserve all possible length, at times it is impossible to salvage any portion of the foot. Once this has been determined or strongly suspected by the primary physician, a surgical consultant with a definite bias toward preservation of locomotor function should be asked to thoroughly review the problem. If the consultant also finds the foot unsalvageable, a prompt transtibial amputation, preserving as much length as possible, should be followed by early prosthetic fitting. In a patient with dry gangrene of the entire foot, there may be no palpable pulses, even at the groin. If the limb below the knee is warm, transcutaneous oxygen mapping of the skin with oxygen challenge will assess healing potential. If skin perfusion is found to be poor (less than 30 mmHg), an *interested* vascular surgeon should determine whether proximal bypass or recanalization is feasible. Even when patches of gangrenous tissue are present distal to the knee at the time of a successful bypass, a short transtibial amputation can often be fashioned using non-standard flaps. The shortest useful transtibial amputation must include the tibial tubercle, to preserve knee extension by the quadriceps. Stable prosthetic socket fitting at this level is greatly enhanced by removal of the fibular head and neck and high transection of the peroneal nerve above the knee. Beyond universal acceptance of this shortest possible functional transtibial level, no agreement has been reached regarding an ideal length for optimum prosthetic function. Experienced amputation surgeons, such as Epps and Moore, however, have strongly endorsed as distal a site as possible in order to minimize the excess energy requirement of prosthetic gait[14,15]. The authors have found that most patients with wet gangrene who have good perfusion will heal at the junction of the proximal two-thirds and distal one-third of the leg. Even in dysvascular cases, healing can often be achieved at the midleg level (for further discussion on optimal length, see Chapter 21).

A different challenge to preservation of the knee joint is presented when a massive closed foot abscess has spread along tissue planes under pressure into the crural compartments. If this occurs, and there is sufficient vascularity, there is no need to amputate above the infection, i.e. at the transfemoral level, so long as the knee joint is uninvolved. Instead, an emergent ankle disarticulation is done. Each crural compartment is then manually stripped from proximal to distal to express any pus. Each involved compartment is then incised longitudinally, beginning distally and extending proximally to the limit of involvement. *All* infected and necrotic tissue is thoroughly excised. The wounds are firmly packed for haemostasis until the next day. Thereafter, they are lightly packed thrice daily with wet-to-dry saline gauze dressings. After 10–14 days, the wounds are usually well-granulated and ready for re-excision and closure at the long transtibial level[13].

Expected Functional Outcome

From a rehabilitation point of view, preservation of the knee joint cannot be overemphasized. Analysis of several studies evaluating the prosthetic rehabilitation of persons with transtibial vs. transfemoral amputations revealed that 75% of transtibial vs. 25% of transfemoral amputees were successfully rehabilitated utilizing a prosthesis[16]. A modern, well-fitted transtibial prosthesis can restore a surprising amount of function, provided that good comfort is achieved in the socket. A dynamic response foot provides good shock absorption at heel contact and gives the amputee a sense of propulsion in late stance. A rotator unit can reduce torsional loads at the stump–socket interface. For a detailed discussion of all aspects of transtibial amputation, including surgical technique, the reader is referred to Chapter 18A of the American Academy of Orthopaedic Surgeons' *Atlas of Limb Prosthetics*, 2nd edn[13].

Knee Disarticulation

When the knee joint cannot be salvaged, knee disarticulation is much to be preferred over transfemoral amputation. Surgically speaking, it is a simpler, less shocking procedure with minimal blood loss and rapid postoperative recovery. The authors advocate the use of a long posterior myofasciocutaneous flap, which includes the full length of the gastrocnemius bellies, thus allowing comfortable direct end-weightbearing[17]. All muscles which crossed the knee joint are sutured to the distal soft tissues, to enhance hip extension. The prosthetic advantages include end-weightbearing through normal proprioceptive pathways and a strong, muscle-balanced lever arm, with the thigh in a normally adducted position. In cases where the patient is permanently bed-and-chair-bound, there is greater bed mobility, including good kneeling and turning ability, as well as better sitting balance and transfer ability, as compared to the transfemoral level.

Transfemoral Amputation

Following transfemoral amputation, only a minority of patients become functional prosthesis users. This is because the excess energy expenditure is 65% or more, far beyond what many patients can safely generate, due to cardiovascular disease. If a transfemoral amputation is unavoidable, however, all length that can be adequately covered with muscle and skin should be saved to minimize this excess oxygen requirement.

On the basis of cadaver studies, Gottschalk calculated that up to 70% of hip adductor power and considerable hip extensor power are lost with division of the adductor magnus muscle, related to its large cross-sectional area and distal attachment at the adductor tubercle. The resulting muscular imbalance between hip abductors and adductors leads to a lurching prosthetic gait, due to a relatively abducted position of the stump in the prosthetic socket. This increase of lateral translation of the body's centre of gravity during gait is one of the major causes of excess energy expenditure at this amputation level. Based on this research, Gottschalk developed a vastly improved technique for transfemoral amputation, which preserves adductor magnus power by reattaching its tendon to the distal-lateral cortex of the femur. The quadriceps muscle, after detachment from the superior pole of the patella, is positioned over the end of the femur and attached to posterior femoral drill holes, thus providing an excellent, stable distal end pad. The hamstrings and the iliotibial band are also re-attached, to assist in hip extension[18].

In summary, this chapter may act as a reliable guide to both beginning and experienced team members in the daunting task of providing the most conservative treatment possible to diabetic patients facing minor or major loss of tissue of the lower limb secondary to infection, dysvascularity or trauma, and various combinations thereof. The bibliography is meant to stimulate further exploration of this often-neglected, but challenging and rewarding, area of care.

ACKNOWLEDGEMENT

The authors wish to express their thanks to Ms Patsy Bain for her expert preparation of this manuscript.

REFERENCES

1. Bowker JH.   Partial foot amputations and disarticulations. *Foot Ankle Clin* 1997; **2**: 153.
2. Lind J, Kramhoff M, Bodker S.   The influence of smoking on complications after primary amputations of the lower extremity. *Clin Orthop Rel Res* 1991; **267**: 211.
3. Janisse DJ.   Pedorthic care of the diabetic foot. In Levin ME, O'Neal LW and Bowker JH (eds), *The Diabetic Foot*, 5th edn. St. Louis, MI: Mosby Year Book, 1993.
4. Grayson JL, Gibbons GW, Balogh K et al.   Probing to bone in infected pedal ulcers. A clinical sign of underlying osteomyelitis in diabetic patients. *J Am Med Assoc* 1995; **273**: 721.

5. Bowker JH. The choice between limb salvage and amputation: infection. In Bowker JH, Michael JW (eds), *Atlas of Limb Prosthetics*, 2nd edn. St. Louis, MI: Mosby Year Book, 1992; 39.

6. Stotts NA, Washington DF. Nutrition: a critical component of wound healing. *AACN Clin Issues* 1990; **1**: 585.

7. Mann RA, Poppen NK, O'Kinski M. Amputation of the great toe. A clinical and biomechanical study. *Clin Orthop Rel Res* 1988; **226**: 192.

8. Durham JR, McCoy DM, Sawchuk AP et al. Open transmetatarsal amputation in the treatment of severe foot infections. *Am J Surg* 1989; **158**: 127.

9. Letts M, Pyper A. The modified Chopart's amputation. *Clin Orthop Rel Res* 1990; **256**: 44.

10. Bowker JH, Bui VT, Redman S et al. Syme amputation in diabetic dysvascular patients. *Orthop Trans* 1988; **12**: 767.

11. Wagner FW Jr. The Syme ankle disarticulation: surgical procedures. In Bowker JH, Michael JW (eds), *Atlas of Limb Prosthetics*, 2nd edn. St. Louis, MI: Mosby Year Book, 1992; 413.

12. Waters RL. The energy expenditure of amputee gait. In Bowker JH, Michael JW (eds), *Atlas of Limb Prosthetics*, 2nd edn. St. Louis, MI: Mosby Year Book, 1992; 381.

13. Bowker JH, Goldberg B, Poonekar PD. Transtibial amputation: surgical procedures and immediate postsurgical management. In Bowker JH, Michael JW (eds), *Atlas of Limb Prosthetics*, 2nd edn. St. Louis, MI: Mosby Year Book, 1992; 429.

14. Epps CH Jr. Amputation of the lower limb. In Evarts MC (ed.), *Surgery of the Musculoskeletal System*, 2nd edn. New York: Churchill Livingstone, 1990; 5121.

15. Moore TJ. Amputations of the lower extremities. In Chapman MW (ed.), *Operative Orthopaedics*, 2nd edn. Philadelphia, PA: Lippincott, 1993; 2443.

16. Bowker JH. Transtibial (below-knee) amputation. *Report of International Society for Prosthetics and Orthotics Consensus Conference on Amputation Surgery.* Copenhagen: International Society for Prosthetics and Orthotics, 1992; 10.

17. Bowker JH, San Giovanni TP, Pinzur MS. An improved technique for knee disarticulation utilizing a posterior myofasciocutaneous flap [Abstract]. In *Conference Book of the Ninth World Congress of the International Society for Prosthetics and Orthotics*. Amsterdam: International Society for Prosthetics and Orthotics, 1998; 373.

18. Gottschalk F. Transfemoral amputation: surgical procedures. In Bowker JH, Michael JW (eds), *Atlas of Limb Prosthetics*, 2nd edn. St. Louis, MI: Mosby Year Book, 1992; 501.

19. Bowker JH. *The Diabetic Foot*, 5th edn. St. Louis, MI: Mosby Year Book, 1993; Chapter 20.

20. Bowker JH. Medical and surgical considerations in the care of patients with insensitive dysvascular feet. *J Prosthet Orthot* 1991; **4**: 23–30.

21. Bowker JH, San Giovanni TP. Amputations and disarticulations. In Hyerson M. (ed.), *Foot and Ankle Disorders*. Philadelphia, PA: Saunders, 2000.

22. Bowker JH, Poonekar PD. *Amputation*. Oxford: Butterworth-Heinemann, 1996; Chapter 31.

20

Rehabilitation after Amputation

ERNEST VAN ROSS and STUART LARNER

Withington Hospital and Manchester Royal Infirmary, Manchester, UK

"Rehabilitation converts a patient into a person."
Lord Holderness

Amputation of an irreparable limb can save life, improve health and, following rehabilitation, allow reintegration into society. All too often, the negative aspects of amputation are emphasized and patients, their families and their doctors consider amputation to be a "failure" of medical and surgical practice. Rather, amputation should be viewed as a therapeutic option to be used judiciously at the most expedient time in the treatment of the patient with diabetes.

Rehabilitation is a planned process with clearly defined objectives, delivered appropriately and efficiently. It aims to maximize the person's physical, psychological, social and vocational functions. Acute medical services concentrate on treatment of the impairment (disturbance in the normal structure and functioning of the body or part of the body). Impairment results in disability (a loss or reduction of functional ability and activity). It is, however, the social and environmental consequences of impairment and disability that cause the person to be at a disadvantage in society. This disadvantage, as compared to his/her fellows, is the "handicap". In most people's perception it is their handicap which is of the greatest concern to themselves and their families. Rehabilitation should address impairments, disabilities and handicaps.

The Foot in Diabetes, 3rd edn. Edited by A. J. M. Boulton, H. Connor and P. R. Cavanagh.
© 2000 John Wiley & Sons, Ltd.

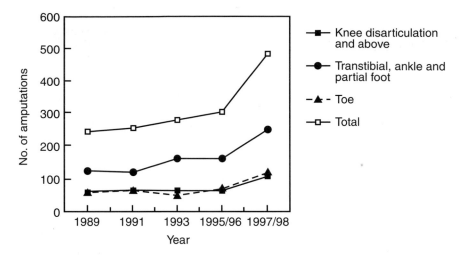

Figure 20.1 Numbers of amputations by level performed on people with diabetes in Scotland. Data from Information and Statistics Division, Edinburgh

THE AMPUTEE POPULATION

There are very few studies of the numbers of amputations performed on a national scale. Most studies relate to clinic-based or hospital-based activities and can only project a small part of the picture. The Information and Statistics Division in Scotland[1] has recorded amputations performed in every Scottish hospital since 1989. These statistics show a steady increase in the numbers of patients with diabetes undergoing amputation. However, other sources, notably the Danish Amputation Register[2], show a reduction of new amputations in people with diabetes.

In the Scottish statistics the levels of amputation have remained broadly similar over the years, with approximately half being performed at the transtibial or ankle level, a quarter being excision of a toe ray and the remaining quarter being at the above-knee level (Figure 20.1). The majority of amputations were performed between the fifth and eighth decade, with a peak in the seventh decade. The male:female ratio was 2:1 when calculated over all ages but was 3:1 in the under-50 age group.

When first seen at the Manchester Artificial Limb Centre, it is estimated that 54% of new referrals have three or more concurrent complications of diabetes[3] that are under medical treatment. All new unilateral amputees show evidence of pathology in the remaining limb—about 30% have pure neuropathy, 20% vascular disease and the remaining 50% neuro-ischaemia (unpublished data).

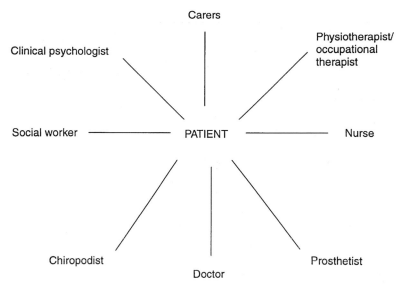

Figure 20.2 Multi-disciplinary team

PATIENT ASSESSMENT AND MANAGEMENT

A comprehensive management programme is best delivered by a well coordinated multidisciplinary team based at a rehabilitation centre[4]. The team (Figure 20.2) should allow every member to have full professional responsibility whilst at the same time giving each of them encouragement to act in concert with other members in order to achieve planned objectives. Patients and their families are very much part of the team and should share all medical information. The team is usually led by a consultant in rehabilitation medicine.

The multidisciplinary team must have good interdisciplinary relationships with those who refer patients from acute medical and surgical specialties and also with primary care clinicians, community rehabilitation teams, social services, benefits agencies and vocational rehabilitation centres. Good communication between various teams allows the patient to receive a seamless package of care.

It is convenient for the purposes of description to divide patient care into pre-amputation, surgical and post-amputation phases of care.

PRE-AMPUTATION PHASE

This phase begins as soon as the decision to amputate has been made by the physicians and surgeons caring for the patient. The reasons for amputation must be made clear to the patient. This is followed by a full medical, psychological and social evaluation of the patient and of the patient's circumstances.

If time allows, and the patient's general health is satisfactory, it is advisable to invite the patient, together with the immediate family, to the artificial limb centre in order to meet the rehabilitation team, see the range of the available prosthetic hardware and get an idea of the rigours of the rehabilitation process. This is the ideal time to begin counselling the patient and the family and it is most helpful to introduce them to a matched patient who has successfully passed through the process.

The patient should be prepared for surgery by improvement in fitness and general health. Muscle exercises and limb joint mobilization will prevent undue muscle wasting and joint contractures.

Patients' psychological perceptions of their medical condition can be gauged by using the "Health Belief Schema"[5]. This provides information on patient satisfaction and motivation and highlights those who will need particular attention in the post-surgical phase.

The family circumstances and home environment should be assessed by the occupational therapist, as this allows time for necessary adaptations to be made to the home and living environment prior to discharge.

SURGICAL PHASE

The objective of amputation surgery is to produce a residual limb (stump) that can accept and work a prosthesis in the most efficient manner, whilst at the same time providing a good cosmetic result. Surgical teams should be proficient with modern operative techniques and knowledgeable of available prosthetic hardware. Close communication with the rehabilitation team is mandatory.

The level of amputation should be chosen not only by the extent of the pathology but also by taking account of the age and physical characteristics of the patient. In general, the more distal the amputation, the greater the advantage—but this must be balanced by the need to produce a stump capable of working a prosthesis. The advantage of preserving a longer residual limb is the lower energy cost of ambulation. Surgeons should be aware that preservation of the knee joint is of the greatest importance to future functionality of the patient (different levels of amputation will be discussed later in the chapter).

The quality of the amputation stump affects the ability of the patient to wear and function with a prosthesis. In one study, surgery performed by more senior surgeons produced better results compared with that performed by junior surgeons[3]. Other factors determining stump quality are length, shape, wound healing, scar quality, swelling or oedema, pain, tenderness and proximal joint mobility.

Adequate analgesia must always be provided around the time of amputation surgery in order to deal with stump pain and phantom phenomena. Nearly all amputees experience either phantom sensation or phantom pain. However, many people with diabetes and peripheral neuropathy have already experienced neuropathic pains. There is some evidence to suggest that peri-operative epidural anaesthesia may have a beneficial affect on post-operative phantom pain[6]. The trials have not been extensive but there is the perception that good peri-operative analgesia has a beneficial affect on post-operative pain.

POST-SURGICAL PHASE

As soon as possible after the patient's health has stabilized following surgery, the physiotherapist should begin a programme of mobilization in order to prevent joint contractures and reduce stump oedema. It is our practice to facilitate early transfer of the patient to the rehabilitation ward. The Amputee Medical Rehabilitation Society recommends that all amputees should be seen at the artificial limb centre within 3 weeks of amputation[7].

Stump dressings have been investigated by a number of research teams. For the transfemoral and knee disarticulation amputation, the traditional wool and crepe bandage dressing is unreliable, difficult to retain and often causes skin pressure necrosis. Use of either a commercially available stump shrinker or elastic stockinette is advised. For the transtibial amputation and Syme amputation, a removable rigid plaster-of-Paris cast dressing is advocated for control of oedema and protection of the wound or, if impractical, a commercial stump shrinker is used[8]. Immediate post-operative mobilization on a prosthesis was advocated by Berlemont[9] in 1961, but has to a large extent been abandoned because the intensive surveillance required to avoid tissue damage could not always be delivered. It is our practice in Manchester to advocate early mobilization on a pneumatic post-amputation mobility (PPAM) aid[10]. This device is easily applied to transtibial, knee disarticulation and standard transfemoral amputation stumps. It gets the patient upright and weightbearing, providing a morale boost to the patient besides being a good assessment tool in deciding the appropriateness of future prescription.

Stump wound healing may be delayed, especially in the more distal amputation. However, with appropriate dressings, antibiotics and sometimes debridement, healing can usually be achieved. Hasty revision surgery and conversion to a higher level amputation in order to achieve quick healing should be avoided unless indicated by unresolving wound infection, severe tissue avascularity or major proximal fixed joint contractures.

Following amputation, the patient may experience two particular types of pain. Stump pain is usually felt around the site of the scar, may be related to the position of the limb remnant and usually responds to simple analgesics. Pain not responding to simple analgesics in the early post-operative period may be a harbinger of infection or haematoma formation. Pain from a neuroma is fairly uncommon and arises about 6–8 weeks following surgery. Phantom phenomena are almost always present, as either a painless phantom sensation or a noxious phantom pain. Phantom feelings come on soon after surgery and can be controlled by physical stimulation, drugs and psychological therapy. Massaging the stump or using a stump shrinker are useful ways of controlling pain. Should it persist, a combination of carbamazepine and amitriptyline is often successful in reducing the pain. Less often, opiate analgesics are indicated.

Additionally, diversionary therapy, or even the process of mobilization, help patients to take their mind off the surgery and concentrate on other aspects of getting well. However, nearly all patients will continue to report episodes of phantom pain for many years after their amputation[11]. Very rarely, patients with recalcitrant pain require referral to a specialist pain clinic.

PSYCHOLOGICAL ASSESSMENT

For many patients with a history of chronic limb ulceration and vascular insufficiency, amputation gives hope for a better quality of life. Even so, there is a high incidence of anxiety and depression following amputation[12], particularly in younger patients who may have lost their limbs through an element of trauma[13]. The Hospital Anxiety and Depression Scale[14] and the Beck Inventory[15] are standardized scales that are useful benchmarks and may be repeated later to monitor the effect of treatment. Psychological treatments using cognitive-behavioural therapy help patients to see that feelings interact with thoughts, fears and behaviour and that all of these are under their own control[16]. Antidepressant medication may be used to supplement this therapy.

Counter-transference is the process whereby the patient's behaviour on the rehabilitation ward may reflect the emotional reactions of the ward staff towards the patient's physical condition[17]. Asking staff what it is about a patient that engenders these feelings in them may sometimes reflect staff members' difficulties—which may need to be addressed. Overprotective ward staff can make the patient enter a state of helplessness which is difficult to correct[18]. The clinical psychologist should encourage the staff to allow the patient to gain as much functional independence as is safely possible.

The "Locus of Control" measures patients' views of their own sense of mastery of the future[19]. Soon after their surgery, many patients have an "external" locus of control and believe they have insufficient power to make any real progress. They accept their fate as being determined by chance or controlled by "powerful others", including the staff. Conversely, patients with an "internal" locus of control have a firm belief in their own powers of rehabilitation and recognize their own responsibilities to the rehabilitation programme. They take charge of their futures and have a plan in mind, believing firmly that progress is up to themselves. Therapeutic approaches in the rehabilitation ward should always aim to foster an internal locus of control among patients.

There are some patients who are quite unrealistic and believe that everything will work out well, even when this is clearly not the case. This group often displays memory impairment, as assessed by the Mini-Mental Score (Folstein) examination or other simple tests[20] (care should be taken in interpreting these results if the patient is on opiate medication or if cognitively impaired from a pre-existing condition). This group requires careful counselling and provision of information on a daily basis, and must be guided by the team into accepting a more realistic pathway of treatment.

Patients' partners and carers should be assessed to determine the effect that surgery and amputation have had on them. Some are obviously overawed and repelled by the limb ablation and project this onto the patient. Likewise, patients may project the amputation stump as the cause of rejection and may anticipate rejection by their partners.

Most partners or carers are concerned for the future and their changing role in the relationship with the patient[21]. The patient's functional limitations may compel the partner to change from being a friend or sexual partner to becoming a nurse. This role change may cause the partner to react with denial, anxiety, disgust, guilt and depression, or to become obsessed with the need for further information. The psychologist must be aware of this change and work with the rehabilitation team to provide support and counselling.

Sexual dysfunction is well documented among people with diabetes. Amputation causes additional physical and psychological difficulties, which should be addressed. If necessary referral should be made for specialist therapy.

The occupational therapist is involved in teaching the skills required to carry out activities of daily living. In particular, this involves good posture, safe transfers, dressing, washing, bathing and general manoeuvrability. Included in the assessment should be the provision of a correctly fitting wheelchair which is stable and takes account of the altered centre of gravity of the patient following limb amputation.

LEVELS OF AMPUTATION

A brief description is provided of the residual limb (stump) and the prosthetic hardware most commonly used.

Partial Foot Amputations

Toe and Toe Ray Excision

These do not greatly influence the biomechanics of walking but significantly affect the pressures under the foot. Appropriate shoes and insoles should be prescribed. Regular surveillance is required to prevent further foot lesions together with on-going patient education regarding foot care.

Transmetarsal Amputations

These require particular attention during surgery in order to achieve a durable stump. A long plantar flap with a dorsally placed scar keeps the stump strong. Metatarsal prominences should be excised in order to prevent undue build-up of pressure in the sole of the foot. The prosthesis may be either a simple Plastazote shoe filler, which may be cosmetically enhanced with a silicone cover, or a full cosmetic silicone cover.

The Transtarsal Amputation

This amputation is performed more proximally in the foot, as in the Chopart and Lisfranc operations, and should only be performed after a thorough pre-amputation review of the patient's requirements. In general, these amputations are more appropriate for the less active patient, where the expectation is of very limited mobility over reasonably flat terrain. The surgeon should aim to provide a long plantar flap with anterior-based scar. In addition, the dorsiflexors of the foot (tibialis anterior and peroneal muscles) should be surgically reconnected in order to avoid the later development of an equinus contracture.

Prosthetic solutions for the transtarsal amputation include the use of customized prosthetic feet with split plastic sockets, or a silicone slip-over prosthesis, used with a surgical overboot (Figure 20.3).

Partial foot amputations are generally associated with longer healing times, lower mortality and increased chances of returning to an independent existence, in comparison with amputations at the above-ankle

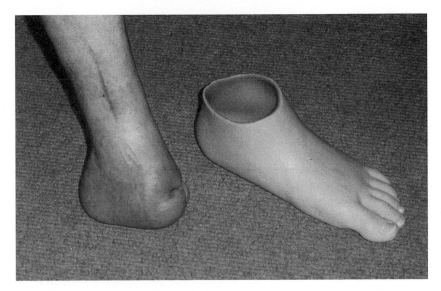

Figure 20.3 Customized silicon prosthesis for use following transtarsal amputation

level[22]. For the younger, fitter patient, the transtarsal amputation may produce a disappointing functional result.

Syme Amputation

The Syme amputation was classically described with bony section just proximal to the ankle joint and using the strong heel pad to cover the bone end. The advantages are a very strong endbearing stump, which may be particularly useful for people living in developing countries or remote areas, where prosthetic technology is not easily available. The major disadvantage is the poor cosmesis resulting from the bulbous distal end of the stump. The Wagner[23] modification, in which the malleoli are excised, has improved the appearance and gives a high level of success in the elderly dysvascular amputee.

The prosthesis required for a Syme amputation consists of a plastic socket extending to the level of the patellar tendon. A vast array of prosthetic feet are available and the prescription should reflect the desired activity level of the patient.

Transtibial (Below-knee) Amputation

The ideal stump should be approximately 15 cm long (although some surgeons advocate a longer stump—see Chapter 19). The long posterior flap method with its variations has been fully described[24]. Preservation of the knee joint is very important: even a stump barely 6 cm long can be fitted with a prosthesis and produce a result functionally superior to the above-knee (transfemoral) amputation. The advantages to the patient of preserving the knee joint are:

1. Lower energy requirement for walking.
2. Improved gait.
3. Ease of donning and doffing the prosthesis.
4. Lighter weight of the prosthesis.
5. Improved functional ability.

The standard prosthesis includes a stump sheath worn inside a customized thermoplastic socket, which is then fitted onto a modular prosthesis. The shank of the prosthesis articulates with a prosthetic foot that is prescribed to match the patient's physique and functional requirements.

Knee Disarticulation (Through-knee) Amputation

This is considered to be a relatively atraumatic surgical procedure that involves no bony surgery. It is indicated especially when the patient's general condition is poor or when a decision has been made that the patient will never be a suitable candidate for prosthetic mobilization—it allows better sitting balance as compared to the transfemoral amputation. The through-knee stump is strong and allows a greater degree of endbearing load. The major disadvantage with this type of amputation is the inadequacy of the prosthetic hardware, which makes it cosmetically and biomechanically mismatched compared with the remaining lower limb. The prosthesis will have a longer thigh section and a proportionately shorter shin section in relation to the remaining lower limb.

Transfemoral (Above-knee) Amputation

The transfemoral amputation should rarely be performed in people with diabetes. When performing this surgery, the surgeon should aim to remove about 12–15 cm of distal femur and resuture the thigh muscles to the bone end in order to avoid muscle retraction and formation of a painful bony prominence under the skin.

The prosthetic prescription should be appropriate to the patient's capabilities. Plastic sockets are the norm, with suspension provided by a soft belt or suction. For the more able patient, a stabilized knee joint with hydraulic or pneumatic swing phase may be used. For the frail, older patient, a locked (rigid) knee is appropriate. The shank of the prosthesis is usually made of lightweight carbon fibre or titanium in an endoskeletal design. The prosthetic foot must match the patient's requirements.

Second Limb (Bilateral) Amputations

The chances of losing the second lower limb are particularly high in people with diabetes. Before undertaking surgery, it is important to assess the patient and agree the rehabilitation goals prior to deciding on the level of amputation. Many patients in this group have multiple co-morbidities and will be unable to walk after surgery. For those unlikely to stand or walk, amputation should aim to allow good sitting balance and transfers, ease of healing and avoidance of painful joint contractures.

ON-GOING MAINTENANCE AND FOLLOW-UP

Rehabilitation demands on-going medical and prosthetic care and psychological support. Physical problems particular to the person with diabetes include the following:

- *Fluctuating stump volume* is associated with the occurrence of nephro-pathy. These patients require regular prosthetic adjustment and review. Using two or more stump socks when measuring for the prosthetic socket allows flexibility in coping with a fluctuating stump volume.
- *Retinopathy.* Diminishing vision, together with neuropathy, make mobilization over uneven surfaces very difficult. Many patients restrict themselves to indoors or only walking outdoors when accompanied.
- *Poor hand function* due to cheiroarthropathy and muscle wasting make donning and doffing the prosthesis difficult. Assistance from family or carers is often required.
- *Peripheral neuropathy* has been associated with impaired balance, which increases the chance of falling[25].

Soon after discharge from hospital the person with an amputation can feel alienated and stigmatized by society. Crowded rooms, such as restaurants, can be quite daunting. The disabled find that acceptance in the world at large is difficult to achieve because of inbuilt reactions and prejudices, which can frequently be stigmatizing. The anniversary of the amputation date is often a major testing time. Psychological treatment, using systematic desensitization and graded exposure with coping responses, can be helpful[26].

An amputee support group is a useful source of information and encourages socializing among patients with amputations. Many who have passed through the rehabilitation programme like to keep in contact and form support groups in the community. These groups are best managed by the client group, with assistance provided by professionals only on request.

The rehabilitation team has a duty to help people to return to work and should not hesitate to liaise with occupational health units and disablement resettlement officers. The rehabilitation team should also provide general advice and assist with amenity planning in the locality, and have input into the design of new public buildings.

Ultimately, people with amputations must have a firm belief in the self, the support of their fellows and the backing of a multidisciplinary team in order to make progress in their new lives.

REFERENCES

1. Information and Statistics Division, Common Services Agency, Trinity Park House, South Trinity Road, Edinburgh. Personal communication, 1998.
2. Ebskov B, Ebskov L. In Murdoch G, Bennett Wilson A Jr (eds), *Epidemiology in Amputation—Surgical Practice and Patient Management*. Oxford: Butterworth-Heinemann, 1996; 23–29.
3. Chakrabarty BK. An audit of the quality of the stump and its relation to rehabilitation in lower limb amputees. *Prosthet Orthot* 1988; **22**: 136–46.
4. Ham R, Regan JM, Roberts VC. Evaluation of introducing the team approach to the care of the amputee: the Dulwich Study. *Prosthet Orthot Int* 1987; **11**: 25–30.
5. Aalto AM, Uutela A. Glycaemic control, self-care behaviours and psychosocial factors among insulin-treated diabetics: a test of an extended belief model. *Int J Behav Med* 1997; **4**: 191–214.
6. Jahangiri M, Jayatunga A, Bradley JW, Dark CH. Prevention of phantom pain after major lower limb amputation by epidural infusion of diamorphine, clonidine and bupivacaine. *Ann R Coll Sur Engl* 1994; **76**: 324–6.
7. Amputee Medical Rehabilitation Society. *Amputee Rehabilitation Recommended Standards and Guidelines*. London: Royal College of Physicians, 1992.
8. Wu Y. Post-operative and preprosthetic management of lower extremity amputations. Capabilities. North Western University Prosthetics Research Laboratory, 1996; **5**(2); 2. Chicago, North Western University's Rehabilitation Engineering Research Programme.
9. Berlemont M. Notre experience de l'appareillage prococe des amputies des membres inferieures aux etablissements. *Ann Med Phys* 1961; **4**: 213.
10. Redhead RG. The early rehabilitation of lower limb amputees using a pneumatic walking aid. *Prosthet Orthot Int* 1983; **7**: 88–90.
11. Sherman RA, Arena JG. Phantom limb pain: mechanisms, incidence and treatment. *Crit Rev Phys Rehabil Med* 1992; **4**: 1–26.
12. Maguire P, Parkes CM. Surgery and loss of body parts. *Br Med J* 1998; **316**: 1086–8.
13. Shakula GD, Sahur SC et al. A psychiatric study of amputees. *Br J Psychiat* 1982; **141**: 54–8.
14. Zigmond AS, Snaith RP. The Hospital Anxiety and Depression Scale. *Acta Psychiat Scand* 1983; **67**: 361–70.
15. Beck AT, Ward C, Mendelson M et al. An inventory for measuring depression. *Arch Gen Psychiat* 1961; **4**: 561–71.

16. Williams JMG. *The Psychological Treatment of Depression.* 2nd edn. London: Routledge, 1992.
17. Laatsch L, Rothke S, Burke WF. Counter-transference and the multiple amputee patient: pit falls and opportunities in rehabilitation medicine. *Arch Phys Med Rehabil* 1993; **74**: 644–8.
18. Frierson RL, Lippmann SB. Psychiatric consultation for acute amputees. *Psychosomatics* 1987; **28**: 183–9.
19. Partridge L, Johnston M. Perceived control of recovery from physical disability: measurement and prediction. *Br J Clin Psychol* 1989; **28**: 53–60.
20. Hodkinson HM. Evaluation of a mental test score for assessment of mental impairment in the elderly. *Age Ageing* 1972; **1**: 233–8.
21. Thompson DM, Haran D. Living with an amputation: the helper. *Soc Sci Med* 1985; **24**: 319–23.
22. Larsson J, Agardh CD, Apelqvist J, Strenstrom A. Long-term prognosis after healed amputation in patients with diabetes. *Clin Orth Rel Res* 1998; **350**: 149–58.
23. Wagner FW. Amputation of the foot and ankle: current status. *Clin Orthop* 1977; **122**: 62–9.
24. Bowker JH. Transtibial amputation. In Murdoch G, Bennett Wilson A (eds), *Amputation, Surgical Practice and Patient Management.* Oxford: Butterworth-Heinemann, 1996; 42–58.
25. Courtemanche R, Teasdale N et al. Gait problems in diabetic neuropathic patients. *Arch Phys Med Rehabil* 1996; **77**: 849–55.
26. Bradbury E. *Counselling People with Disfigurement.* Leicester: British Psychological Society, 1996.

21

The International Consensus and Practical Guidelines on the Diabetic Foot

KAREL BAKKER*

International Working Group on the Diabetic Foot, Amsterdam,
The Netherlands

THE NEED FOR A CONSENSUS

Many disciplines are involved in the care of diabetic patients and various strategies are needed for prevention and treatment. Several studies have shown that a multidisciplinary approach, with a well-structured organization and appropriate facilities, can reduce the risk of development and progression of diabetic foot disorders. Concerted action by all people working with diabetic patients is required for such an approach to be effective, and specific guidelines are needed to realize a uniform high standard of diabetic foot care. Currently there are still many different strategies applied in diabetic foot care, not only between different countries but also within the same country, and a uniformly high standard has not been achieved.

In the last decade, guidelines on the prevention, diagnosis and management of diabetic foot problems have been formulated in several countries. However, the contents of these guidelines have often been mutually inconsistent.

*On behalf of the Editorial Board of the International Working Group: K. Bakker, W. H. van Houtum, N. C. Schaper, J. Apelqvist and M. H. Nabuurs-Franssen

The Foot in Diabetes, 3rd edn. Edited by A. J. M. Boulton, H. Connor and P. R. Cavanagh.
© 2000 John Wiley & Sons, Ltd.

Incompatibilities have arisen for various reasons. In some cases, the group compiling the guidelines has not been fully representative of all the disciplines involved in diabetic foot care; some have been intended for one group of users but not for others, and ambiguities have resulted from a lack of clear definitions of what constitutes "an ulcer", "an amputation" and other terminology. Furthermore, there were no guidelines addressed specifically at policy makers who allocate resources for health care. Discussion following a diabetic foot meeting in Malvern, UK, in 1996, convinced many of those present of the need for an international set of definitions and guidelines on prevention and management, and this led to the formation of an International Working Group on the Diabetic Foot.

THE INTERNATIONAL WORKING GROUP
ON THE DIABETIC FOOT

The 15 members of the Working Group met in January 1997 to discuss the feasibility of creating a consensus text on the diabetic foot, for world-wide circulation to diabetic clinics and primary care practitioners with an interest in diabetes mellitus, and to agree upon the consensus procedure to be followed, the aims of the guidelines and items that should be addressed.

The goal of the Working Group was to develop evidence-based guidelines, augmented by expert opinion, in order to reduce the impact of diabetic foot disease, by means of cost-effective quality health care. The text was to delineate how and when actions should be taken and by whom. Finally, the organization of care and implementation of the guidelines were to be addressed.

It was decided that the Consensus Document should be written for three target groups: policy makers in health care; general health care professionals; and foot care specialists. Therefore, three separate documents were to be created.

The Text for Policy Makers was to contain elements essential for policy makers involved in planning and allocating health care resources. This document would focus on the socio-economic impact of the diabetic foot and the potential for reducing this impact by well-targeted intervention strategies.

The second document to be created was the actual Consensus Document. This text would address all the essential elements encountered in the field of the diabetic foot. It was to be mainly evidence-based information, augmented where necessary with expert opinion. The target group was every specialist involved in diabetic foot care, and it was to be comprehensive and accurate, with chapters on: definitions and criteria; epidemiology; socio-economics; pathophysiology; neuropathy; peripheral vascular disease; biomechanics and footwear; ulcers; infection; the Charcot foot; amputation; prevention; organization; and regional overviews. This international Consensus Document was to serve as the source reference for the third document, called the *Practical Guidelines*.

In the *Practical Guidelines* the basic principles of prevention and treatment were described. Depending upon local circumstances, these principles would have to be adapted and translated for local use, taking into account regional differences in socio-economics, accessibility to health care and cultural factors. The *Practical Guidelines* were aimed at health care workers involved in the care of diabetic patients.

Given the very broad scope of the problem, it was thought crucial to have an early consensus on what should be included and what should be excluded from the three documents. Every participant was asked to allocate a priority marking to each of 128 possible topics, and the results were circulated before the first meeting of the Working Group. During the meeting, consensus was reached on these topics and on the chapters. For each chapter, one or more specialists were assigned as primary writers and an editorial board was set up to oversee the project.

In this process, several lessons were learned. The aims of the Consensus Document text and the *Practical Guidelines* were sometimes confusing. More importantly, evidence-based information was lacking in several areas and this was particularly apparent when seeking evidence for clear and unequivocal practical guidelines. For instance, there are few thorough studies of the diagnostic strategies used in daily practice, on optimal wound treatment, on antibiotic treatment, on how and when patients should be educated, or on optimum frequency of foot screening examinations. Expert opinion was therefore accepted in these areas of uncertainty. In this process, the work of the International Editorial Board facilitated the process, as they met on several occasions to discuss the texts with the original writers. Furthermore, every time a text had been edited it was redirected to the original writer and the members of the International Working Group for further comments. In this process, all participants had many opportunities to express their ideas or criticisms.

THE FULL WORKING PARTY

After the initial phase a preliminary text was produced, which was sent for comment to a group of 45 experts from 23 countries, representing all continents and all specialties involved in the diabetic foot. This "Full Working Party" included primary care physicians; diabetologists; podiatrists; diabetes nurses; general, vascular and orthopaedic surgeons; internists; and neurologists. The Full Working Party met in January 1998 in Heemskerk, The Netherlands, to discuss, adjust and improve the preliminary Consensus text.

After this meeting, the preliminary Consensus Document text was rewritten by the original authors, sometimes in collaboration with members of the Full Working Party. Subsequently, every member of the Full Working Party was given the opportunity to comment on the revised texts. The Editorial Board reviewed all these further comments, adjusting the text where necessary, and the final documents were then produced. All the members of the Full Working Party then agreed on the final text.

The Consensus Document, entitled *International Consensus on the Diabetic Foot*, and the *Practical Guidelines* were launched during the Third International Symposium on the Diabetic Foot in Noordwijkerhout, The Netherlands, May 5–8 1999.

Implementation

The important next step is to implement the *Practical Guidelines*. Useful strategies, as described in the Consensus Document, include the use of influential local people or groups, outreach visits, care plans or structured prompts in medical records, and regular audit. If the *Guidelines* are to be effective, they must be adapted to suit local circumstances. National representatives are therefore being appointed to organize local meetings to implement the Consensus Document on a world-wide basis. The *Guidelines* have been developed in close association with the World Health Organization and endorsed by the International Diabetes Federation. Endorsement will also be sought from national and regional diabetes associations.

The implementation process is a continuous one, and national representatives will be invited to report their experiences at a meeting in 2003, at which time new evidence-based information will be evaluated by the Working Group and, if valid, incorporated into a second edition. In this way both the Consensus Document and the *Practical Guidelines* will be continuously updated in the light of both experience and evidence.

Funding

Financial support is essential to enable this independent and non-profit-making programme to function to its best potential. Until now, Johnson & Johnson, Dermagraft Joint Venture (Advanced Tissue Sciences/Smith & Nephew) and the Dutch EASD Fund have donated generously, but more donations are needed for the implementation programme.

PRACTICAL GUIDELINES

Practical Guidelines are reproduced below (pp. 327–344). Copies of the Consensus Document can be obtained from the International Working Group on the Diabetic Foot, PO Box 9533, 1006 GA Amsterdam, The Netherlands. E-mail: diabetic-foot@mail.com

Practical Guidelines

on the Management and the prevention
of the Diabetic Foot

Based upon the International Consensus on the Diabetic Foot
prepared by the International Working Group on the Diabetic Foot

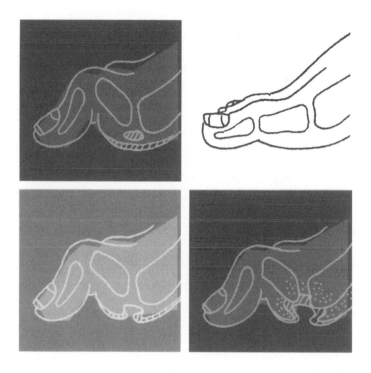

© Copyright 1999 by The International Working Group on the Diabetic Foot
ISBN 90-9012716-x

Introduction

Foot complications are one of the most serious and costly complications of diabetes mellitus. Amputation of (part of) a lower extremity is usually preceded by a foot ulcer. A strategy which includes prevention, patient and staff education, multi-disciplinary treatment of foot ulcers and close monitoring can reduce amputation rates by 49-85%. Therefore, several countries and organizations, such as the World Health Organization and the International Diabetes Federation, have set goals to reduce the rate of amputations by up to 50%.

In these guidelines the basic principles of prevention and treatment will be described, based upon the document entitled "International Consensus on the Diabetic Foot". Depending upon local circumstances these principles have to be translated for local use, taking into account regional differences in socio-economics, accessibility to healthcare and cultural factors.

The "Practical Guidelines" are aimed at healthcare workers involved in the care of diabetic patients. For more details and information on treatment by specialists in foot-care, the reader is referred to the International Consensus document.

Pathophysiology

Pathophysiology

Although the spectrum of foot lesions varies in different regions of the world, the pathways to ulceration are probably identical in most patients. Diabetic foot lesions frequently result from two or more risk factors occurring together. In the majority of patients diabetic peripheral neuropathy plays a central role; up to 50% of type 2 diabetic patients have neuropathy and at-risk feet. Neuropathy leads to an insensitive and subsequently deformed foot, with possibly, an abnormal walking pattern. In neuropathic patients minor trauma, caused for example by ill-fitting shoes, walking barefoot or an acute injury, can precipitate a chronic ulcer. Loss of sensation, foot deformities, and limited joint mobility can result in abnormal biomechanical loading of the foot. As a normal response callus is formed, but finally the skin breaks down, frequently preceded by subcutaneous hemorrhage. Whatever the primary cause, the patient continues walking on the insensitive foot, impairing subsequent healing *(see figure 1)*. Peripheral vascular disease, usually in conjunction with minor trauma, may result in a painful, purely ischemic foot ulcer. However, in patients with both neuropathy and ischemia (neuro-ischemic ulcer), symptoms may be absent despite severe peripheral ischemia. Micro-angiopathy should not be accepted as a primary cause of an ulcer.

Fig 1. Illustration of ulcer due to repetitive stress

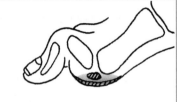

1. Callus formation

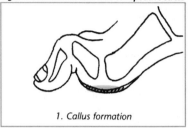

2. Subcutaneous hemorrhage

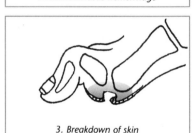

3. Breakdown of skin

4. Deep foot infection with osteomyelitis

Cornerstones of the management of the diabetic foot

Five cornerstones of the management of the diabetic foot

• Regular inspection and examination of the foot at risk   **1**

• Identification of the foot at risk   **2**

• Education of patient, family and healthcare providers   **3**

• Appropriate footwear   **4**

• Treatment of non-ulcerative pathology   **5**

1   **Regular inspection and examination of the foot at risk**

All diabetic patients should be examined at least once a year for potential foot problems, and patients with demonstrated risk factor(s) should be examined more often (every 1-6 months). The absence of symptoms does not mean that the feet are healthy, since the patient can have neuropathy, peripheral vascular disease or even an ulcer without any complaints. The feet should be examined with the patient lying down and standing up, and the shoes and socks should also be inspected.

History and examination

History	Previous ulcer/amputation, previous foot education, social isolation, poor access to healthcare, bare-foot walking
Neuropathy	Symptoms, such as tingling or pain
	Loss of sensation
Vascular status	Claudication, rest pain, pedal pulses
	Discoloration (rubor) on dependency
Skin	Color, temperature, edema
	Nail pathology (e.g. ingrown nails), wrongly cut nails
	Ulcer
	Callus, dryness, cracks, interdigital maceration
Bone/joint	Deformities (e.g. claw toes, hammer toes) or bony prominences
	Loss of mobility (e.g. hallux rigidus)
Footwear/stockings	Assessment of both inside and outside.

3

Sensory loss due to diabetic polyneuropathy can be assessed using the following techniques:

Pressure perception	Semmes-Weinstein monofilaments *(10 gram, see addendum)*
	The risk of future ulceration can be determined with a 10 gram monofilament
Vibration perception	128 Hz tuning fork *(hallux, see addendum)*
Discrimination	Pin prick (dorsum of foot, without penetrating the skin)
Tactile sensation	Cotton wool (dorsum of foot)
Reflexes	Achilles tendon reflexes

2   **Identification of the foot at risk**
Following examination of the foot, each patient can be assigned to a risk category, which should guide subsequent management.

Progression in risk categories

Sensory neuropathy and/or foot deformities or bony prominences and/or signs of peripheral ischemia and/or previous ulcer or amputation

Sensory neuropathy

No sensory neuropathy

Areas at risk

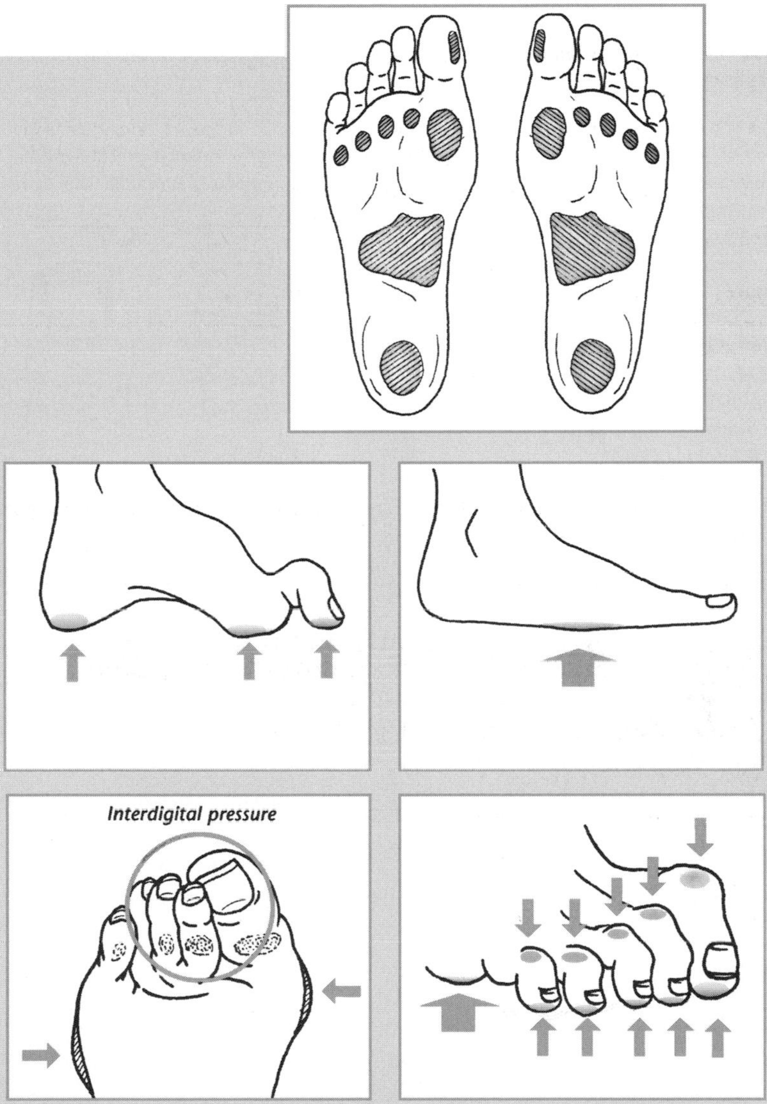

Fig 2. Risk areas for foot ulcers in diabetic patients

5

3 **Education of patient, family and healthcare providers**

Education, presented in a structured and organized manner, plays an important role in prevention. The aim is to increase motivation and skills. The patient should be taught how to recognize potential foot problems and what action should be taken. The educator must demonstrate the skills, e.g. how to cut nails appropriately. Education should be provided in several sessions over time and preferably a mixture of methods should be used. It is essential to evaluate whether the patient has understood the message, is motivated to act and has sufficient self-care skills. An example of instructions for the high risk patient and family is given below. Furthermore, physicians and other healthcare professionals should receive periodic education to improve the care delivered to high risk individuals.

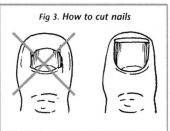

Fig 3. How to cut nails

Items which should be covered when instructing the high-risk patient

- Daily feet inspection, including areas between the toes.
- If the patient cannot inspect the feet, someone else should do it.
- Regular washing of feet with careful drying, especially between the toes.
- Temperature of the water should always be less than 37° C.
- Avoidance of barefoot walking in- or outdoors and wearing of shoes without socks.
- Chemical agents or plasters to remove corns and calluses should not be used.
- Daily inspection and palpation of the inside of the shoes.
- If vision is impaired, the patient should not try to treat the feet (e.g. nails) by themselves.
- Lubricating oils or creams should be used for dry skin, but not between the toes.
- Daily change of stockings.
- Wearing of stocking with seams inside out or preferably without any seams at all
- Cutting nails straight across *(See figure 3).*
- Corns and calluses should not be cut by patients, but by a health care provider.
- The patient must ensure that the feet are examined regularly by a health care provider.
- The patient should notify the healthcare provider at once if a blister, cut, scratch or sore has developed.

4 Appropriate footwear

Inappropriate footwear is a major cause of ulceration. Appropriate footwear (adapted to the altered biomechanics and deformities) is essential for prevention. Patients without loss of protective sensation can select off-the-shelf footwear by themselves. In patients with neuropathy and/or ischemia extra care must be taken with the fitting, particularly when foot deformities are also present. The shoe should not be too tight or too loose *(see figure 4)*. The inside of the shoe should be 1-2 centimeters longer than the foot itself. The internal width should be equal to the width of the foot at the site of the metatarsal phalangeal joints and the height should allow enough room for the toes. The fitting must be evaluated with the patient in standing position, preferably at the end of the day. If the fitting is too tight due to deformities or if there are signs of abnormal loading of the foot (e.g. hyperemia, callus, ulceration) patients should be referred for special footwear (advice and/or construction), including insoles and orthoses.

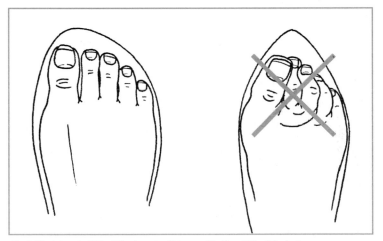

Fig 4. The internal width of the shoe should be equal to the width of the foot.

5 Treatment of non-ulcerative pathology

In a high risk patient callus, nail and skin pathology should be treated regularly, preferably by a trained foot-care specialist. If possible, foot deformities should be treated non-surgically (e.g. with an orthosis).

Foot ulcer

Foot ulcer

A standardized and consistent strategy of evaluating wounds is essential and will guide further therapy. The following items must be addressed:

The cause of ulcer

Ill-fitting shoes are the most frequent cause of an ulcer, even in patienst with "pure" ischemic ulcers. Therefore, the shoes should be examined meticulously in all patients.

The type of ulcer

Most ulcers can be classified as neuropathic, ischemic or neuro-ischemic. This will guide further therapy. Assessment of the vascular tree is essential in the management of a foot ulcer.

If pedal pulses are absent and/or the ankle brachial index is <0.9, or if an ulcer does not improve despite optimal treatment, more extensive vascular evaluation should be performed. If a major amputation is under consideration, the option of revascularization should be considered first. Measurement of the ankle pressure is the most widely used method to diagnose and quantify peripheral vascular disease. However, ankle pressures may be falsely elevated due to calcification of the arteries.

Alternative methods are compared in *figure 5*.

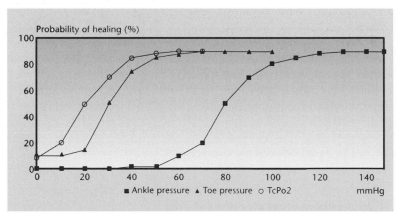

Fig 5. A schematic estimate of the probability of healing of foot ulcers and minor amputations in relation to ankle blood pressure, toe blood pressure and transcutaneous oxygen pressure (TcPo2) based on selected reports.

The site and depth

Neuropathic ulcers frequently occur on the plantar surface of the foot, or in areas overlying a bony deformity. Ischemic and neuro-ischemic ulcers are more common on the tips of the toes or the lateral border of the foot.

The depth of an ulcer can be difficult to determine due to the presence of overlying callus or necrosis. Therefore, neuropathic ulcers with callus and necrosis should be debrided as soon as possible. This debridement should not be performed in ischemic or neuro-ischemic ulcers without signs of infection. In neuropathic ulcers the debridement can usually be performed without (general) anesthesia.

Signs of infection

Infection in a diabetic foot presents a direct threat to the involved limb and should be treated promptly and aggressively. Signs and/or symptoms of infection, such as fever, pain or increased white blood count/ESR, are often absent. But, if present, substantial tissue damage or even development of an abscess is likely.

The risk of osteomyelitis should be determined. If it is possible to place a probe down to the bone before initial debridement, there is an increased risk of the presence osteomyelitis.

A superficial infection is usually caused by Gram-positive bacteria. In cases of (possible) deep infections Gram stains and cultures from the deepest tissue involved are advised (no superficial swabs); these infections are usually polymicrobial, involving anaerobes and Gram positive/negative bacteria.

Ulcer treatment

Ulcer treatment

If treatment is based on the following principles healing rates of 80-90% can be attained. The best wound care cannot compensate for continued injury, ischemia or infection. Patients with an ulcer deeper than the subcutis should be treated aggressively and, depending on local resources and infrastructure, hospitalization must be considered.

Principles of ulcer treatment

Relief of pressure

- Non weight bearing is essential
  - Limitation of standing and walking
  - Crutches, etc.
- Mechanical unloading
  - Total contact casting/other casting techniques
  - Temporary footwear
  - Individually molded insoles.

Restoration of skin perfusion

- Arterial revascularization procedures (results do not differ from non-diabetic patients, but distal bypass-surgery is needed more frequently)
- The benefits of pharmacological treatment to improve perfusion have not yet been established
- Treat smoking, hypertension and dyslipidemia.

Treatment of infection

- Superficial ulcer with extensive cellulitis
  - Debridement with removal of all necrotic tissue and oral antibiotics aimed at Staphylococcus aureus and streptococci
  - No topical antibiotics
- Deep (limb-threatening) infection
  - Surgical drainage as soon as possible (emergency referral) with removal of necrotic or poorly vascularized tissue, including infected bone
  - Revascularization if necessary
  - Broad-spectrum antibiotics intravenously, aimed at Gram-positive and negative micro-organisms, including anaerobes.

Metabolic control and treatment of comorbidity

• Optimal diabetes control, if necessary with insulin
  (blood glucose < 10 mmol/l or < 180mg/dl)
• Treat edema and malnutrition.

Local wound care

• Frequent wound debridement (with scalpel, e.g. once a week)
• Frequent wound inspection
• Absorbent, non-adhesive, non-occlusive dressings
• Growth factors have been shown to be effective in plantar neuropathic ulcers,
  but their exact place in treatment has yet to be determined
• The following treatments are still experimental   - Bio-engineered tissue
                                                     - Hyperbaric oxygen treatment
• Footbaths are contra-indicated as they induce maceration of the skin.

Instruction of patient and relatives

• Instruction should be given on appropriate self-care and how to recognize and report signs
  and symptoms of (worsening) infection, such as fever, changes in local wound conditions
  or hyperglycemia.

Determining the cause and preventing recurrence

• Determine cause as ulceration is a recurrent disease
• Prevent ulcers on contralateral foot and give heel protection during bed rest
• Patient must be included in a comprehensive foot-care program with life-long observation.

11

Organization

Effective organization requires systems and guidelines for education, screening, risk reduction, treatment and auditing. Local variations in resources and staffing will often determine the ways in which care is provided. Ideally, a foot-care program should provide:

Foot-care program provisions

- Education of patients, carers and healthcare staff in hospitals, primary healthcare and the community
- A system to detect all patients at risk, with annual foot examination of all known patients
- Measures to reduce risk, e.g. podiatry and appropriate footwear
- Prompt and effective treatment
- Auditing of all aspects of the service, to ensure that actual practice meets standards determined by local implementation of these guidelines
- An overall structure which is designed to meet the needs of patients requiring chronic care, rather than simply responding to acute problems when they occur.

In all countries at least three levels of foot-care management are needed:

Levels of foot management	
Level 1	General practitioner, diabetic nurse and podiatrist
Level 2	Diabetologist, surgeon (general and/or vascular and/or orthopedic), diabetic nurse and podiatrist
Level 3	Specialized foot center

Setting up a multidisciplinary foot-care team has been found to be accompanied by a drop in the number of amputations. If it is not possible to create the full team from the outset, the team should be built up step by step, introducing the various different disciplines at different stages. This team must work in both primary and secondary care settings.

Ideally a foot-care team would consist of a diabetologist, surgeon, podiatrist, orthotist, educator, and plaster technician, in close collaboration with an orthopedic, podiatric and/or vascular surgeon and dermatologist.

Sensory foot examination

Neuropathy can be detected using the 10g (5.07 Semmes-Weinstein) monofilament, tuning fork (128 Hz), and/or cotton wisp.

Semmes-Weinstein monofilament

- Sensory examination should be done in a quiet and relaxed setting. First apply the monofilament on the patient's hands (or elbow, or forehead) so the patients know what to expect.
- The patient must not be able to see if and where the examiner applies the filament. The three sites to be tested on both feet are indicated in *figure 6*.

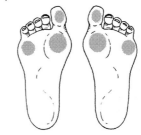

Fig 6. Sites to be tested with the monofilaments

- Apply the monofilament perpendicular to the skin surface *(figure 7a)*.
- Apply sufficient force to cause the filament to bend or buckle *(figure 7b)*.
- The total duration of the approach, skin contact, and removal of the filament should be approximately 2 seconds.
- Apply the filament along the perimeter of and not on an ulcer site, callus, scar or necrotic tissue. Do not allow the filament to slide across the skin or make repetitive contact at the test site.
- Press the filament to the skin and ask the patient IF they feel the pressure applied (yes/no) and next WHERE they feel the pressure applied (left/right foot).
- Repeat this application twice at the same site, but alternate this with at least one "sham" application, in which no filament is applied (total three questions per site).

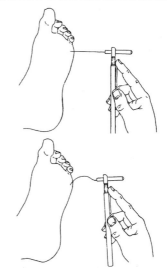

Fig 7a and 7b. Application of the monofilaments

- Protective sensation is present at each site if the patients correctly answers two out of three applications. Protective sensation is absent with two out of three incorrect answers, and the patient is then considered to be at risk of ulceration.
- Encourage the patients during testing.

Tuning fork

- The sensory exam should be done in a quiet and relaxed setting. First apply the tuning fork on the patient's wrists (or elbow, or clavicula) so the patient knows what to expect.
- The patient must not be able to see if and where the examiner applies the tuning fork. The tuning fork is applied on a bony part on the dorsal side of the distal phalanx of the first toe.
- It should be applied perpendicularly with a constant pressure *(figure 8)*.
- Repeat this application twice, but alternate this with at least one "sham" application, in which the tuning fork is not vibrating.
- The test is positive if the patient correctly answered at least two out of three applications, and negative ("at risk for ulceration") with two out of three incorrect answers.
- If the patient is unable to sense the vibrations at the big toe, the test is repeated more proximally (malleolus, tibial tuberositas).
- Encourage the patient during testing.

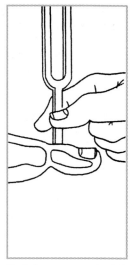

Fig 8. How to use a tuning fork

Easy to use foot screening assessment sheet for clinical examination

The foot is at risk if any of the below are present	
Deformity or bony prominences	Yes / No
Skin not intact (ulcer)	Yes / No
Neuropathy	
- Monofilament undetectable	Yes / No
- Tuning fork undetectable	Yes / No
- Cotton wool undetectable	Yes / No
Abnormal pressure, callus	Yes / No
Loss of joint mobility	Yes / No
Foot pulses	
- Tibial posterior artery absent	Yes / No
- Dorsal pedal artery absent	Yes / No
Discoloration on dependency	Yes / No
Any others	
- previous ulcer	Yes / No
- amputation	Yes / No
Inappropriate footwear	Yes / No

Actions to be taken	
Action recommended	Yes / No
Referral	Yes / No

15

Address

International Working Group on the Diabetic Foot
PO Box 9533
1006 GA Amsterdam
The Netherlands

E-mail: diabetic-foot@mail.com

22

The Foot in Leprosy—Lessons for Diabetes

GRACE WARREN

Westmead Hospital, Sydney, NSW, Australia

"The diabetic foot" is a term that implies impaired physiological function that may result in damaged tissues, ulceration, deformity, destruction and amputations. Many of these problems are the result of neuropathy, which is slowly progressive and may be fibre-selective, with pain fibres frequently affected early, well before there is clinical loss of touch or pressure sensation. It is often unaccompanied by definite symptoms, so that many patients do not realise that a neural deficit is developing until they are confronted with ulceration or other resultant problems.

A similar problem may occur in leprosy, in which the nerves are parasitized early without any symptoms. Over a period of many years there may be increasing fibrosis and slow loss of neural function until the limb is totally neuropathic, motor and autonomic as well as sensory. The sensory neuropathy is the main problem, allowing the possibility of unnoticed and hence untreated trauma because the patient does not have enough pain perception to demand care. The resultant problems are virtually the same as those seen in diabetes. In leprosy, as in diabetes, the autonomic involvement causing altered skin physiology makes the skin more prone to trauma from stress, bumps or dehydration.

Together with many other neuropathies, these diseases have several problems in common. The most important is the so-called "non-healing ulcer". In 1877 John Hilton[1] wrote: "pain was made the prime therapeutic agent . . . After injury, pain suggested the necessity of, and indeed compelled

The Foot in Diabetes, 3rd edn. Edited by A. J. M. Boulton, H. Connor and P. R. Cavanagh.
© 2000 John Wiley & Sons, Ltd.

man to seek for, rest". Because of the damage to sensory nerve pain fibres, these patients lack the natural sparing reflex that makes man seek for that rest.

In the middle of the twentieth century, large institutions provided prolonged outpatient care for thousands of leprosy patients and residential care for hundreds who lived in these institutions for many years. This provided an excellent opportunity for studying the effects of all degrees of neuropathy and of observing the results of neglect and the effects of methods of management.

Previously, it was assumed that the ulcers of leprosy patients were part of the disease and would never heal. However, with the introduction of effective bactericidal drug therapy, it was realised that these ulcers were not part of the disease itself but were mainly due to the loss of pain perception. Dr Paul Brand, working at the Christian Medical College Hospital in Vellore, South India, in the late 1940s, was challenged with the question, "Why do ulcers continue to occur when the disease is cured?" He did not know; no-one knew. He gathered around him a group of researchers who played a major role in identifying the reason for continuing ulcers and determining methods of management that literally save hands and feet, not only of leprosy patients, but of persons with neuropathy from any cause. The story of the battle to understand the problem of "no pain" is a fascinating one of how many people, working together, eventually solved the problem of why neuropathic ulcers appear not to heal[2]. The understanding we now have, and the methods that we have been using for leprosy for over 40 years, stem from this research. In the last 40 years I have been asked to treat neuropathy from many causes and I have found that the same methods are effective, irrespective of the cause of the neuropathy[3]. The principles laid down by Dr Brand and his colleagues are still applicable world-wide in saving limbs and improving the quality of life of those who have damaged nerve function from *any* cause.

In diabetes, as in leprosy, there are often no characteristic symptoms that indicate that a nerve deficit is developing. Hence, the patient may not realise that the ability to feel pain has been lost until some accident occurs that results in a lesion that is surprisingly painless. This may be a burn, a blister or a fracture. The common factor is that a lesion caused by trauma is neglected because it is painless and the patient does not automatically respond by protecting the traumatized area, and hence the lesion may become a non-healing ulcer. However, in leprosy it had been shown that if an affected limb was completely rested, ulcers healed[4] as quickly as similar lesions in a sensate limb. This understanding resulted in the use of total contact casts[5], which encouraged healing by preventing excess pressure on the traumatized areas but enabled the patient to continue walking.

Special testing of nerve function is often requested following examination of the patient. Nerve conduction studies may show the speed with which an impulse travels along a nerve, but do not tell what information those impulses pass to the brain. Many patients with neuropathy have paraesthesiae, but what do those paraesthetic feelings indicate? Is the body trying to indicate what a person with normal sensation would interpret as pain? It is the ability of perceiving pain as pain that is the important factor. Hence, electrical testing may give false ideas of the patient's ability to protect him/herself. Loss of pain perception is the biggest problem. The use of Semmes–Weinstein monofilaments[6] to test skin sensation is helpful to chart variations in neural function. But it is *not* a measure of protective sensation, as it does not test for pain perception. A patient may have normal perception of a 10 g fibre but have no discomfort when a sliver of glass cuts the foot. The wisest rule is to treat any patient with any suspicion of neuropathy as though there was complete loss of sensory perception and to start teaching the patient self-care as soon as neuropathy is suspected.

Leprosy patients may show marked motor and autonomic nerve dysfunction, even when there is little obvious sensory deficit[5]. It is advised that multiple neuropathies be assumed to be present whenever any neural deficit is detected. Over the past 40 years the writer has managed patients with neuropathy from many causes, using the same principles as those indicated by Coleman and Brand[7]. *Teach the patient how to protect the limbs as though there was no sensation at all.* The patient may say that feeling is present, but who can know exactly what that patient means by "feeling". Is it paraesthesia, numbness or one of a multitude of feelings, such as "burning", "cutting", or "compression" that do not include protective sensation and do not provide the stimulus needed for the patients to protect themselves? Many patients say they have pain but describe what may be "tingling", or "pins and needles" that may be due to abnormal nerve activity and may even indicate regrowth of damaged nerves. Young patients may call this "pain" because they have no previous experience of real pain. It is advisable to inquire into the quality of "pain" and perhaps record the feelings as discomfort rather than pain. If deformity and disability are to be prevented, it is essential that the patient realises that there is a deficiency in sensory perception.

Our work with leprosy patients brought to our attention other problems arising from nerve deficits that may be relevant to diabetic patients. The involvement of motor nerves may result in clawing of the toes which, in turn, causes excessive pressures over proximal interphalangeal joints and on the plantar surface of the metatarsal heads. In diabetic patients this is often dealt with by orthoses and moulded shoes. These have also been used in leprosy patients, but it was found that surgery[8], such as that for correcting clawed toes or a dropped foot, could correct the problem permanently. This could eliminate the constant need for new footwear by straightening the toes yet leaving them mobile, flexing the metatarsal joints and so spreading the stresses of weightbearing. It reduces the risk of ulceration. The excessive stresses caused by muscle imbalance in the lower limbs may stimulate excessive callus formation and may result in ulceration. In leprosy, many of the consequences of muscle imbalance are minimized by tendon surgery and, in my experience, these procedures are just as effective in neuropathy from other causes[9] and have often resulted in the salvage of a limb that might otherwise have been amputated. Unfortunately, it is uncommon for diabetic patients to benefit from this type of surgery, although for the diabetic patients on whom I have performed reconstructive surgery, the results have been well worthwhile[3].

In leprosy patients a large proportion of ulcers originate under callus or scarred skin. This callus, if not regularly removed, builds up and forms a thick mass, some of which dehydrates and becomes very hard. If on the sole, this may cause excessive pressures in the deeper tissues during walking and result in ulceration. A similar situation exists in diabetes[10] and other neuropathies[9]. After removal of the callosity, leprosy patients are taught to rub oil into the area on a daily basis, which keeps moisture in the skin, preventing dehydration[3]. Skin treated in this way improves in texture and resilience and, by becoming less fragile, is better able to withstand trauma. The same principles have been applied to patients with diabetes presenting with dry, fragile skin. Regular rehydration and oiling results in improved smoothness and suppleness and ability to withstand the stresses of daily use. Rehydration and oiling help to compensate for the effect of autonomic neuropathy on the sweat and sebaceous glands when the secretion of both sets of glands may be greatly reduced or completely lost. Brand[4] observed that feet that sweat normally rarely become ulcerated and that rehydration is possible. In 1966, Harris and Browne[11] published observations showing that the application of cosmetic moisturisers alone did not improve skin quality, but soaking in water, followed by oil, was effective as long as it was continued regularly. Tovey[10] suggested that, for diabetic patients, oilatum emulsion be added to the water used for soaking dry skin and aqueous cream be rubbed into the skin afterwards.

There are an estimated 15 million people affected by leprosy in the world, mostly in areas where there are minimal medical facilities, and it was necessary to devise treatment plans that patients could do themselves at minimal cost. The following daily routine has been taught in many areas so that the patient provides his/her own home care[3].

DAILY CARE FOR PERSONS WITH NEUROPATHIC LIMBS

It is important to teach all patients who are suspected of having neuropathy to start daily care as soon as possible in order to maintain the affected areas, especially the feet, in good condition. This teaching should be given by demonstration. Do not just tell the patients; show them how and then get them to do it themselves so that they really know how to continue at home[3]. As the feet are the most likely areas to be affected, the care of the feet will be described but the principles can be adapted to other areas of the body.

1. *LOOK* at their own feet every day, preferably at night, so that any wounds can be treated that night. If they cannot see the sole of the foot they can use a mirror or arrange for a partner or carer to do it for them. Their feet and shoes should be inspected by a staff member *every* time they attend clinic. This helps to impress importance of foot care upon the patients and their relatives and may reveal trauma that has been considered unimportant. Many patients have stated, "my feet are fine", yet painless lesions are found on removal of shoes and socks.

2. *SOAK* the feet and legs in plain water every day. This remains a controversial point in diabetes but is used by some clinicians treating diabetes[10]. In leprosy, as stated above, it has been shown time and time again that soaking is beneficial[5]. Dryness is very obvious when people walk barefoot or wear open sandals, and a dry atmosphere constantly increases the dehydration of the skin. In leprosy clinics it has been observed that healing occurs more rapidly on ulcerated feet that are soaked daily and in which dehydration is prevented by oiling, than in those feet that are left dry. The application of moisturising creams and lotions does not actually rehydrate the deeper layers of dry skin. They may improve hydration of superficial layers and reduce further dehydration, hence they keep in what water there is and make the skin feel moist for a period.

3. *SCRAPE off* hard, dry or rough callus that may irritate or increase local pressure: smooth dry hard callus splits and cracks, traumatizing tissues. Most patients can learn to keep callus under control themselves at home (in the case of those visually impaired, a relative can do it for them). However, this is controversial and not all authorities recommend self-care of callus in neuropathic patients. If the clinician or podiatrist commences by removing the excessive amounts of callus, it should be possible for the patient to prevent a new build-up of callus. However, it is still advisable for the patient to visit the podiatrist regularly to ensure that new masses of callus do not build up. Many patients have used a pumice stone or nylon pot scraper which, to be effective, needs to be rough. Other commitments often mean there may be long intervals between visits, allowing excessive amounts of callus to develop unless the patient can help by doing a little every day.

The first time a patient is seen with an ulcer surrounded or covered by callus, it is essential that the callus be removed in order to determine the size and severity of the ulcer[3]. The pressures caused by localized masses of callus are one of the most likely causes of ulceration in the insensate limb and the patient needs to understand that thick, dry, hard, irregular or cracked callus causes problems.

4. *OIL* the skin to keep the water in. Any oil or moisturising cream will be adequate to help prevent evaporation and dehydration. There is evidence that fish oil or animal oil, such as lanoline, may be absorbed and improve the quality of the skin as well as keeping it hydrated, and these oils are often rubbed in regularly to improve quality of scars after burns.

5. *DRESS WOUNDS* with simple dressings to keep them clean. Expensive dressings have no advantage over saline, simple ointment, Ungvita or Magnoplasm[3]. Most neuropathic wounds will heal with anything on them except the patient's weight! It is not the dressing that heals the ulcer. The ulcer will heal if it is kept clean and protected from further trauma. Pressure on an ulcer causes local anoxia and this damages the healing tissues.

6. *PROTECT* from trauma. If there is no wound or ulcer on the limb, proper protection would be the wearing of suitable footwear and the use of other protective appliances. If there is trauma or an ulcer on a vulnerable site, some form of splinting or other protection should be instituted once the dressing is in place.

7. *EXERCISE* to maintain mobility of ankles, toes and hands, and to gain optimal efficiency of any functioning muscle.

THE ORIGIN AND TREATMENT OF ULCERS

How do ulcers start[7]? The initial ulcer is usually the result of primary trauma. It may be due to:

1. Sudden very high pressure, as when jumping from a height, or stepping on a sharp object.
2. Lower pressure occurring intermittently for a long period, as in walking.
3. Low pressure occurring continuously, as with bed sores, or when wearing tight shoes.
4. Burns, cuts, bruises and friction.

Once an ulcer has healed, an area of scar will remain that will be more prone to trauma than normal tissue.

Most ulcers need only to be kept clean and rested and they will heal. The ideal is that an ulcer on a weightbearing surface should not be walked on[7].

The best method of treating an ulcer is *"REST and PROTECT—NOT ONE STEP PER DAY"* on the ulcer unless it is protected in a suitable walking cast. Ulcers on neuropathic feet will heal as rapidly as would a similar ulcer on a sensate foot, *if* adequately rested and protected. The provision of healing shoes does encourage ulcers to heal more quickly than they would in a normal shoe, but while walking in a shoe they will heal more slowly than if fully rested. In leprosy it was found that the use of total contact walking casts resulted in the healing of most ulcers within 6 weeks, although very gross ulcers may take much longer.

However, many clinicians are not prepared to "hide" an ulcer under a cast for 6 weeks. Hence, total contact casting has now been modified by bivalving the total contact cast, as shown in Figure 22.1[3], so that it can be removed, as needed, for dressings. When replaced correctly and held firmly by Velcro or bandages, it still functions as a total contact cast and eliminates stress and friction on the wounds, by spreading the patient's weight over the whole inside of the cast while allowing the patient to walk. These casts are worn 24 hours a day and, in many patients, it is best that they are removed only for inspection or dressings, i.e. not removed regularly for bathing or at night. These casts have proved popular with patients and staff and are very effective in obtaining healing of "non-healing ulcers"[3]. A total contact cast enables the patient to have full rest of the ulcerated area and yet be at home and mobile. It is *not* the dressing that heals the ulcer. The "rest and protect" allows the body to proceed with healing without the constant interruption of repeated trauma.

Diabetic patients with "non-healing" ulcers are frequently sent to a vascular surgeon: however, there may be no deficiency in the blood supply. The autonomic nerve damage results in a warm limb, which is also very common in leprosy patients[7,10,11]. The capacity of increased flow in the presence of infection is as great as normal, producing the normal signs of inflammation when appropriate.

Special shoes are often prescribed to provide relief of pressures on the ulcer[4]. If these are total contact shoes and correctly made they will assist in healing the ulcer, but healing will be slower than in a total contact walking cast (TCC). In a special shoe the area of weightbearing is much less, so pressures are greater. Also, patients remove shoes at night, when trauma can occur. One step is enough to undo any healing that has occurred during that day. If a moulded insole is provided and the shoe is not correctly fitted to the foot, it may do more harm than good as peak pressure points may fall on incorrect areas of the traumatized foot. A dressing on the ulcer may destroy the fit of the shoe, causing increased pressure to occur at the site of the dressing, and this may increase the anoxia and tissue breakdown at that

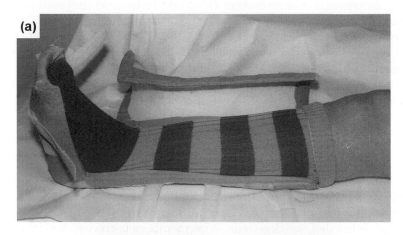

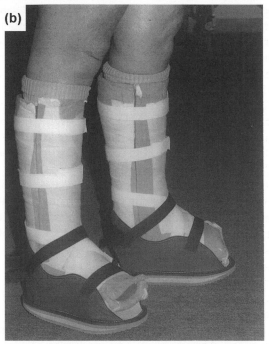

Figure 22.1 A total contact cast that has been bivalved. (a) The use of a football sock as a liner to replace the minimal padding used to make the cast. This padding is discarded when the cast is bivalved. The two halves of the cast are side-by-side, ready to be closed round the leg. (b) The two pieces of the cast held firmly by Velcro. The patient was able to walk well even though both feet required casting

site or elsewhere. A foot which is still basically anatomically normal does not require a moulded sole[4].

The so called "non-healing ulcer" is usually an ulcer that has not been given the opportunity to heal. It has not been adequately rested and trauma still continues to damage the healing tissues. The non-healing ulcer is a compromised ulcer; either the clinician has not offered the best treatment or the patient has not complied[3].

HOT SPOTS

A common presenting symptom of patients with neuropathy is altered temperature perception. Yet that limb is still able to become warmer than normal as a response to inflammation. The natural response to inflammation from any cause is heat, redness, swelling and pain. In the neuropathic limb the ability to appreciate pain is frequently defective, so we must teach patients to depend on heat, redness and swelling to inform themselves of any form of inflammation and to make the patients think how to deal with the problem and prevent it becoming worse. For practical purposes we term this a "hot spot", and the patient with neuropathy needs to look for "hot spots" every day during foot examination and know how to deal with them without delay[3].

A hot spot indicates the presence of some tissue pathology[3]. It may be a sprain or a torn ligament or tendon, an infection either superficial or deep, soft tissue inflammation or osteomyelitis, or a fracture that, if neglected, may result in bone disintegration. Unfortunately, when many clinicians see a warm swollen painless foot, either they do nothing or they diagnose osteomyelitis, even when there is no other evidence of infection (Figure 22.2). A full examination and history are mandatory. If a hot spot persists for days or weeks it should be regarded as serious. If it settles rapidly while the patient is resting, it is obviously not osteomyelitis. However, if it returns as soon as use is resumed—beware. The oedema of travel or heart failure is not usually hot. A patient with a neuropathic foot may feel no pain on slipping or twisting a foot, so usually there is no known history of trauma[9]. A hot spot on the sole of the foot usually indicates incipient blistering or ulceration, and if that foot is rested at once it may be possible to prevent a blister or an ulcer occurring. Many hot spots that indicate potential ulceration will completely resolve in a week of total rest or in a total contact cast. If the hot spot occurs on the dorsum of the foot, without obvious signs of infection, it is more likely to indicate a lesion of neuropathic bone—such as a fracture or neuropathic disintegration. These lesions will settle very quickly on complete rest but return within 24 hours on resumption of normal activity. A radiograph may not show any bone lesion initially, as also happens with a stress fracture. The latter often requires 6–8 weeks

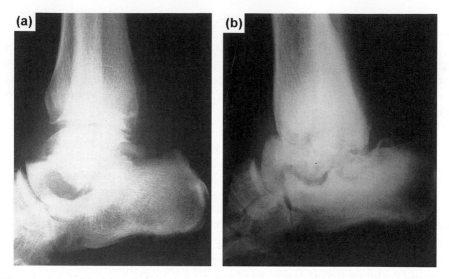

Figure 22.2 This diabetic patient had a history of at least twelve months duration of a warm swollen painless foot, a "hot spot". She was admitted and treated as osteomyelitis although no proof of that diagnosis was forthcoming. (a) Lateral radiograph showing marked variations in the density of calcification of the talus and some lucencies. There is also bone haziness of the posterior tubercle of the talus. The AP view showed a crack in the talus that was not reported but was present 12 months earlier. The patient was treated with prolonged antibiotics but the foot was never casted or protected. (b) The same view, taken 12 months later, shows some dense bone but is dominated by the collapsing talus and loss of ankle joint space. This case is typical of the progressive deformities that result from neuropathic bone disintegration

before there is enough osteoporosis to make the fracture obvious. If it is considered that it may be a neuropathic bone lesion, it is best to immobilize in a total contact cast for 6–8 weeks and then review with new radiographs. To allow the patient unprotected walking at this time is to risk bone disintegration and increasing deformity.

BONE LESIONS

Neuropathic bone lesions are relatively common problems in the neuropathic foot[12]. They are usually secondary to trauma and not to infection, although infection may be present when the disintegration is secondary to the osteopenia that occurs in association with an ulcer or infected lesion. In adults it is rare to find blood-borne osteomyelitis affecting an ulcer-free area. Hence, a "painless hot spot" on a neuropathic non-ulcerated foot should be considered to be neuropathic bone disintegration (NBD), unless proved otherwise. The treatment for NBD is a fixed total contact cast for a prolonged period[3]. To give antibiotics "just in case of osteomyelitis" will not do any harm to the NBD if it is in a total contact cast, but to treat the hot spot with antibiotics alone, assuming osteomyelitis, and not provide a protective cast is asking for increasing deformity and disability.

Patients should be taught to examine their feet every day looking for heat and swelling. If any is found at night then check again in the morning. Heat and swelling that persist overnight are warnings of trouble. Radiographs should be taken as soon as definite symptoms or signs occur, and inform the radiologist that you suspect a bone problem at such and such a point. If the hot spot persists and there is no obvious fracture, it is advisable to apply a total contact walking cast for 6–8 weeks and then re-X-ray. That time will allow the more simple things like sprains and twists to heal uninterrupted. It will also allow the osteoporosis around the fracture to develop until it can be seen. If the patient does not wear a total contact cast, there is danger of wearing away the osteoporotic bone and the fracture will turn into bone disintegration which, if allowed to progress without restriction, may eventually develop into a neuro-arthropathic foot. The observation of many leprosy patients has enabled us to say that many neuro-arthropathic feet are really neuropathic disintegration that started as a neglected fracture because of little or no pain (see Figure 22.3)[3]. Some show no real disintegration but are deformed because an undiagnosed fracture displaced, and then healed producing a deformity that caused an ulcer-prone stress point.

In the neuropathic foot, any fracture must be treated adequately. Because of the lack of pain perception the patient will not limp to spare the traumatized limb and may cause displacement of the fragments, impaction or disintegration that results in a deformed limb, which then becomes ulcer-prone. Our experience suggests that the limb requires total immobilization (which can be in a total contact walking cast once the swelling has subsided) for two or three times as long as would be required for the normal sensate foot[3]. In neuropathy there appears to be a normal ability to heal but, because of the lack of pain perception, the patient overstresses the healing tissue too early and fractures it. Hence, for a midtarsal fracture it is recommended that the foot be immobilized for 8–12 months before a trial of free walking is allowed. The foot shown in Figure 22.4 indicates the typical ability to heal.

There is no place for surgical interference in early true disintegration without displacement, but in diabetic patients the displacement of fractures in the Lisfranc area is common and, if seen early enough, it may be advisable to internally fix them, if this can be done adequately, rather than allow displacement. Prolonged supported immobilization is still essential to obtain bone healing. Where NBD has resulted in marked deformity, it is advisable to treat in a total contact cast for 6 months or until the bones have

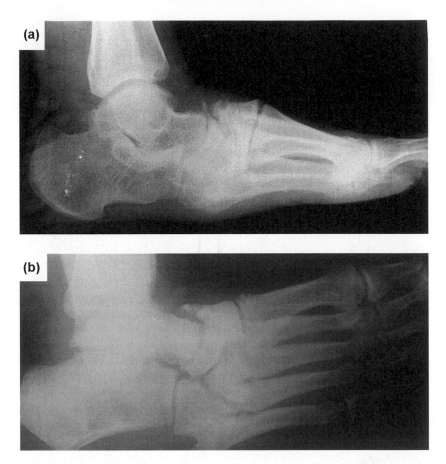

Figure 22.3 This diabetic patient presented with a painless, warm swollen foot. (a) Radiograph showing a fracture of the navicular, which was reported as a "Charcot foot". The surgeon stated that a Charcot foot would not respond to treatment, but the patient should wear an orthopaedic shoe. The patient attempted to do this, but the condition of the foot deteriorated. Six months later he presented with an ulcer over the cuboid, and radiograph (b) shows impaction of the head of the talus into the navicular, producing a boat-shaped deformity. The bone did heal in a total contact cast, after which the deformity was corrected

reconstituted, and then to perform wedge osteotomies or other surgery to reconstruct a functional shape[3] as shown in Figure 22.5 (for further discussion of this somewhat controversial area, see Chapters 17 and 18).

Neuropathic bone disintegration and the effects of chronic infection, such as osteomyelitis, frequently leave local pressure points that are predisposed to ulceration. It is practical to consider ostectomies to remove such bumps, rough bones and irregular periosteum that may predispose to further

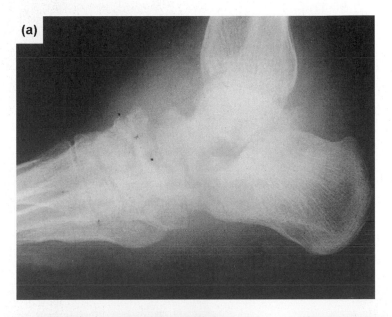

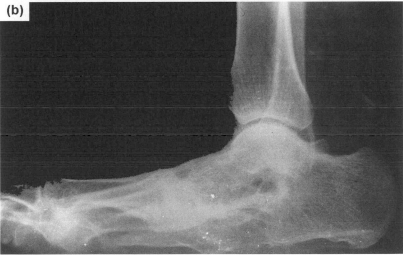

Figure 22.4 (a) Radiograph of a painless foot that had been hot and swollen for many months and shows generalized marked osteoporosis and a midtarsal fracture. Complete immobilization in a fixed total contact walking cast for 12 months resulted in union of all the bony fragments. Most of the joints fused into one solid bone mass. (b) Radiograph taken 4 years after full healing had occurred

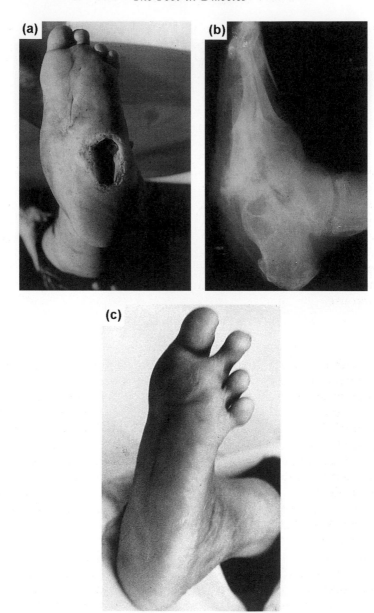

Figure 22.5   (a) This woman presented with a chronic ulcer. (b) This ulcer was seen on radiograph to be over the point of a "boat-shaped foot" that had resulted from impaction of a fracture involving the dorsal surface of the foot. A mid-tarsal osteotomy to realign the foot resulted in a functional non-ulcerating foot that could be shod with a normal shoe. An extra resilient insole ensured no recurrence of the ulceration. (c) Photograph taken about 4 years after the surgery

ulceration in the future. Basic surgical principles should be strictly observed and all incisions on the weightbearing surface should be kept to a minimum[3]. Moreover, as much good-quality weightbearing surface as possible must be preserved in order to spread the load of body weight as widely as possible.

TRIAL WALKING

Whenever a patient with neuropathy resumes free walking, such as after removal of a cast or a prolonged period of rest in bed without walking, it is advisable that a trial of walking is undertaken[3]. This is a slowly graded daily increase in the duration of walking allowed, starting with only 3–5 minutes at a time, with the foot checked for hot spots 2 hours after the walk. If there is no heat and swelling, the duration of walking can be regularly increased until the patient is walking for 40 minutes at a time without problems. Persistent heat and swelling will indicate that the bones have not fully healed or that the newly healed scars are not strong enough to withstand use.

FOOTWEAR

Patients with neuropathy frequently have muscle wasting and, as a result, may develop clawed toes and prominent metatarsal heads. There are many "extra-depth" shoes to accommodate the clawed toes, and it is essential that they have a resilient insole to compensate for the lack of normal padding[3,4]. Poron, which is a material commonly used by podiatrists, does not offer enough resilience for an insensate foot. Brand[4] showed in leprosy that a material of 15 degrees Shore provided a excellent insole to minimize pressure points. Alternatively, moulded shoes can be made to accommodate the deformities[9]. When these are used it is essential that the patient *always* wears the shoes for every step and that they are always worn fastened up. Moulded shoes, when not firmly fixed to the correct place on the foot, can do more harm than good. For some patients the best solution is to "make the foot fit the shoe" by surgery—in other words, remove rough bones and bumps and correct gross deformities so that the patient does not need moulded shoes. Even then, the patient will be better off if wearing resilient insoles in adequately large shoes and wearing them all the time.

It is not what you use but how you use it that counts. Brand showed that a suitably resilient insole will reduce the rate of ulceration by 50%, without any other measure, in a foot that still has basically normal anatomy[4]. There are suitable insoles that can be added to convert less ideal soles into reasonable ones, providing there is adequate depth. It is important to ensure that you know how to check that your patients have adequate resiliency in their footwear, so that you can teach them how to check when they buy new shoes. It is not softness but *resiliency* that counts[3,4]. In many Asian countries leprosy patients with totally anaesthetic feet are kept ulcer-free by routine daily care; looking, soaking, scraping, oiling, exercising and the wearing of sandals with micro-cellular rubber (MCR) insoles of 15 degrees Shore.

SURGICAL CONSIDERATIONS

The neuropathic foot may have involvement of sensory, motor and autonomic nerves. Motor nerve problems in diabetes usually affect only the intrinsic muscles. In many patients the intrinsics have already atrophied through disuse and a degree of clawing has resulted even before diabetes was diagnosed. The risk of ulceration on the plantar surface of the metatarsal heads, as well as over the proximal interphalangeal joints where they tend to rub the shoe uppers, increases as the toes become progressively more flexed and stiff. It is not uncommon for patients to have a toe removed because of such problems. However, if this deformity is seen while the toes are still mobile, it is very easy to perform a Girdlestone[3] procedure and transfer the long flexor of each toe to the dorsum of its own toe, so that the long flexor replaces the lumbrical as the flexor of the metatarsophalangeal joint[3]. This brings the distal phalanges back into contact with the ground, and so increases the weightbearing surface and decreases the amount of stress on the high-pressure points of the sole. This simple procedure reduces the chance of ulceration by both friction and pressure and increases the weightbearing surface, so the final result is a reduced tendency to ulceration and other trauma. When doing this transfer, it is advisable to deal with any other deformities present at the same time, to reduce the need for further reconstructive surgery in the near future.

When joints are deformed, arthroplasty may be indicated to increase the weightbearing surfaces and eliminate pressure points. Even in the elderly with cardiovascular problems, it has been found that carefully conducted conservative surgery, with adequate rest and protection, will be successful as long as there is a reasonable capillary return in the toes. Any major amputation is a traumatic procedure and in the elderly often means the patient will never walk again. There are some special procedures, like the Pirogoff amputation and the Boyd modification[13], that retain a weightbearing heel while removing the ulcerated forefoot. For years these operations have kept many patients mobile and independent. They are preferable to a Syme amputation, in which the terminal portion frequently becomes hypermobile and is easily displaced inside the prosthesis. This is a real problem with the insensate stump as it may remain folded on itself in the prosthesis for a prolonged period, and so be traumatized by painless ischaemia. The patient must never walk on the stump without a prosthesis. Hence a Syme amputation should not be advised for those with crippled hands or those who cannot easily attach a prosthesis.

CONCLUDING REMARKS

From leprosy we have learned that patients need to understand, at an early stage, what their problems are and how to apply regular daily care to maintain their limbs in good condition. All patients must know that ulcers will heal if adequately rested and protected, and must realise that disability can be prevented and that if it does occur then much can be done to reduce it. The patient must be able to apply suitable first aid after any trauma to prevent complications. Many hours of tuition may be needed before a patient becomes proficient. The patient's whole future is in their own hands. If patients look after themselves they can maintain a satisfactory lifestyle for the rest of their lives.

NOTE

This chapter has been heavily edited by Professors Boulton and Cavanagh in line with the rest of the volume, therefore the views expressed are not necessarily those of the author.

REFERENCES

1. Hilton J. *Rest and Pain*. London: George Bell and Sons, 1877; 4.
2. Brand PW, Yancey P. Chapters 7, 9 and 13. In *Pain: The Gift Nobody Wants*. New York: Harper Collins, 1993.
3. Warren G, Nade S. *The Care of Neuropathic Limbs. A Practical Handbook*. Carnforth: Parthenon, 1999.
4. Brand PW. *Insensitive Feet. A Practical Handbook on Foot Problems in Leprosy*, revised edn. London: The Leprosy Mission, 1977; 16–47.
5. Brand PW, Fritschi EP. Rehabilitation in leprosy. In Hastings RC (ed.), *Leprosy*. New York: Churchill Livingstone, 1985; 300–2.
6. Klenerman L, McCabe CJ, Cogley D et al. Screening for patients at risk of diabetic foot ulceration in a general diabetic outpatient clinic. *Diabet Med* 1996; **13**: 561–3.
7. Coleman WC, Brand PW. The diabetic foot. In *Ellenberg and Rifkin's Diabetes Mellitus*, 5th edn. Amsterdam: Elsevier, 1997; 1159–82.
8. Warren G. The surgery of leprosy. In King M et al (eds), *Primary Surgery*, vol 1, *Non-trauma*. Oxford: Oxford Medical Publications, 1990; 518–25.
9. Brand PW. Management of sensory loss in the extremities. In Omer GE Jnr, Spinner M, Van Beek AL (eds), *Management of peripheral nerve problems* 2nd edn. Philadelphia, PA: Saunders, 1998.
10. Tovey FI. Care of the diabetic foot. *Pract Diabet* 1986; 130–4.
11. Harris JR, Browne SG. The management of dry skin in leprosy patients. *Lancet* 1966; **i**: 1011–12.

12. Harris JR. Brand PW. Patterns of disintegration of the tarsus in the anaesthetic foot. *J Bone Joint Surg* 1966; **48B**.
13 Warren G. Conservative amputation of the neuropathic foot—the Pirogoff Procedure. *Oper Orthop Traumatol* 1997; **9**: 49–58.

23

Conclusions

HENRY CONNOR, ANDREW J. M. BOULTON*
and PETER R. CAVANAGH†

County Hospital, Hereford, UK, *Manchester Royal Infirmary, Manchester,
UK and †Pennsylvania State University, University Park, PA, USA

In the second edition of this book, the Editors noted that there had been many improvements in the provision of diabetic foot care in recent years, but that there was still much to be done[1]. Much has happened in the last 6 years, but has significant progress been made? Are we any nearer to achieving the reduction of 50% in the numbers of amputations, which was the target set in the St Vincent Declaration[2] in 1990? Regrettably, the answer has to be "No". In this context it is essential to consider only those studies which have examined amputation rates using defined geographical populations, rather than clinic populations, as the denominator. While there have been reports of reductions in amputation rates in health districts in Sweden[3] and Holland[4], a study from Germany found no change between 1990 and 1995[5], and one from England reported a 50% increase between 1990 and 1994[6]. Statistics from national data are even less encouraging, with reports of a 45% increase in total numbers of diabetic amputations in England between 1990 and 1994[7], and a similar increase in Scotland between 1993 and 1998 (Figure 20.1). Increases in total numbers (as opposed to rates) of amputations may be partly attributable to better documentation and to an increase in the prevalence of diabetes but, in percentage terms, they are of an order of magnitude greater than increases in the prevalence of diabetes. Given that the increase in the prevalence of diabetes is expected to continue[8], we must expect a concomitant increase in the numbers of amputations and thus progress toward achieving the objective set in the St Vincent Declaration becomes even more imperative.

The Foot in Diabetes, 3rd edn. Edited by A. J. M. Boulton, H. Connor and P. R. Cavanagh.
© 2000 John Wiley & Sons, Ltd.

In Chapter 1, Ward reminds us that the problems posed by diabetic foot disease in wealthy countries pale almost into insignifance compared with those faced in the poorer countries, and yet it is in the latter that the greatest increases in the prevalence of diabetes are to be expected[8]. Even in the wealthiest countries, as pointed out by Harkless and Armstrong from the USA (Chapter 8), the provision of foot care and footwear may be limited to those who can afford them or is otherwise restricted by bureaucratic processes. In the UK, where all diabetic patients have theoretically equal access to care from a National Health Service, there is evidence that "wealthy means healthy"[9]. These results require not only medical but also political solutions, as was recognized by the initiators of the St Vincent Declaration and, more recently, by the members of the International Working Group on the Diabetic Foot, who have included material aimed specifically at "policy makers" in their Consensus Document (Chapter 21). Much more effort will be required if we are to achieve equity of access to care for our patients.

The organization of services to provide foot care is a recurring theme throughout this book (Chapters 6, 7, 9, 20 and 21). Nikolai Pirogoff, who organized the Russian medical services in Sebastopol during the Crimean war of 1854–1856, recognized that "not medicine but administration plays the major role in the task of helping the wounded and sick on the battlefield". His genius for organization produced a system which allowed his staff to carry out amputations at a rate of 14 per hour[10]. We need systems of organization that can *prevent* amputation rates of the same order of magnitude because, if the amputation rates in Scotland during 1996–1998 (Figure 20.1) were applicable to the world population, the current global rate of amputations in people with diabetes would be 55 each hour. Systems for prevention must be population-based and not clinic-based because, even in a wealthy country like the UK, only about 40% of patients who come to amputation have been currently attending a specialist diabetic clinic[6]. Good organization of district-based systems of care, as described in Chapter 6, will ensure that we maximize the effectiveness of available resources.

Better organization is essential, but we also need to ensure that our clinical practice is effective. All too often the evidence on which we base our clinical practice is either weak or totally lacking. Chantelau (Chapter 11) has described the methodological shortcomings in many studies of diabetic footwear. Cullum and her colleagues (Chapter 13) and others[11,12] paint a similarly sorry picture of the problems which bedevil many of the reports on management of foot ulcers (Table 23.1). We must ensure that future studies are adequately powered (a lesson that we should have learned from the DCCT and UKPDS reports), that there are agreed universal definitions of what constitutes an ulcer or an amputation[13], and that we achieve a consensus on length of follow-up intervals and on the

Table 23.1 Common defects in clinical trials of diabetic foot disease

1. Inadequate sample sizes (important in diabetic foot disease where there are many confounding variables), with lack of pre-existing power calculations based on expected differences in healing rates
2. Inadequate description of randomization methods, and of withdrawals and drop-outs from the trials
3. Follow-up intervals
   - Of too short duration to allow for complete healing in a reasonable proportion of cases or to allow for early recurrences
   - Variable intervals within the same trial, with results expressed as mean or median
4. Outcome measures imprecisely defined
5. Variability in choice of outcome measures
   - Time to healing/time to reduce ulcer size
   - Percentage of patients completely healed/percentage achieving a degree of wound closure

Inconsistencies in all these variables reduces possibilities for meta-analysis (see text, reference 11 and Chapter 13 for discussion).

universal criteria for what constitutes healing or cure. For example, calculating "wound-free time" during a 12 month period after entry into a study might be a better outcome measure than "percentage of ulcers healed" or "time to healing"[11].

The principles of management which allow ulcers to heal are well established: neuropathic ulcers must be unloaded, infection must be treated, and ischaemic feet must be revascularized. Most ulcers can be healed, but far too many patients suffer a recurrence at the same or at another site. Even in those clinics with a special interest in diabetic foot disease, the recurrence rates after 1–2 years are approximately 30% in those who continue to wear their own shoes[14,15] and the overall figure at 5 years may be as high as 70%[16]. Footwear and education should provide the key to prevention of recurrence, but our evidence base in both of these areas is still weak. Even if the footwear we provide were universally effective, about one-third of patients choose not to wear it regularly[6,14]. We do not know to what extent this is because patients find the shoes unacceptable or how far it is due to a failure of our educational efforts. Certainly we must recognize, as Spraul reminds us in Chapter 9, that "education is more than knowledge transfer" and that our educational programmes must be constructed in line with accepted principles of adult education. Our teaching must take into account the barriers to behavioural change described by Spraul and elaborated by Vileikyte in Chapter 10. Rethinking our approach to education and learning to understand more about how our patients perceive what seems obvious to us may not be as exciting or glamorous as the advances in revascularization or the potential benefits of new biological wound dressings, but unless we tackle the former effectively our patients are unlikely to derive full benefit from the latter.

In conclusion, therefore, the "end-of-term report" for this third edition of *The Foot in Diabetes* must be: much achieved—could do better—much still to be done.

REFERENCES

1. Boulton AJM, Connor H, Cavanagh PR. *The Foot in Diabetes*, 2nd edn. Chichester: Wiley, 1994; 241–3.
2. Diabetes Care and Research in Europe: the St Vincent Declaration. *Diabet Med* 1990; **7**: 360.
3. Larsson J, Apelqvist J, Agardh C-D, Strenström A. Decreasing incidence of major amputation in diabetic patients: a consequence of a multi-disciplinary foot care approach? *Diabet Med* 1995; **12**: 770–6.
4. Bakker K, Dooren J. Een gespecialiseerde voetenpolikliniek voor diabetes-patienten vermindert het aantal amputaties en is kostenbesparend. *Ned Tijdschr Geneeskd* 1994; **138**: 565–9.
5. Stiegler H, Standl E, Frank S, Mendler G. Failure of reducing lower extremity amputations in diabetic patients: results of two subsequent population based surveys 1990 and 1995 in Germany. *VASA* 1998; **27**: 10–14.
6. Anonymous. An audit of amputations in a rural health district. *Pract Diabet Int* 1997; **14**: 175–8.
7. Hewitt D. Data currently available to the Department of Health on diabetes. In Dawson A, Ferrero M (eds), *Chronic Disease Management Registers*. London: HMSO, 1996; 34–8.
8. Amos AF, McCarty DJ, Zimmet P. The rising global burden of diabetes and its complications: estimates and projections to the year 2010. *Diabet Med* 1997; **14**(suppl 5): S25–34.
9. Ward JD. Wealthy means healthy: diabetes and social deprivation. *Diabet Med* 1994; **11**: 334–5.
10. Sorokina TS. Russian Nursing in the Crimean War. *J R Coll Physicians Lond* 1995; **29**: 57–63.
11. Kaltenthaler E, Morrell CJ, Booth A, Akehurst RL. The prevention and treatment of diabetic foot ulcers: a review of clinical effectiveness studies. *J Clin Effect* 1998; **3**: 99–104.
12. De P, Scarpello JHB. What is the evidence for effective treatment of diabetic foot ulceration? *Pract Diabet Int* 1999; **16**: 179–84.
13. Connor H. Diabetic foot disease—where is the evidence? *Diabet Med* 1999; **16**: 799–800.
14. Chantelau E, Leisch A. Footwear: uses and abuses. In Boulton AJM, Connor H, Cavanagh PR (eds), *The Foot in Diabetes*, 2nd edn. Chichester: Wiley, 1994; 99–108.
15. Uccioli L, Faglia E, Monticone G, Favales F et al. Manufactured shoes in the prevention of diabetic foot ulcers. *Diabet Care* 1995; **18**: 1376–8.
16. Apelqvist J, Larsson J, Agardh CD. Long-term prognosis for diabetic patients with foot ulcers. *J Intern Med* 1993; **233**: 485–91.

Index

Note: Page references in *italics* refer to Figures; those in **bold** refer to Tables

Index compiled by Annette Musker